CASE REVIEW
General and Vascular Ultrasound

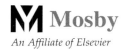
Mosby
An Affiliate of Elsevier

William D. Middleton, MD, FACR
Professor of Radiology
Mallinckrodt Institute of Radiology
Washington University School of Medicine
St. Louis, Missouri

CASE REVIEW

General and Vascular Ultrasound

CASE REVIEW SERIES

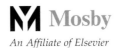

Editor: Stephanie Smith Donley
Manuscript Editor: Jeffrey L. Scheib
Production Manager: Guy Barber
Illustration Specialist: Robert F. Quinn

Permissions may be sought directly from Elsevier's Health Sciences Rights Department in Philadelphia, USA: phone: (+1)215-238-7869, fax: (+1)215-238-2239, email: healthpermissions@elsevier.com. You may also complete your request on-line via the Elsevier Science homepage (http://www.elsevier.com), by selecting 'Customer Support' and then 'Obtaining Permissions'.

Mosby, Inc.
An Affiliate of Elsevier
11830 Westline Industrial Drive
St. Louis, Missouri 63146

Printed in the United States of America.

Library of Congress Cataloging-in-Publication Data

Middleton, William D.
      General and vascular ultrasound: case review/William D. Middleton.
         p. ; cm.
      ISBN 0–323–00736–8
      1. Diagnosis, Ultrasonic—Case studies. 2. Blood-vessels—Ultrasonic imaging—Case studies. I. Title.
      [DNLM: 1. Ultrasonography—methods—Examination Questions.
2. Ultrasonography—methods—Problems and Exercises. 3. Vascular Diseases—ultrasonography—Examination Questions. 4. Vascular Diseases—ultrasonography—Problems and Exercises. WN 18.2 M629g 2002]
      RC78.7.U4 M53 2002
      616.07°543—dc21   2001044156

04 05 06 07 08   WBS/MV   9 8 7 6 5 4

To my students. This book is for the current, past, and future sonographers, residents, and fellows whom I have worked with and helped to train. Their intellectual curiosity has kept me stimulated, and their passion for learning has rewarded me throughout my career.

To my teachers. They are too many to name, but their efforts were instrumental in guiding my career and inspiring me to accomplish all that I could.

To my mother and father. They are both retired teachers, and any ability I have in education is in large part due to their influence.

To my children. They kept me happy and entertained, and focused my priorities throughout the process of writing this book.

To my wife. She is the love of my life and, once again, she has recognized the importance of this project and sacrificed some of our time together so that I could complete this book.

As radiologists we must maintain the high standards for image generation, relevant interpretations, effective communication, and outstanding patient service. This is particularly true in general and vascular ultrasound, where patient interaction is essential and where the value of a high-quality examination and interpretation often guides clinical management. This book will help you become a greater sonographer. Ping!

Dr. Middleton has embodied the principles of the Case Review Series in this volume on general and vascular ultrasound. Just as he and Al Kurtz have written a masterpiece in the *Ultrasound: The Requisites* volume, so too has Dr. Middleton hit a home run in this Case Review book. It is refreshing to read his preface, which so embodies the goals of this series: "to provide an affordable, useful, and enjoyable learning tool for sonographers, residents, and practicing physicians." The fact that nearly every case was personally selected and scanned by Dr. Middleton attests to his commitment to the case review mode of teaching. I believe that the reader will sense that dedication as he or she reviews Dr. Middleton's wonderful volume.

The philosophy of the Case Review Series is to review each specialty in a challenging, interactive way. Each book in the series has gradations of difficulty so that the reader can assess his or her proficiency and can use this self-evaluation to guide continued education. Since each case in the book is distinct, this is the kind of text that can be picked up and read at any time in your day, in your career.

I am very pleased to welcome Dr. Middleton's *General and Vascular Ultrasound* edition to the ever-expanding Case Review Series, which includes *Musculoskeletal Imaging,* by Joseph Yu, *Obstetric and Gynecological Ultrasound,* by Al Kurtz and Pam Johnson, *Spine Imaging,* by Brian Bowen, *Thoracic Imaging,* by Phil Boiselle and Theresa McLoud, *Genitourinary Imaging,* by Ron Zagoria, William Mayo-Smith, and Glenn Tung, *Gastrointestinal Tract Imaging,* by Peter Feczko and Robert Halpert, *Brain Imaging,* by Laurie Loevner, and *Head and Neck Imaging* by me.

David M. Yousem, M.D.
Case Review Series Editor

Writing a book is never easy and rarely enjoyable. Nevertheless, when I was first told of the plans for this book and informed of the format to be used, I was excited. I recalled as a medical student and a radiology resident that the knowledge gained from textbooks was fleeting unless it was reinforced with lessons learned at the patient's bedside or at the viewbox. And as painful as it sometimes was, the things I remembered best came from the questions I was forced to answer. Now that I am a teacher, it is clear to me that didactic lectures do not transmit information as effectively as engaging a group with a series of questions. For these reasons I was enthusiastic about participating in the Case Review Series.

In preparing this book, I have tried to select cases that cover all the material typically shown for board examinations. These sorts of cases are included primarily in the first two sections of the book. However, I believe it is nearsighted to focus intellectual energy on simply passing a test. It is much more important to learn the things that will aid your patients once exams are over. So in the third section, I have included many cases that will never appear on a board exam, but may be seen eventually in real life. I recognize that some conditions have been left out. That is unavoidable when the length of the book is limited and the topic is as broad as ultrasonography is. Nevertheless, I have tried to include a broad range of cases, realizing that the final selection undoubtedly reflects a bias based on the type of exams that are performed at the Mallinckrodt Institute of Radiology.

Once the case topics were decided, I had to accumulate images to display those conditions or to illustrate specific technical points. For me, this was the most enjoyable aspect of preparing the book. All of the images in the book came from patients I scanned myself, and I made a prospective effort to obtain images that were specifically focused on displaying important findings. For the past three years, whenever I took a little extra time scanning a patient, the sonographers and residents knew it was destined to become another "textbook case." Whenever possible, I have also tried to broaden the exposure of the reader by including images from different patients who have the same condition. Although I am pleased with the way the book turned out in general, I am particularly proud of the images.

A vexing problem that is unique to ultrasound texts is reproduction of color images. Although color Doppler is critical, in order to keep the cost of the book affordable, all of the color images had to be grouped together as color plates. Therefore, cases that contain color are displayed in black and white, with a reference to a particular color plate located in the front of the book. I apologize for this inconvenience and hope that it does not prove to be too annoying.

After selecting the cases and images, the next task was developing questions. I wanted to emphasize the most important aspect of sonography and the things that I stress as an oral board examiner. That is: identifying the important findings, establishing a reasonable differential diagnosis, narrowing the differential, and recommending appropriate further workup. Although this sequence mirrors what we do daily in clinical practice, the organization into a series of questions proved to be harder than I anticipated. The major dilemma was asking questions that did not give away the diagnosis. To accomplish this, the diagnosis could not be mentioned in any of the questions. This unfortunately creates the situation where the reader may have to answer questions about a condition without having determined what the condition is. In preceding volumes, many authors have decided to mention the diagnosis early in the case questions to avoid this latter problem. I decided that the latter problem was less critical than the former. So I did my best to keep the diagnosis in doubt and accepted the fact that with some cases, the reader may be forced to turn the page for the diagnosis before all the questions can be answered.

I also tried to present a range of questions. When I interact with residents and sonographers, I am gratified and proud when they know the answers to my questions. Nevertheless, I know that I have taught them more if I find a question that they can't answer correctly. So even for the cases where the diagnosis may be easy, I have tried to include some questions that are more of a challenge.

Finally, the Comments to each case were written with the intention of providing at least the basic information necessary to deal with patients who suffer from the conditions illustrated. Where room permitted, I tried to go into more detail to satisfy the more curious reader. References have been provided for those who want to learn more about a condition. In most cases, the references are review articles that cover a topic in detail. Cross-references to the *Requisites* Series have also been provided for conditions that were covered in that series.

In summary, the goal for this book was to provide an affordable, useful, and enjoyable learning tool for sonographers, residents, and practicing physicians. I hope that all of these groups will benefit as much from reading the book as I did from writing it.

William D. Middleton, M.D.

Most importantly, I would like to acknowledge all of the anonymous patients whose images are used throughout this book to teach future doctors and sonographers. There are certain inconveniences that patients have to deal with when they are cared for in an academic facility, and I thank them for their understanding. I would also like to thank the sonographers who worked with me while I was writing this book. I know I slowed down the schedule as I took extra time to get that perfect image, and I appreciate their patience. I am indebted, as always, to my secretaries, Sue Day and Pam Schaub. They provided their unique expertise when I faced word processing problems and handled all the mundane issues that surface periodically when completing a task such as this. I am grateful to the residents who proofread segments of the manuscript, and especially to my wife, Dr. Mary Middleton, who critiqued the entire thing. I thank Dr. David Yousem for conceiving the idea and including me as part of it. Liz Corra from Mosby guided the initial production of this series and should be credited with getting the ball rolling. Finally, Dr. Yousem and Stephanie Donley have organized the completion of the series and have been encouraging, supportive, and understanding throughout the sometimes drawn-out process of completing the book.

William D. Middleton, M.D.

COLOR PLATES

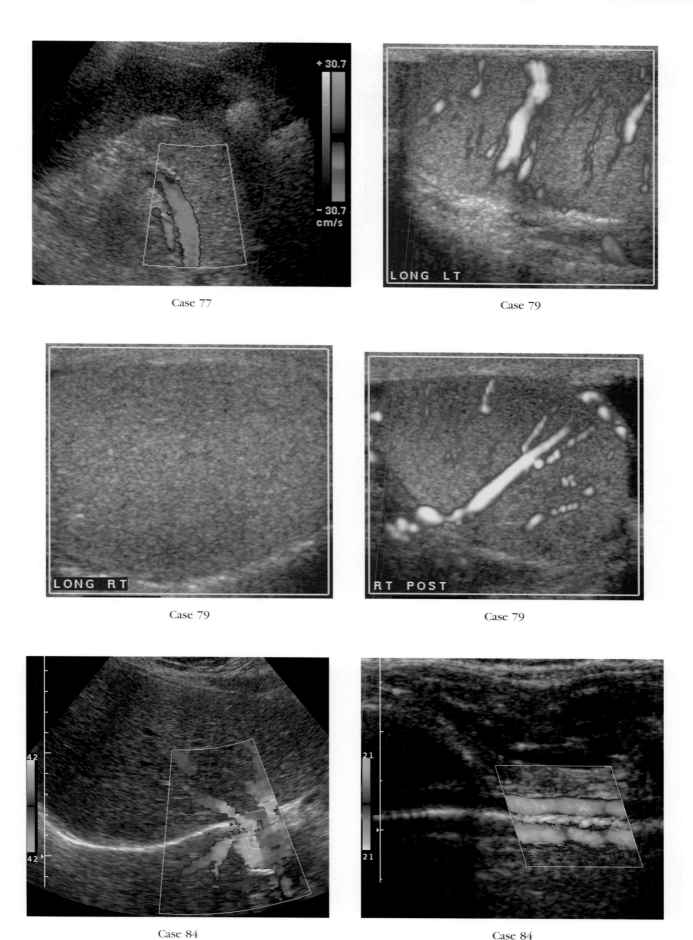

Case 77

Case 79

LONG LT

LONG RT

Case 79

RT POST

Case 79

Case 84

Case 84

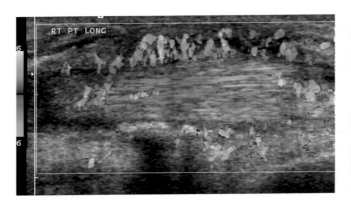

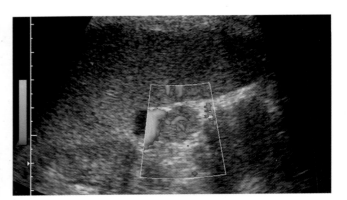

Case 85

Case 94

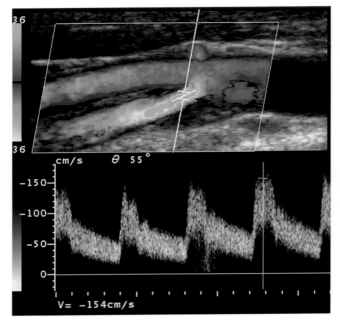

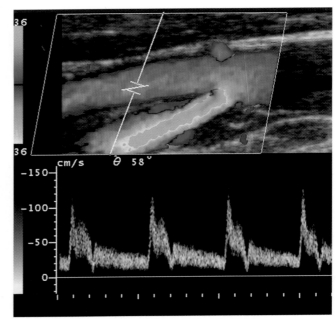

Case 97

Case 97

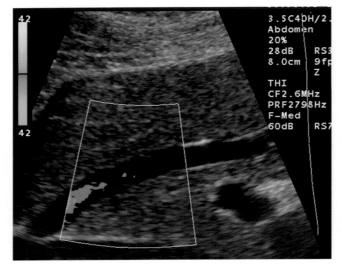

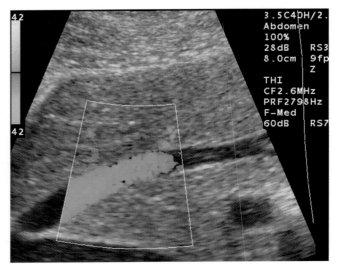

Case 98

Case 98

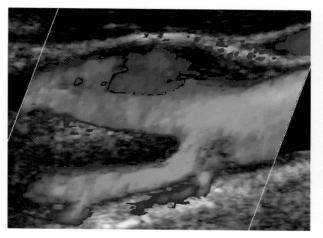

Case 40

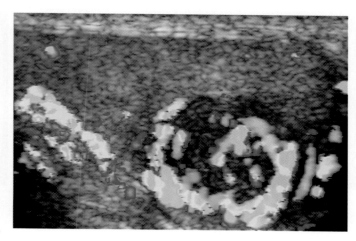

Case 41

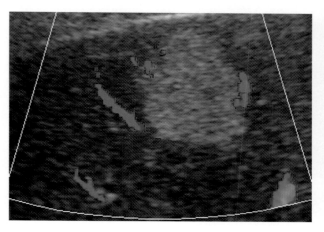

Case 49

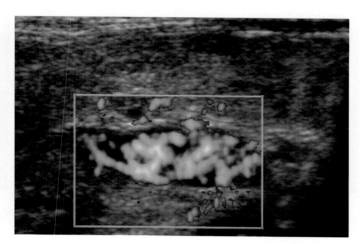

Case 53

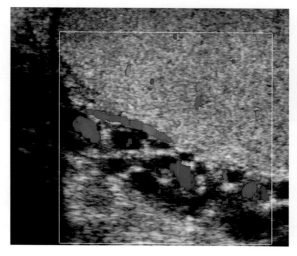

Case 61

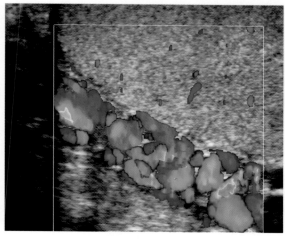

Case 61

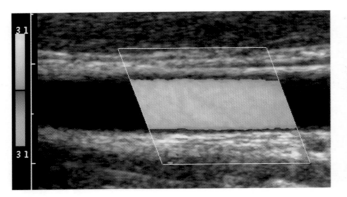

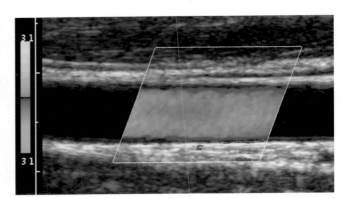

Case 62

Case 62

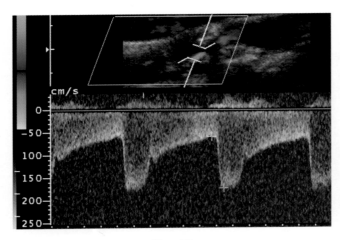

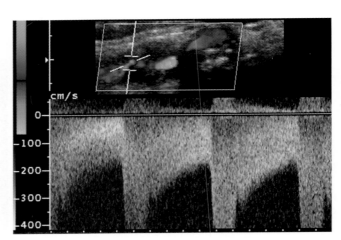

Case 73

Case 73

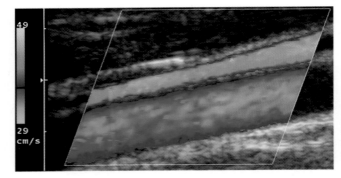

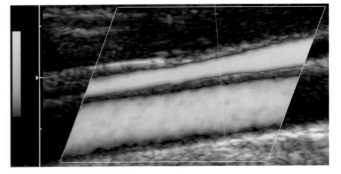

Case 74

Case 74

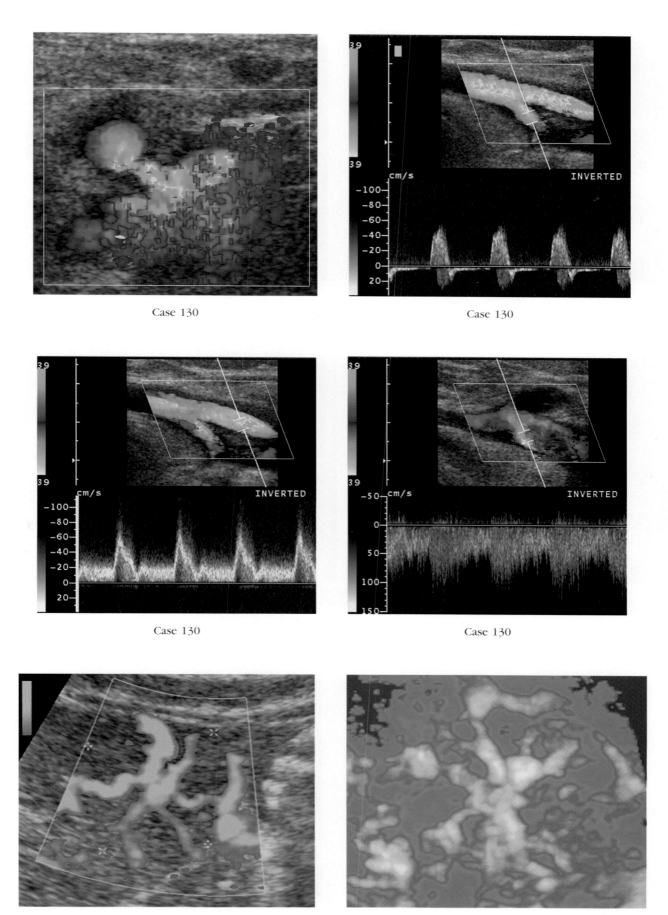

Case 130

Case 130

Case 130

Case 130

Case 145

Case 145

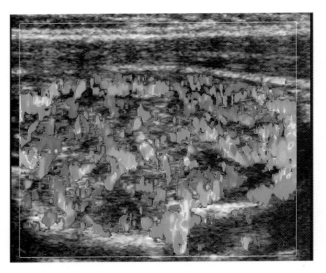

Case 146

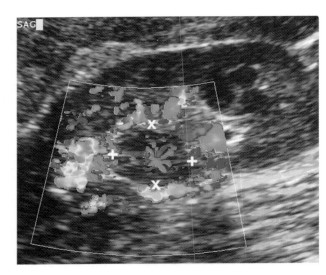

Case 150

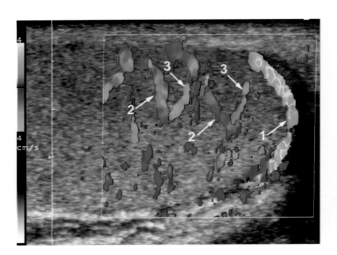

Case 153

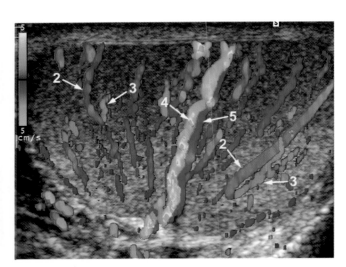

Case 153

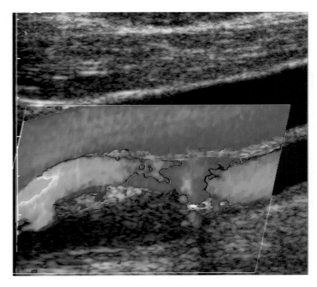

Case 154

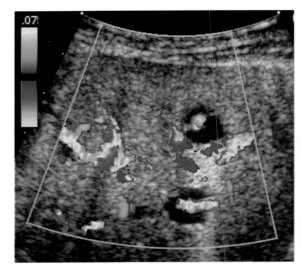

Case 159

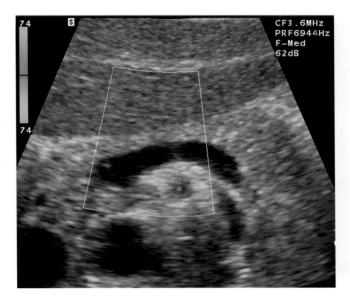

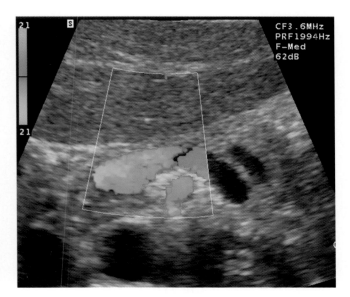

Case 104

Case 104

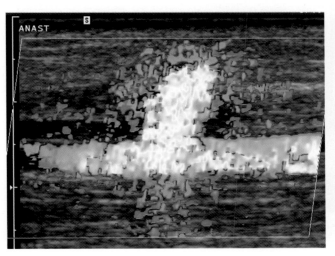

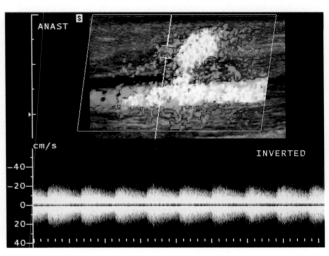

Case 105

Case 105

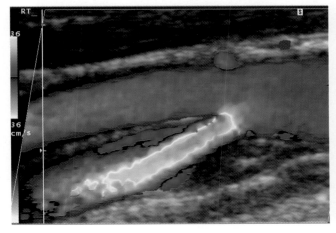

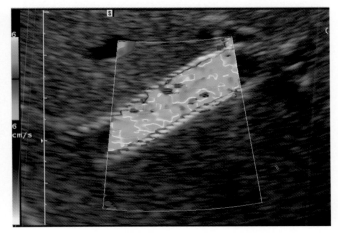

Case 116

Case 116

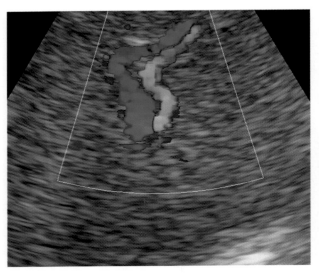

Case 117

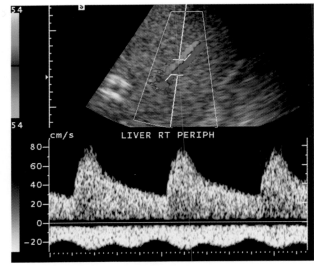

Case 117

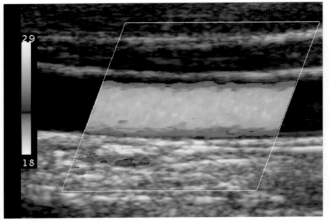

Case 124

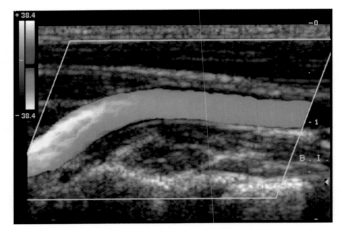

Case 124

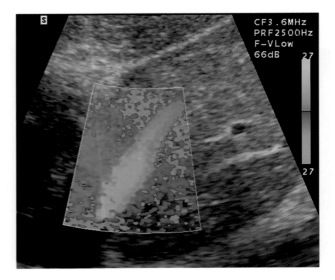

Case 125

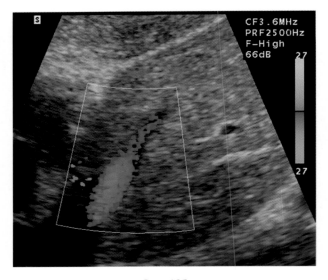

Case 125

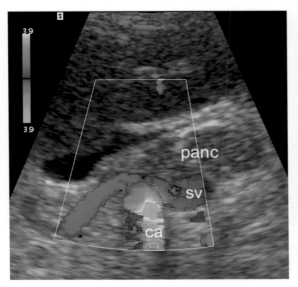

Case 171

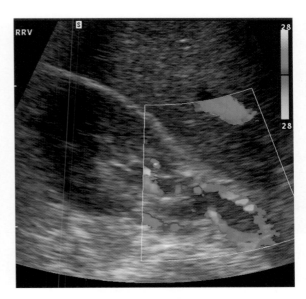

Case 174

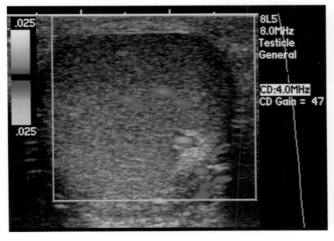

Case 175

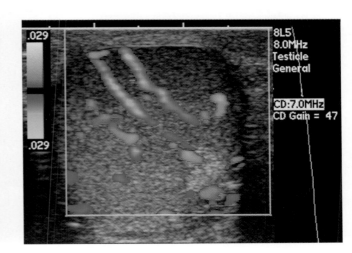

Case 175

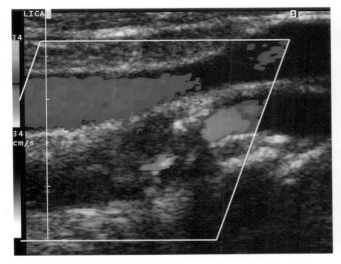

Case 182

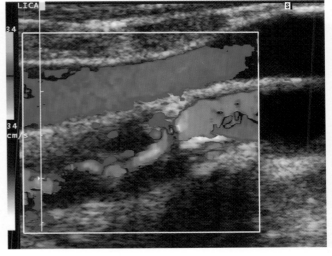

Case 182

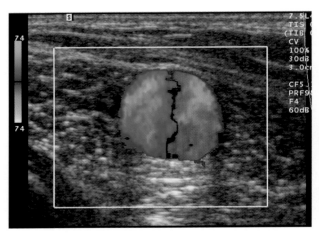

Case 183

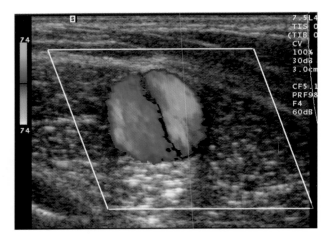

Case 183

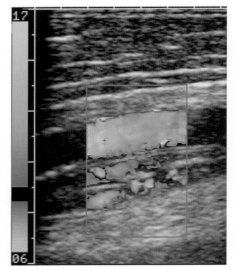

Case 188

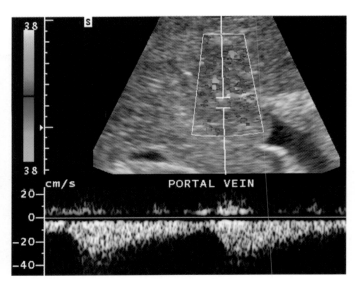

PORTAL VEIN

Case 189

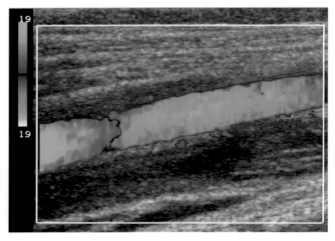

Case 194

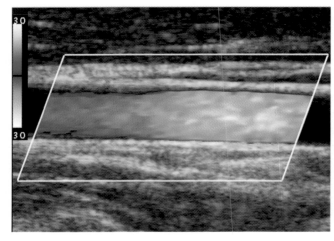

Case 194

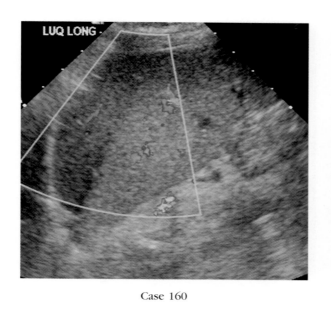

Case 160

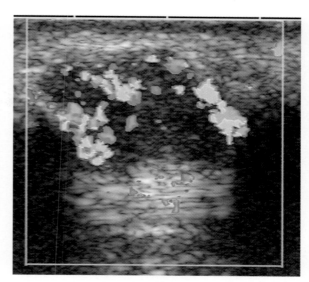

Case 162

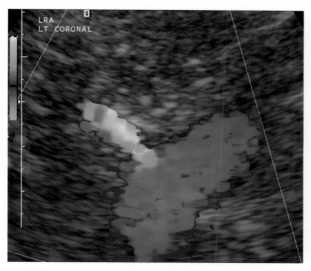

Case 165

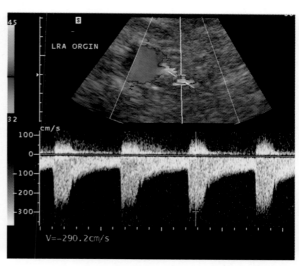

Case 165

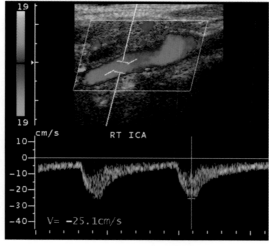

Case 166

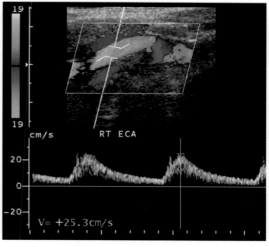

Case 166

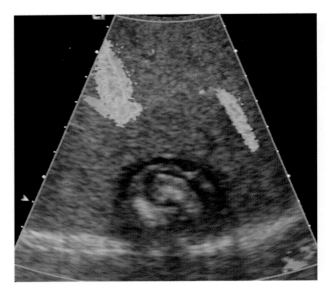

Case 168

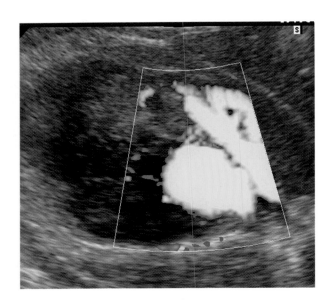

Case 167

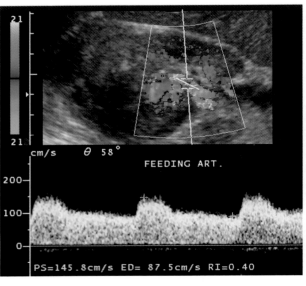

Case 167

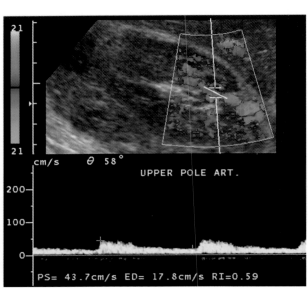

Case 167

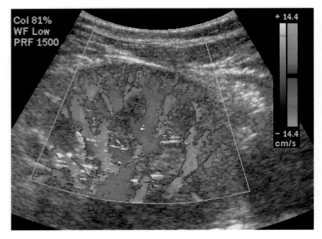

Case 170

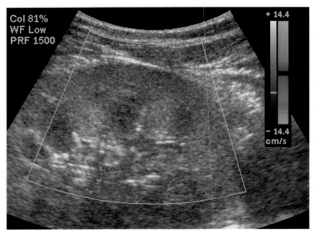

Case 170

CASE REVIEW
General and Vascular Ultrasound

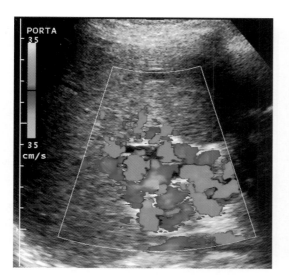

Case 195

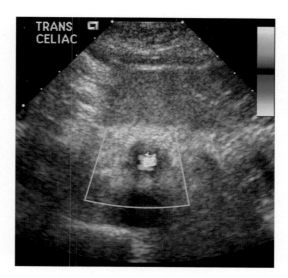

Case 196

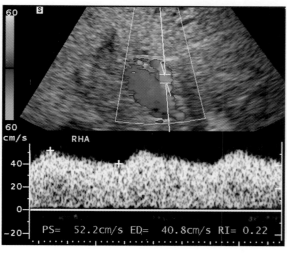

Case 200

PS= 52.2cm/s ED= 40.8cm/s RI= 0.22

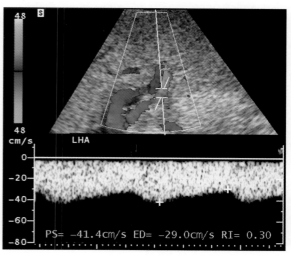

Case 200

PS= -41.4cm/s ED= -29.0cm/s RI= 0.30

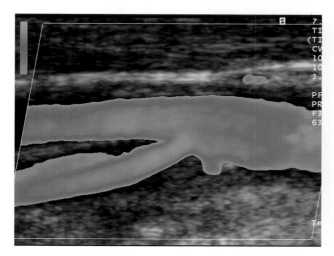

Case 201

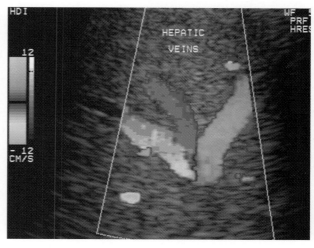

Case 205

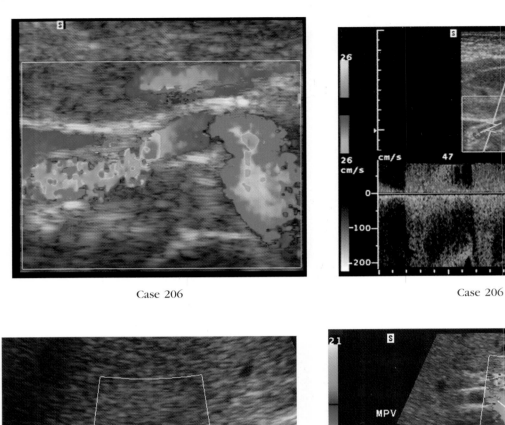

Case 206

Case 206

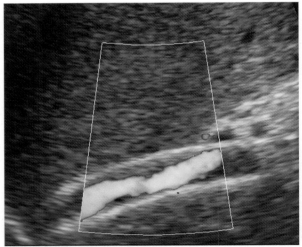

Case 210

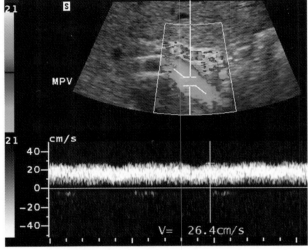

Case 210

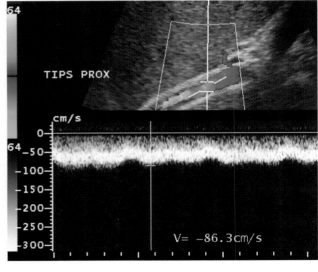

Case 210

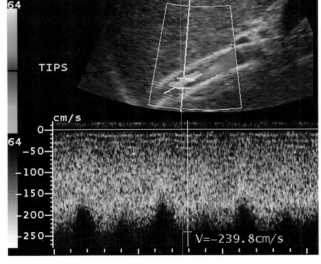

Case 210

I Opening Round

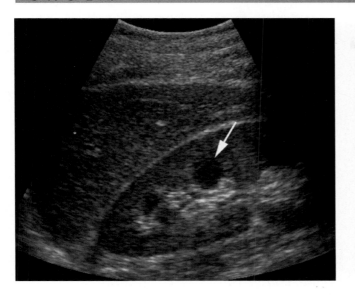 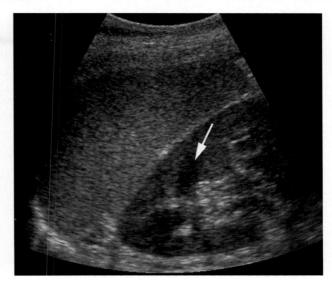

Longitudinal views of the kidneys from the same patient.

1. Do these kidneys appear normal or abnormal?
2. Which is the right kidney and which is the left?
3. What are the arrows pointing to in the kidneys?
4. What is the normal length for an adult kidney?

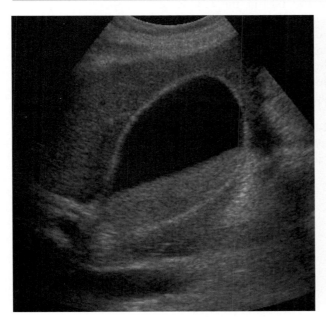 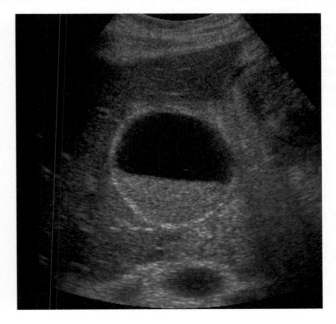

Longitudinal and transverse views of the gallbladder.

1. Should the abnormality shown on these images move when the patient rolls?
2. What causes the echogenicity of the bile in this condition?
3. Is surgery indicated?
4. What less common causes are there for this sonographic appearance?

Normal Kidneys

1. The kidneys shown in this case are normal.

2. The first image is the right kidney and the second image is the left kidney. The only way to tell the difference is to compare the echogenicity of the adjacent liver and spleen. The normal liver is usually similar or slightly more echogenic than the right kidney. The spleen is considerably more echogenic than the left kidney.

3. The arrows are pointing to the renal pyramids.

4. The normal adult kidney is approximately 11 cm ± 2 cm.

Reference

Thurston W, Wilson SR: The urinary tract. In Rumack CM, Wilson SR, Charboneau JW (eds): *Diagnostic Ultrasound,* 2nd ed. St. Louis, Mosby, 1998, pp 329–399.

Cross-Reference

Ultrasound: THE REQUISITES, pp 73–77.

Comment

Unlike most of the other solid organs in the abdomen, the kidneys have a relatively complex sonographic appearance. The central renal sinus contains a combination of fat and soft tissue and appears echogenic. The renal parenchyma, on the other hand, is hypoechoic. In many patients, including the one shown in this case, it is possible to visualize the renal pyramids as structures even slightly less echogenic than the renal cortex. Normally, the renal parenchyma is the least echogenic solid organ in the upper abdomen, followed by the liver, the spleen, and the pancreas.

When performing scans of the kidneys, it is important to compare their echogenicity to that of the liver and the spleen. This allows for detection of abnormally echogenic kidneys, as well as abnormalities in hepatic and splenic echogenicity. Therefore, views including a portion of the liver and spleen, such as those shown in this case, are important to obtain. Given the size of the liver, it is typical to view the right kidney using the liver as a window, so comparison of the right kidney with the liver is generally easy. Since the spleen is much smaller than the liver, comparison of the spleen with the left kidney is more difficult. Nevertheless, a high posterior and lateral approach with the patient supine will work for almost all patients except those with unusually small spleens. It is also helpful to scan both kidneys from a posterior and lateral approach without using the liver or spleen as windows, since this will provide a closer approach to the kidneys and in some cases will allow you to identify abnormalities that might otherwise be overlooked.

Gallbladder Sludge

1. Sludge should move to the dependent portion of the gallbladder when the patient changes position.

2. The echogenicity of sludge is due to crystals, especially cholesterol and calcium bilirubinate.

3. Sludge will usually resolve without any complications, so surgery is usually not indicated.

4. Blood and pus can simulate sludge.

Reference

Middleton WD: The gallbladder. In Goldberg BB (ed): *Diagnostic Ultrasound.* Baltimore, Williams & Wilkins, 1993, pp 116–142.

Cross-Reference

Ultrasound: THE REQUISITES, pp 40–41.

Comment

Gallbladder (GB) sludge consists of viscous bile that contains cholesterol crystals and calcium bilirubinate granules. It appears as echogenic material in the lumen of the GB. Since it is not attached to the GB wall, sludge should be mobile. However, if the bile is very thick and viscous, mobility may be very slow. Usually, sludge will layer into the dependent portion of the GB, and a straight line will form between the sludge and the rest of the bile in the GB. In some patients, sludge will completely fill the lumen of the GB. Sludge is usually homogeneous but occasionally will contain areas of heterogeneity. Blood and pus both can simulate sludge but are much less common. Unlike GB stones, sludge does not shadow. If even slight shadowing is detected within sludge, it indicates the presence of associated stones.

The clinical significance of sludge is not well established. In most instances, it is asymptomatic and resolves spontaneously. In some cases, it progresses to gallstone formation.

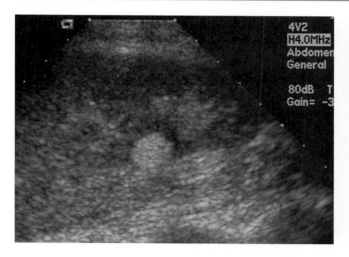

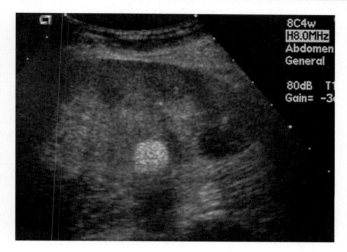

Two longitudinal views of the lower pole of the same kidney.

1. What important finding is seen on the second image but not on the first?
2. Why doesn't the first image show this important finding?
3. Does this lesion require further evaluation?
4. What is the major complication of this lesion?

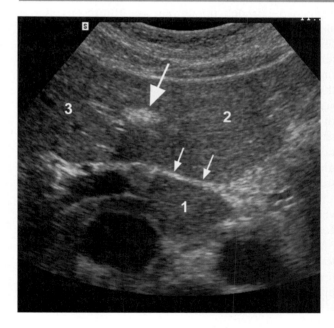

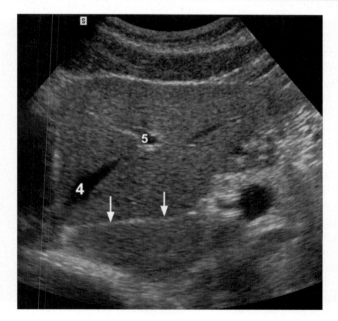

Transverse and longitudinal views of the liver.

1. What structure is the large arrow pointing to in the first image?
2. What structure are the small arrows pointing to in both images?
3. What embryologic remnant travels in the structures indicated by the arrows?
4. What liver segments are indicated by the numbers 1, 2, and 3 in the first image, and what vessels are indicated by the numbers 4 and 5 in the second image?

Angiomyolipoma

1. Both images show a hyperechoic mass, but the second image also shows slight posterior shadowing. These findings are typical of an angiomyolipoma (AML).

2. The shadowing is not seen on the first image because it was taken with a lower frequency transducer (4 MHz versus 8 MHz).

3. Further evaluation of a lesion such as this is controversial. However, since renal cell carcinoma is occasionally similarly hyperechoic, it is not unreasonable to recommend either a noncontrast CT or MRI to prove that the lesion contains fat, or follow-up sonography to prove stability.

4. The major complication of an AML is bleeding.

Reference

Siegel CL, Middleton WD, Teefey SA, McClennan BL: Angiomyolipoma and renal cell carcinoma: Ultrasound differentiation. *Radiology* 1996;198:789–793.

Cross-Reference

Ultrasound: THE REQUISITES, pp 93–94.

Comment

AML is a benign renal tumor that contains fat, smooth muscle, and vessels. These tumors can occur either sporadically or in association with tuberous sclerosis. Sporadic AMLs typically occur in middle-aged women and are solitary. On the other hand, AMLs associated with tuberous sclerosis are usually multiple, small, and bilateral and show no gender predilection.

The great majority of AMLs are asymptomatic. Large AMLs (>4 cm) may cause bleeding into the subcapsular or perinephric space. This bleeding may be related in part to the abnormal vessels and microaneurysms that are present in these tumors. Some urologists advocate removal of these large lesions.

The sonographic appearance of an AML is usually very typical. In approximately 80% of cases, an AML appears as a homogeneous hyperechoic mass similar in echogenicity to renal sinus or perinephric fat. A small percentage of AMLs are less echogenic than fat but more echogenic than renal parenchyma.

Although the usual appearance of an AML is very characteristic, it does overlap with the appearance of renal cell cancer (RCC). Approximately 10% of all RCC appears echogenic enough to simulate an AML. This is even more common in small RCC. Some features can help in the differentiation of echogenic RCC and AML. If any cystic elements or a hypoechoic halo or calcification are seen, then the mass is much more likely to be RCC. On the other hand, if there is attenuation of the sound so that there is slight posterior acoustic shadowing, then the mass is much more likely to be an AML than RCC.

Normal Anatomy of the Liver

1. The large arrow is pointing to the ligamentum teres.

2. The small arrow is pointing to the fissure for the ligamentum venosum.

3. The umbilical vein remnant travels in the ligamentum teres, and the ductus venosus travels in the fissure for the ligamentum venosum.

4. 1 = Caudate segment, 2 = Left lateral segment, 3 = Left medial segment. 4 = Left hepatic vein, 5 = Branch of the left portal vein.

Reference

Withers CE, Wilson SR: The liver. In Rumack CM, Wilson SR, Charboneau JW (eds): *Diagnostic Ultrasound,* 2nd ed. St. Louis, Mosby, 1998, pp 87–154.

Cross-Reference

Ultrasound: THE REQUISITES, pp 3–5.

Comment

The ductus venosus is the embryologic vessel that provides communication between the umbilical vein and the inferior vena cava. It runs between the umbilical segment of the left portal vein and the most superior aspect of the inferior vena cava. It is embedded in the liver via a deep fissure that can be seen on both longitudinal and transverse images of the left lobe of the liver. This fissure separates the caudate lobe from the lateral segment of the left lobe. Whenever the fissure for the ligamentum venosum is seen, the portion of the liver seen anteriorly must be the lateral segment of the left lobe. Therefore, in the longitudinal view, the portal vein branch and hepatic vein branch that are seen must be branches of the left portal vein and hepatic vein that supply the lateral segment.

The ligamentum teres is the remnant of the umbilical vein. On transverse views such as those shown in this case, it appears as a round, echogenic structure that often produces some posterior shadowing. It attaches to the most anterior aspect of the left portal vein. In the fetus, blood flow from the umbilical vein travels into the liver, through a short segment of the left portal vein, and then into the ductus venosus. The segment of the left portal vein that connects the umbilical vein to the ductus venosus is called the umbilical segment of the left portal vein. The ligamentum teres and the umbilical segment of the left portal vein both separate the medial and lateral segments of the left lobe.

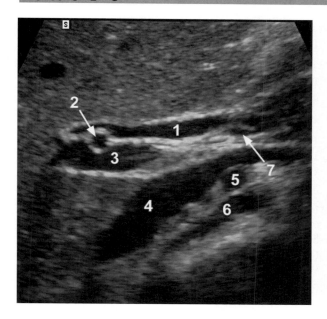
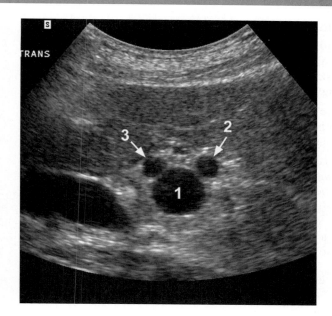

Longitudinal and transverse views of the porta hepatis.

1. Name the numbered normal structures on the longitudinal view.
2. Name the numbered normal structures on the transverse view.
3. Are measurements of the common duct obtained from the inner wall or the outer wall?
4. What segment of the bile duct is usually the largest?

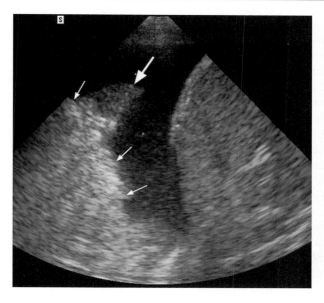
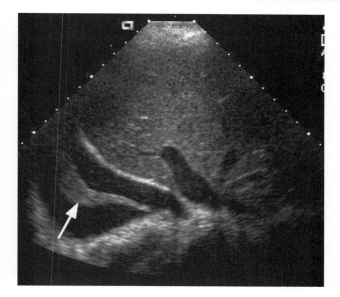

Longitudinal view of the right posterior hemithorax and transverse view of the right upper quadrant obtained in two patients.

1. What is the diagnosis in these two patients?
2. To what is the large arrow pointing?
3. To what are the small arrows pointing?
4. When the abdomen is scanned, is this abnormality easier to detect on the right side or on the left side?

Normal Anatomy of the Common Bile Duct

1. 1 = Common bile duct, 2 = Right hepatic artery, 3 = Portal vein, 4 = Inferior vena cava, 5 = Right renal artery, 6 = Crus of the right diaphragm, 7 = Cystic duct insertion.

2. 1 = Portal vein, 2 = Proper hepatic artery, 3 = Common hepatic duct.

3. Bile duct diameter is measured from inner wall to inner wall. This is done to allow for better correlation with measurements taken during cholangiography.

4. The bile duct diameter is usually greatest in its mid segment (i.e., between the porta hepatis and the pancreatic head).

Reference

Middleton WD: The bile ducts. In Goldberg BB (ed): *Diagnostic Ultrasound.* Baltimore, Williams & Wilkins, 1993, pp 146–172.

Cross-Reference

Ultrasound: THE REQUISITES, pp 55–57.

Comment

The left and right hepatic ducts join each other to form the common hepatic duct. The common hepatic duct joins the cystic duct to form the common bile duct. Although it is visualized in this case, the insertion of the cystic duct is usually difficult to visualize. Therefore, it is usually not possible to precisely determine where the junction of the common hepatic duct and the common bile duct is located. For this reason, many ultrasonologists refer to the common hepatic duct and the common bile duct together as the "common duct."

In most views of the porta hepatis, it is easy to identify the portal vein and to identify tubular structures anterior to the portal vein that represent the hepatic artery and the common duct. The common hepatic artery arises from the celiac axis. Following the takeoff of the gastroduodenal artery, it ascends into the porta hepatis as the proper hepatic artery. Therefore, the proper hepatic artery is usually what is visualized in the porta hepatis.

As shown in this case, the proper hepatic artery is usually more to the left and the common duct to the right. This can be easily remembered, since the artery arises from the aorta (which is to the left of the midline) and the common duct arises from the liver (which is to the right of the midline). After the proper hepatic artery bifurcates into the right and left hepatic arteries, the right hepatic artery crosses between the portal vein and the common duct. This produces the classic view showing the bile duct in long axis, the right hepatic artery in short axis, and the portal vein in an oblique axis, which is shown in the first image.

Pleural Effusion

1. Both patients have pleural effusions.

2. The large arrow is pointing to atelectatic lung floating in the pleural fluid.

3. The small arrows are pointing to aerated lung and the posterior shadow.

4. Pleural effusions are easier to see on the right side because the liver provides a better window to the costophrenic angle than does the spleen.

Reference

Brant WE: The thorax. In Rumack CM, Wilson SR, Charboneau JW (eds): *Diagnostic Ultrasound,* 2nd ed. St. Louis, Mosby, 1998, pp 575–598.

Cross-Reference

Thoracic Radiology: THE REQUISITES, p 491.

Comment

Pleural effusions are frequently seen as incidental findings on abdominal scans. Normally, the aerated lung is closely applied to the diaphragm, so that sound cannot penetrate to the posterior structures of the chest. Pleural effusions displace aerated lung enough to provide a window to the posterior surface of the costophrenic sulcus. When the effusion is small, this produces a triangular-shaped collection. When the effusion is larger, there is usually associated compressive atelectasis of the lung, producing a mobile, curvilinear soft-tissue structure floating within the fluid. Aerated lung, appearing as hyperechoic tissue with dirty posterior shadowing, is often seen above the atelectatic lung. Perihepatic ascites is easily differentiated from pleural effusions, since ascites will displace the diaphragm from the liver, making the diaphragm appear as a separate structure. In addition, the bare area of the liver prohibits ascites from extending to the posterior medial aspect of the liver. Pleural effusions typically do extend to the most medial aspect of the liver, near the vena cava.

As shown on the first image, pleural effusions can also be seen by scanning directly over the chest wall in the region of the effusion. This scanning is commonly done when performing ultrasound-guided thoracentesis. The fluid is seen separating the parietal and visceral layers of the pleura. In the longitudinal plane, the ribs are seen as shadowing echogenic structures and the parietal pleura as a smooth, linear reflection deep to the ribs. Pleural effusions that appear simple on sonography may be either transudative or exudative. Complex effusions that contain septations and/or internal floating reflectors are usually exudative.

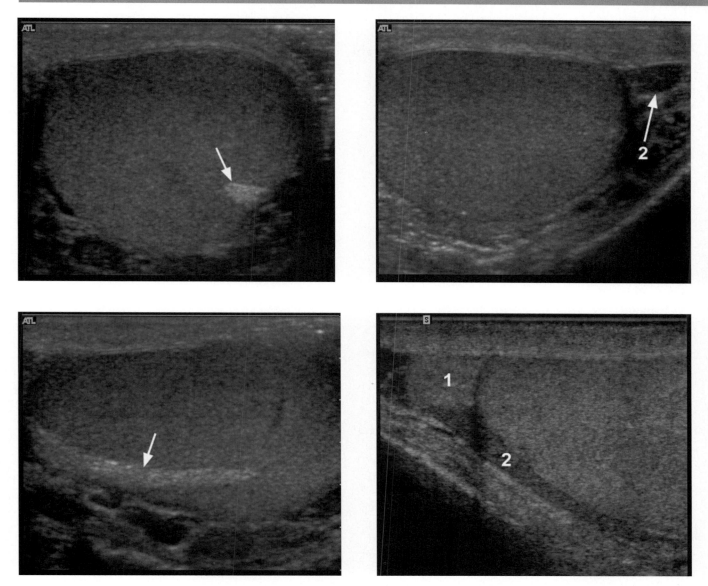

Two transverse and two longitudinal views of the scrotum.

1. What is the normal echogenic structure (arrow) shown on the first transverse view and the first longitudinal view?

2. What are the normal peritesticular structures labeled 1 and 2 on the second transverse view and the second longitudinal view?

3. What is the normal relative echogenicity of the testis and of the head of the epididymis?

4. What is the normal relative echogenicity of the testis and of the body of the epididymis?

Normal Scrotal Anatomy

1. The peripheral echogenic structure is the mediastinum of the testis.

2. 1 = Head of the epididymis, 2 = Body of the epididymis.

3. The head of the epididymis is normally isoechoic to the testis.

4. The body of the epididymis is normally hypoechoic to the testis.

Reference

Feld R, Middleton WD: Recent advances in sonography of the testis and scrotum. *Radiol Clin North Am* 1992;30:1033–1051.

Cross-Reference

Ultrasound: THE REQUISITES, pp 435–436.

Comment

The testes are paired ovoid organs residing within the two halves of the scrotum. Six scrotal layers (the skin, dartos, external spermatic fascia, cremasteric muscle, internal spermatic fascia, the tunica vaginalis) surround them and the testicular capsule called the tunica albuginea. The two scrotal sacs are divided by a midline median raphe.

Each testis is divided into approximately 300 lobules. Each lobule contains up to four extremely convoluted seminiferous tubules. As they converge to exit the testis, the seminiferous tubules join together to form the straight tubules. The straight tubules then join to form a plexus of channels called the rete testis that is located within an infolding of the tunica albuginea called the mediastinum. The mediastinum is the hilum of the testis. The rete testes empty into the head of the epididymis via 10 to 15 efferent ductules. In the head of the epididymis, the efferent ductules join together to form a single convoluted ductus epididymis. The epididymis is a crescent-shaped structure that rests on the surface of the testis near the mediastinum. It is divided into the head superiorly, the tail inferiorly, and the body in between.

The normal testis has a low- to medium-level echogenicity and a homogeneous echotexture. It measures approximately 4 cm in length and 2 cm in width and thickness. In most testes the mediastinum is seen as an echogenic structure at the periphery of the testis that runs from the upper third to the lower third of the testis. The epididymal head rests on the upper pole of the testis and has an echogenicity similar to that of the testis. During real-time scanning, the epididymal head can usually be followed into the body of the epididymis, which is slightly less echogenic than the testis. The location of the epididymal body is variable because the testis itself is somewhat mobile within the scrotal sac. Most often, the epididymal body is seen along the anterior and lateral aspect of the testis, as shown on the second transverse image. In some patients the epididymal body is located posterior to the testis, as shown on the second longitudinal image. A small amount of fluid is often seen in the scrotal sac, usually around the epididymal head.

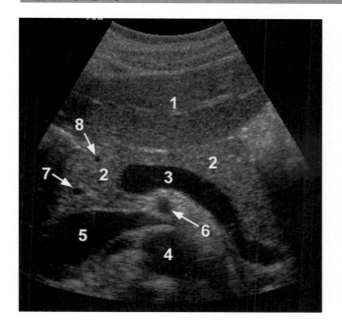
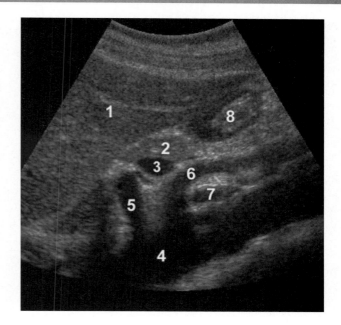

Transverse and sagittal views of the upper abdomen.

1. Name the normal numbered structures on the transverse scan.
2. Name the normal numbered structures on the sagittal scan.
3. Is the pancreatic body normally round or oval-shaped on sagittal scans?
4. Is the superior mesenteric artery or vein closer to the pancreas?

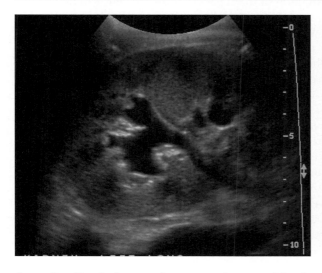
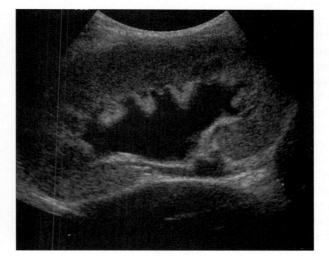

Longitudinal views of two patients with the same abnormality.

1. What is wrong with these kidneys?
2. Under what circumstances is this a medical emergency?
3. How would you grade the abnormality shown here?
4. In what plane are these images acquired?

Normal Peripancreatic Anatomy

1. 1 = Left lobe liver, 2 = Pancreas, 3 = Portosplenic confluence, 4 = Aorta, 5 = Inferior vena cava (IVC), 6 = Superior mesenteric artery (SMA), 7 = Common bile duct (CBD), 8 = Gastroduodenal artery.

2. 1 = Left lobe liver, 2 = Pancreas, 3 = Splenic vein, 4 = Aorta, 5 = Celiac axis, 6 = SMA, 7 = Left renal vein, 8 = Gastric antrum.

3. The pancreatic body is oval on sagittal scans.

4. The superior mesenteric vein is immediately adjacent to the head and uncinate process of the pancreas. The SMA is separated from the pancreas by a ring of echogenic fibrofatty tissue.

Reference

Schneck CD, Dabezies MA, Friedman AC: Embryology, histology, gross anatomy, and normal imaging anatomy of the pancreas. In Friedman AC, Dachman AH (eds): *Radiology of the Liver, Biliary Tract, and Pancreas.* St. Louis, Mosby, 1994, pp 715–742.

Cross-Reference

Ultrasound: THE REQUISITES, pp 122–124.

Comment

The pancreas is one of the more difficult organs to visualize with ultrasound. Knowledge of the peripancreatic vessels aids greatly in localizing the gland. The most useful landmark is the portosplenic venous confluence. On transverse scans, this appears as a tadpole-shaped hypoechoic to anechoic structure posterior to the body of the pancreas. The head of the pancreas wraps around the right lateral aspect of the portal vein at the level of the portomesenteric confluence, and the uncinate process extends posterior to the superior mesenteric vein. All of the peripancreatic veins are immediately adjacent to the pancreas without any intervening fatty tissue. On the other hand, the peripancreatic arteries are surrounded by echogenic fibrofatty tissue and do not make direct contact with the pancreas. The celiac axis typically arises at the superior aspect of the pancreas. The body of the pancreas can be seen by scanning just below the origin of the proper hepatic artery and splenic artery. The SMA arises from the aorta immediately posterior to the pancreas and the portosplenic confluence. A characteristic hyperechoic ring of fibrofatty tissue surrounds the SMA.

The CBD travels in the most posterior aspect of the pancreas. In fact, it often appears immediately anterior to the IVC. The gastroduodenal artery arises from the common hepatic artery and descends along the anterior aspect of the head of the pancreas. These two structures often appear as two small anechoic dots on transverse views of the pancreatic head.

Hydronephrosis

1. The renal collecting system is dilated.

2. If the kidney is infected and obstructed.

3. This is referred to as grade 2 hydronephrosis.

4. Coronal or semicoronal.

Reference

Ellenbogen PH, Scheible FW, Talner LB, Leopold GR: Sensitivity of gray scale ultrasound in detecting urinary tract obstruction. *AJR Am J Roentgenol* 1978;130:731–733.

Cross-Reference

Ultrasound: THE REQUISITES, pp 77–81.

Comment

Sonographic detection of urinary obstruction depends on identification of a dilated collecting system, which appears as anechoic spaces within the echogenic central renal sinus. Under most circumstances, it is easy to document that the cystic spaces communicate with each other and with the renal pelvis. This confirms that the fluid is in the collecting system.

Hydronephrosis is graded into different levels of severity. Grade 0 refers to a normal sonogram. Grade 1 refers to minimal separation of the central echogenic renal sinus. Grade 2 refers to obvious distention of the renal collecting system. Grade 3 refers to marked distention of the renal collecting system with associated cortical thinning.

Whenever hydronephrosis is detected, the next task is to determine the level and cause of obstruction. When the hydronephrosis is bilateral, the obstruction is often at the level of the bladder, and this is usually easy to document sonographically. Prostatic hypertrophy is easy to identify in men, and pelvic tumors are usually easy to identify in women. Primary bladder tumors are often easily identified in both genders. Unilateral obstruction of the ureter at a level above the bladder is more difficult to sort out with ultrasound. Depending on the patient, it may be possible to follow the ureter over its entire course and document the transition point. However, the mid ureter is often not visible, and unless the obstruction is caused by a sizable mass, the source of mid-ureteral obstruction may not be visible sonographically. In such cases, sonography should be followed by further imaging tests, such as intravenous urography, CT, or retrograde pyelography.

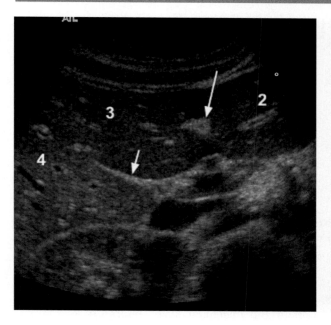
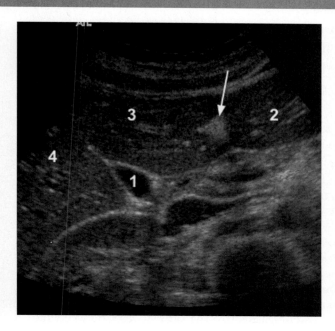

Transverse views of the liver.

1. What is the echogenic structure indicated by the long arrow?
2. What is the linear structure indicated by the short arrow?
3. What is the fluid-filled structure indicated by the number 1?
4. What liver segments are indicated by the numbers 2, 3, and 4?

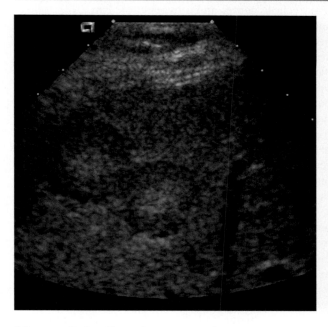
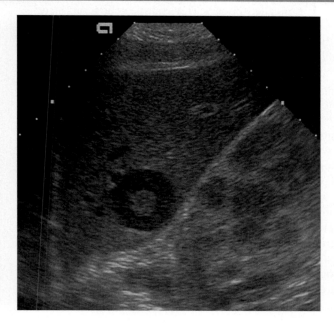

Views of the liver in two patients.

1. Are these lesions most likely benign or malignant?
2. What is the differential diagnosis?
3. What does the peripheral hypoechoic region represent?
4. Is the differential diagnosis the same for a lesion that is hypoechoic centrally and has a hyperechoic peripheral ring?

Normal Liver and Gallbladder Anatomy

1. The long arrow is pointing at the ligamentum teres.

2. The short arrow is pointing at the interlobar fissure.

3. The number 1 is identifying the gallbladder.

4. Numbers 2, 3, and 4 are in the left lateral, left medial, and right anterior segments, respectively.

Reference

Middleton WD: The gallbladder. In Goldberg BB (ed): *Diagnostic Ultrasound.* Baltimore, Williams & Wilkins, 1993, pp 116–142.

Cross-Reference

Ultrasound: THE REQUISITES, pp 35–38.

Comment

The normal gallbladder (GB) is located along the inferior and posterior aspect of the liver. It rests between the right and left lobes and serves as a valuable landmark to help separate the right and left lobes. In most fasting patients, the GB is readily identified simply by moving the transducer along the right inferior costal margin while visualizing the lower margin of the liver. In cases where the GB is difficult to find, it is helpful to use hepatic landmarks. Start by finding the ligamentum teres between the medial and lateral segments of the left lobe. It typically appears as a round, echogenic structure, often with some posterior shadowing. Then look to the right for the interlobar fissure. This fissure is a shallow indentation on the posterior-inferior aspect of the liver that appears as an echogenic line extending from the porta hepatis into the liver parenchyma. The interlobar fissure separates the left lobe (medial segment) and right lobe (anterior segment). The GB is located immediately adjacent to the interlobar fissure. In some patients, the interlobar fissure is not visible sonographically. This most often occurs when the GB is well distended. Fortunately, the interlobar fissure is usually easiest to see in those situations when the GB is contracted and harder to see.

The GB is usually well distended in a patient after an overnight fast. The upper limit of normal for GB size, even in a fasting patient, is 4 cm in the transverse plane. The transverse diameter is a better indicator of overdistention than the longitudinal diameter. Nevertheless, most GBs will be less than 8 cm in length. The GB wall thickness should not exceed 3 mm. When the GB is contracted, the wall may seem thick and the muscle layer may become apparent as a hypoechoic layer deep to the mucosa. However, even in the contracted state, it is unusual for the wall to measure more than 3 mm.

Hepatic Target Lesions

1. Target lesions are much more likely to be malignant.

2. The differential diagnosis includes metastases, hepatocellular cancer, lymphoma, and abscess. Benign lesions such as focal nodular hyperplasia or hepatic adenomas are possible but much less likely.

3. The hypoechoic halo is usually viable tumor but may occasionally be compressed liver parenchyma.

4. Reverse targets are much less likely to be malignant.

References

Kruskal JB, Thomas P, Nasser I, et al: Hepatic colon cancer metastases in mice: Dynamic in vivo correlation with hypoechoic rims visible at US. *Radiology* 2000;215:852–857.

Wernecke K, Vassallo P, Bick U, et al: The distinction of benign and malignant liver tumors on sonography: Value of the hypoechoic halo. *AJR Am J Roentgenol* 1992;159:1005–1009.

Cross-Reference

Ultrasound: THE REQUISITES, pp 7–9.

Comment

The lesions shown in these figures have an isoechoic or hyperechoic center and a hypoechoic rim. This appearance is referred to as a target lesion, and the great majority of these lesions are malignant. Liver metastases are most common, but hepatocellular carcinoma and lymphoma can also have a target appearance and should be considered in the proper clinical setting. Initial discussions of target lesions stated that the hypoechoic rim represented compressed liver parenchyma. This may be true when the hypoechoic halo is thin. However, more recent reports show that in most cases, the rim represents viable tumor. In fact, when performing percutaneous biopsy of these lesions, the highest yield is from the hypoechoic rim.

It is very uncommon to see target lesions from benign etiologies. Hepatic adenomas and focal nodular hyperplasia rarely appear as target lesions, but they are much less common than hepatic metastases. Hemangiomas are extremely common liver tumors, but it is rare for them to have a hypoechoic rim. It is important to recognize that reverse target lesions (lesions with an isoechoic or hypoechoic center and a hyperechoic rim) are unlikely to be malignant. In fact, this is a relatively typical appearance for a hemangioma.

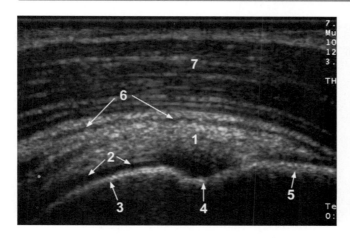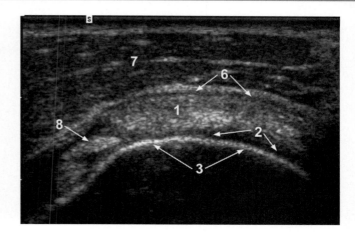

Longitudinal and transverse views of the shoulder.
1. Identify the numbered normal structures in the two figures above.
2. The rotator cuff is composed of how many tendons?
3. What structure separates the subscapularis from the supraspinatus?
4. Is the normal rotator cuff compressible?

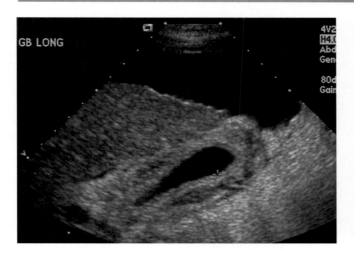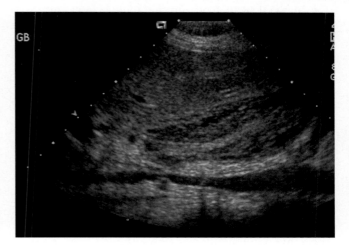

Longitudinal images of the gallbladder in two patients.
1. Do these patients have anything in common?
2. What is the differential diagnosis?
3. What do you think is the cause of the abnormality in these two patients?
4. Are any measurements useful in detecting this abnormality?

C A S E 1 2

Normal Anatomy of the Shoulder

1. 1 = Rotator cuff (RC), 2 = Cartilage, 3 = Humeral head, 4 = Anatomic neck, 5 = Greater tuberosity, 6 = Subdeltoid bursa, 7 = Deltoid, 8 = Biceps tendon.

2. The rotator cuff is composed of four tendons and muscles, the subscapularis, the supraspinatus, the infraspinatus, and the teres minor.

3. The intra-articular portion of the biceps tendon separates the subscapularis and the supraspinatus.

4. The normal rotator cuff is not compressible.

Reference
Middleton WD, Teefey SA, Yamaguchi K: Sonography of the shoulder *Semin Musculoskeletal Radiol* 1998; 2:211–221.

Cross-Reference
Ultrasound: THE REQUISITES, pp 455–457.

Comment
The RC is a band of conjoined tendons that covers the humeral head. The anterior tendon (subscapularis) crosses the glenohumeral joint and attaches to the lesser tuberosity. The superior tendon (supraspinatus) attaches to the greater tuberosity just posterior to the biceps tendon groove. The intra-articular portion of the long head of the biceps tendon separates these two tendons. Anatomic studies have shown that the supraspinatus tendon measures approximately 1.5 cm in width. Behind and inferior to the supraspinatus tendon is the infraspinatus tendon, which also inserts on the greater tuberosity. A minor tendon located just inferior to the infraspinatus is the teres minor.

Sonograms of the shoulder display multiple structures in a series of layers. The deepest structure is the humeral head, which appears as a strong, curvilinear reflection. On longitudinal views, the concave anatomic neck separates the humeral head and the greater tuberosity. Immediately on top of the humeral head is a thin layer of anechoic or hypoechoic articular cartilage. The next layer is the RC, which appears as a thick (4 to 6 mm) band of tissue. In most patients the RC appears hyperechoic compared to the overlying deltoid muscle. In elderly patients, the RC and the deltoid may appear more similar in echogenicity. Superficial to the RC is a thin, hypoechoic layer that represents the subdeltoid bursa. Superficial to this is a thin, hyperechoic layer that represents peribursal fat. The deltoid muscle is the final layer. Like other muscles, it is hypoechoic.

The outer surface of the normal RC is convex. Conversion to a concave contour is an important sign of a full-thickness RC tear. In addition, the normal RC is not compressible. The ability to compress the RC is another sign of a full-thickness tear.

C A S E 1 3

Gallbladder Wall Thickening

1. Both patients have thick gallbladder (GB) walls. The first image also shows ascites and a nodular liver consistent with cirrhosis. The second image also shows a completely contracted GB lumen.

2. The causes of a thick GB wall include heart failure, hypoproteinemia, edema-forming states, hepatitis, cirrhosis, portal hypertension, lymphatic obstruction, GB cancer, adenomyomatosis, and cholecystitis.

3. The nodularity of the liver surface in the first image is consistent with cirrhosis, and this is the cause of the GB wall thickening. The lumen of the GB is completely contracted in the second image, and this finding should raise the possibility of hepatitis.

4. The upper limit of normal for GB wall thickness is 3 mm.

Reference
Middleton WD: The gallbladder. In Goldberg BB (ed): *Diagnostic Ultrasound.* Baltimore, Williams & Wilkins, 1993, pp 116–142.

Cross-Reference
Ultrasound: THE REQUISITES, pp 49–50.

Comment
A large number of processes can cause thickening of the GB wall. Most of the etiologies are not related to intrinsic GB disease. These non-biliary causes produce thickening of the GB wall as a result of edema. In general, the most pronounced GB wall thickening is usually due to one of these non-biliary causes. Acute hepatitis in particular can cause extensive GB wall thickening. Hepatitis may also result in contraction of the GB lumen to the point that the lumen is completely collapsed. As shown in the second image, a collapsed lumen is seen as a linear reflection from the apposed walls of the lumen.

In most cases, marked GB thickening is manifested by irregular or striated intramural sonolucencies, as is seen in this case. When this pattern is noted, it usually means that the thickening is not related to cholecystitis. However, if this pattern is identified in a patient with well-established clinical and sonographic evidence of cholecystitis, then it usually indicates more advanced disease.

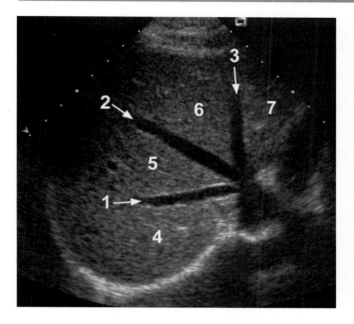
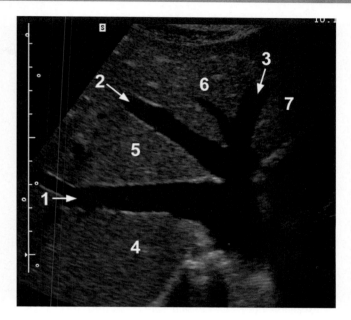

Transverse view of the liver.

1. What are the vascular structures indicated by the numbers 1, 2, and 3?

2. What segments of the liver, indicated by the numbers 4, 5, 6, and 7, do these vessels separate?

3. How can you distinguish the hepatic veins and portal veins on a static grey-scale view of the liver?

4. To what vein does the caudate lobe drain?

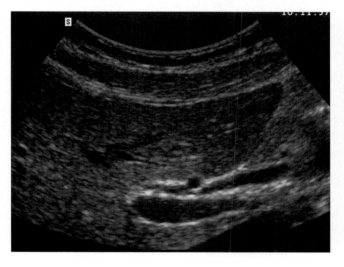
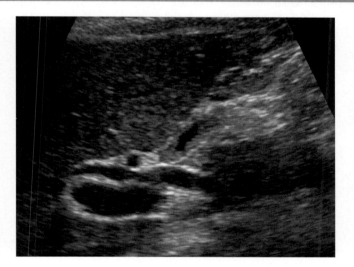

Longitudinal views of the porta hepatis in two patients.

1. Where is the common duct in these patients?

2. In what percentage of patients is the duct located as shown here?

3. Which is straighter, the bile duct or the hepatic artery?

4. Which varies more in caliber, the bile duct or the hepatic artery?

Normal Hepatic Venous Anatomy

1. The three vessels are the hepatic veins. 1 = Right, 2 = Middle, 3 = Left. This view is usually obtained from an epigastric approach with the transducer angled superiorly.

2. The right hepatic vein separates the anterior (5) and posterior (4) segments of the right lobe. The middle hepatic vein separates the anterior segment of the right and the medial segment (6) of the left lobe. The left hepatic vein separates the left lateral (7) and the left medial segments.

3. Unlike the portal veins, the hepatic veins are not surrounded by fibrofatty tissues and therefore have much less echogenic walls. In fact, under most circumstances, the wall of the hepatic vein is not visible sonographically. The exception is when the hepatic vein is viewed with the walls perpendicular to the direction of the sound. In this situation, the wall produces a specular reflection and appears as a thin, echogenic line. This is well demonstrated in the right hepatic vein on the first image.

4. The caudate lobe drains into the vena cava via small veins that are separate from the three main hepatic veins. This is the reason the caudate veins function as collaterals in patients with Budd-Chiari syndrome.

Reference
Schneck CD: Embryology, histology, gross anatomy and normal imaging anatomy of the liver. In Friedman AC, Dachman AH (eds): *Radiology of the Liver, Biliary Tract, and Pancreas.* St. Louis, Mosby, 1994, pp 1-25.

Cross-Reference
Ultrasound: THE REQUISITES, pp 3-5.

Comment
Three major veins drain hepatic blood flow into the vena cava. The main hepatic veins travel between the segments of the liver and therefore are used as landmarks for identifying the segments. The middle and left hepatic veins usually join together before emptying into the inferior vena cava. In most patients, the right hepatic vein is best imaged from an intercostal approach near the midaxillary line. This not only allows for visualization on grey-scale but also provides a good angle for Doppler imaging. The left hepatic vein is best imaged from a midline subxiphoid approach. The middle hepatic vein is best seen from an approach somewhere between the right and left vein.

In addition to the three main hepatic veins, a variable number of smaller dorsal hepatic veins may drain directly into the vena cava from the posterior right lobe and the caudate lobe. These dorsal veins often act as collaterals when the three main veins are obstructed.

Variant Relationship of Right Hepatic Artery and Bile Duct

1. In both cases the bile duct is located between the portal vein and the right hepatic artery. Normally the right hepatic artery is located between the portal vein and the bile duct.

2. This variant occurs in up to 20% of patients.

3. The bile duct is straighter than the artery.

4. The bile duct is more variable in diameter than the artery.

Reference
Middleton WD: The bile ducts. In Goldberg BB (ed): *Diagnostic Ultrasound.* Baltimore, Williams & Wilkins, 1993, pp 146-172.

Cross Reference
Ultrasound: THE REQUISITES, pp 55-56.

Comment
Anatomic variations around the porta hepatis are relatively common. The variant shown in this case, where the right hepatic artery crosses anterior to the duct, is reported to occur in up to 20% of individuals. However, it is not documented that commonly on sonography. Since the hepatic artery may cross in front of the bile duct, or the bile duct may pass in front of the hepatic artery, identification of the bile duct can sometimes be confusing. One clue that is helpful is that the bile duct is usually straighter than the hepatic artery. Therefore, it is easier to get a view of the bile duct that shows it over several centimeters, whereas the hepatic artery is too tortuous to see over a significant length. In addition, the hepatic artery maintains a fairly constant diameter, while the bile duct varies in diameter from proximal to distal. In many patients, the hepatic artery will indent the bile duct, but the bile duct never indents the artery.

In addition to the right hepatic artery, occasionally the cystic artery (the artery that supplies the gallbladder) can be seen near the common bile duct. This artery usually arises from the right hepatic artery to the right of the common duct. When it arises to the left of the common duct, it must cross the common duct on its way to the gallbladder. In some patients it passes in front and in others it passes behind the common duct. Therefore, it is possible to see two arteries behind the duct, an artery in front of and behind the duct, and two arteries in front of the duct.

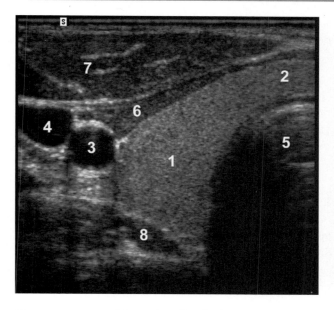
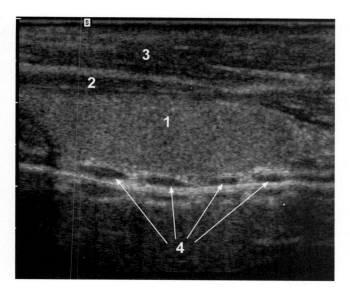

Transverse and longitudinal views of the thyroid.

1. Name the normal numbered structures on the transverse scan of the right side of the neck.

2. Name the normal numbered structures on the longitudinal scan of the neck.

3. How can the carotid artery be distinguished from the jugular vein on grey-scale scans of the neck?

4. Can the normal parathyroid glands be seen on ultrasonography?

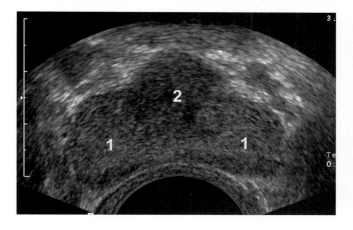
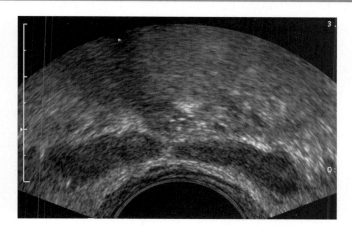

Transverse views of the prostate from a transrectal approach. The second image was obtained slightly superior to the first.

1. What zone of the prostate is indicated by the numbers 1 and 2?

2. What structures are shown in the second image?

3. What zone is the largest, and how does this vary with age?

4. What is the normal value for prostate-specific antigen (PSA)?

CASE 16

Normal Anatomy of the Thyroid

1. 1 = Right thyroid lobe, 2 = Thyroid isthmus, 3 = Carotid, 4 = Jugular, 5 = Trachea shadow, 6 = Strap muscles, 7 = Sternocleidomastoid muscle, 8 = Longus coli muscle.

2. 1 = Thyroid, 2 = Strap muscles, 3 = Sternocleidomastoid muscle, 4 = Cartilage rings of trachea.

3. The carotid artery is circular, the jugular vein is oval. The carotid is more medial and deep, the jugular is more lateral and superficial. The carotid is noncompressible, the jugular is easily compressible. The diameter of the carotid is constant, the diameter of the jugular varies.

4. The normal parathyroids are too small to be seen on sonography.

Reference

Solbiati L, Livraghi T, Ballarati E, et al: The thyroid. In Solbiati L, Rizzatto G (eds): *Ultrasound of Superficial Structures*. Edinburgh, Churchill Livingstone, 1995, pp 49–86.

Cross-Reference

Ultrasound: THE REQUISITES, pp 448–449.

Comment

The normal thyroid gland consists of a left and a right lobe connected by a thin isthmus. It is located in the inferior aspect of the neck on both sides of the trachea. A minority of patients have a thin pyramidal lobe that extends superiorly from the isthmus and can be seen in childhood. In adults, the normal thyroid is 4 to 6 cm long and 13 to 18 mm in anteroposterior diameter. It has a homogeneous medium-level echogenicity. Normally, the thyroid is more echogenic than the overlying strap muscles and the sternocleidomastoid muscles.

The parathyroid glands typically measure 4 × 3 × 1 mm in size, with the long axis oriented in a craniocaudal direction. The two superior glands are usually located behind the mid aspect of the thyroid, and the two inferior glands are located behind or just inferior to the lower pole of the thyroid. Approximately 20% of inferior parathyroid glands are located within 4 cm of the lower pole of the thyroid. A fifth gland, usually associated within the thymus, is present in approximately 13% of patients.

CASE 17

Normal Prostate

1. Number 1 indicates the peripheral zone. Number 2 indicates the central gland, which includes the central zone and the transitional zone.

2. The second image is taken slightly superior to the first and shows the paired seminal vesicles.

3. In young men the peripheral zone is the largest. Because of the effects of benign prostatic hypertrophy (BPH), the central gland is the largest in older men.

4. The normal PSA is less than 4 ng/ml.

Reference

Kaye KW, Richter L: Ultrasonographic anatomy of the normal prostate gland: Reconstruction by computer graphics. *Urology* 1990;35:12–17.

Cross-Reference

Ultrasound: THE REQUISITES, pp 458–460.

Comment

The prostate is divided into several zones. The peripheral zone is the largest in normal prostates. It is located posteriorly and laterally and extends inferiorly to the prostate apex. The central zone accounts for approximately 25% of normal prostate volume, while the transitional zone accounts for 5%. The central zone is located in the middle of the base (superior aspect) of the prostate. There is also a nonglandular area anteriorly called the fibromuscular stroma. On sonography, the transitional zone and the central zone cannot be distinguished, so they are referred to jointly as the central gland. The surgical capsule separates the peripheral zone from the central gland. The normal prostate in a young man weighs approximately 20 g. A gland weighing more than 40 g is considered enlarged in older men. Prostate volume is calculated based on the equation for an elliptical-shaped structure. A simplified equation is length times width times height divided by 2.

Superior to the base of the prostate are the paired seminal vesicles. They appear as oval shaped and taper toward the midline. They are normally less echogenic than the prostate gland.

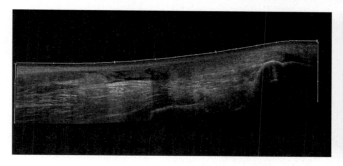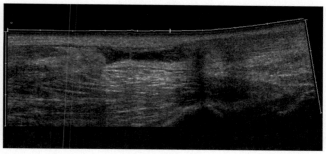

Two longitudinal, extended-field-of-view scans of the Achilles tendon. The first image covers a 15-cm length from the distal calf to the calcaneus, and the second covers a 9-cm length of the distal calf.

1. Describe the abnormality.
2. Should the Achilles tendon be scanned in plantarflexion or in dorsiflexion?
3. In what part of the tendon does this condition normally occur?
4. What muscles contribute to the Achilles tendon?

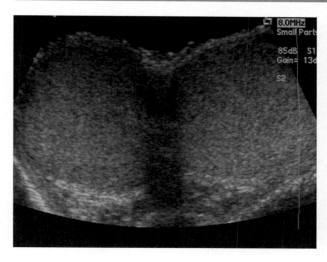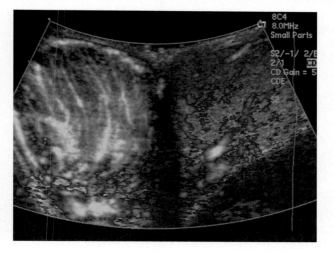

Transverse grey-scale and power Doppler view of the scrotum in a patient with testicular pain.

1. Which testis is abnormal, and what is the likely diagnosis?
2. With what condition is this testicular abnormality most often associated?
3. Which is most sensitive for this diagnosis, grey-scale or color Doppler?
4. Is this typically diffuse or focal?

Complete Tear of the Achilles Tendon

1. Both scans show a complete gap in the normal continuity of the tendon located approximately 6 cm proximal to the calcaneus. This is the most common location and appearance of a complete tear of the Achilles tendon.

2. In a patient with a complete tear of the Achilles, the tendon should be scanned in both plantarflexion and dorsiflexion.

3. Tears usually occur 2 to 6 cm proximal to the insertion.

4. The gastrocnemius and soleus muscles form the Achilles tendon.

Reference

Fessell DP, Vanderschueren GM, Jacobson JA, et al: US of the Ankle: Technique, anatomy, and diagnosis of pathologic conditions. *Radiographics* 1998;18:325–340.

Cross-Reference

Ultrasound: THE REQUISITES, p 455.

Comment

The Achilles tendon is the thickest and strongest in the body. It is composed of fibers from the soleus and gastrocnemius muscles. As these fibers descend toward the insertion on the posterior surface of the calcaneus, they spiral approximately 90 degrees, so that the fibers that start in a medial location end up in a superficial location. This arrangement conveys some elastic property to the tendon.

Despite its size and strength, the Achilles tendon is the most commonly injured tendon in the ankle. It can tear when it is exposed to unusual stresses, when it is exposed to chronic low-grade stresses, or with age-related attritional changes. Because the Achilles is easy to palpate, complete tears are usually easy to diagnose clinically. Most complete tears can be managed effectively without imaging of any type.

On sonography, complete tears of the Achilles tendon appear as a focal total disruption of the normal fibrillar pattern. This disruption usually occurs in a relatively hypovascular zone 2 to 6 cm proximal to the Achilles insertion. In the acute setting, there is a heterogeneous, often solid- and cystic-appearing hematoma at the site of the tear. This is seen in this case. The retracted tendon ends may lose their fibrillar appearance, at least partially, because they are no longer stretched and the fibers are not straight. In the chronic setting, scar tissue and granulation tissue develop in the tear and are distinguished from normal tendon by their lack of fibrillar architecture.

One useful role of sonography in patients with complete Achilles tears is to measure the gap between the proximal and distal fragments. When the fragments are closely apposed during plantarflexion, the tear can be treated conservatively with casting. When the gap is large, surgical repair is necessary.

Orchitis

1. Blood flow to the right testis is dramatically increased. This degree of hyperemia is usually due to orchitis. Normal flow is present in the left testis.

2. Orchitis is usually associated with epididymitis.

3. Color Doppler shows increased blood flow to the testis before any grey-scale changes are apparent.

4. Orchitis usually affects the entire testis in a diffuse manner.

Reference

Horstman WG, Middleton WD, Melson GL: Scrotal inflammatory disease: Color Doppler ultrasonographic findings. *Radiology* 1991;179:55–59.

Cross-Reference

Ultrasound: THE REQUISITES, pp 445–447.

Comment

Orchitis typically occurs as a secondary event in patients with primary epididymitis. However, it can also be isolated, such as with mumps orchitis or other viral infections. Regardless of its cause, orchitis is manifest clinically as an enlarged and painful testis.

On sonography, orchitis appears as a hypoechoic, enlarged testis. On color Doppler, an inflammatory hyperemia will appear as increased blood flow to the affected side. Generally, the changes in blood flow precede the changes in testicular morphology. Therefore, color Doppler is more sensitive to the diagnosis than is grey-scale sonography.

In most cases, the entire testis is involved. When focal orchitis occurs, it appears as a focal area of decreased echogenicity and increased vascularity. This sonographic appearance can overlap with the appearance of testicular tumors. The easiest way to distinguish a tumor from focal orchitis is on clinical grounds. Tumors will usually be readily palpable and nontender, while focal orchitis is nonpalpable and tender. On sonography, it is helpful to look at the epididymis. Focal orchitis will usually be associated with epididymitis, and an enlarged hyperemic epididymis will be apparent. Testicular tumors usually do not involve the epididymis. It is also useful to look in the retroperitoneum, since detectable adenopathy makes a tumor much more likely than a benign testicular process.

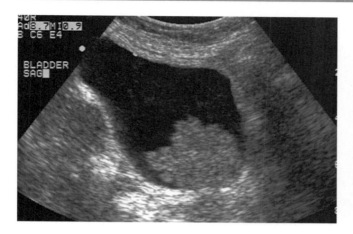
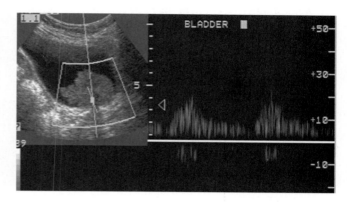

Longitudinal grey-scale view of the bladder and similar view with pulsed Doppler analysis.

1. Describe the abnormality.

2. What is the likely diagnosis?

3. Is this abnormality easier to detect on the anterior or posterior wall?

4. What is the most common location of this type of lesion?

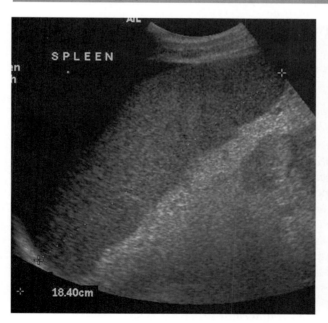
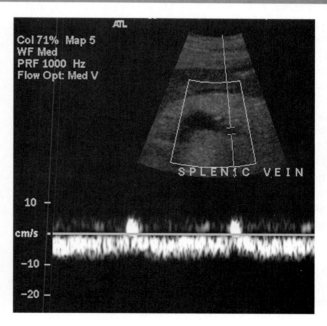

Longitudinal view of the spleen and transverse view of the epigastrium with pulsed Doppler waveform of the splenic vein.

1. What is the upper limit of normal for spleen length?

2. Is the flow in this patient's splenic vein normal?

3. What is the likely cause of this patient's splenic abnormality?

4. Does the spleen normally extend below the left kidney?

Transitional Cell Carcinoma of the Bladder

1. A soft-tissue mass in the base of the bladder with internal arterial flow.

2. The most likely diagnosis is transitional cell carcinoma (TCC).

3. Tumors on the posterior wall are easier to detect sonographically. Near-field reverberation artifact can obscure anterior wall masses.

4. TCC of the bladder typically occurs on the lateral and posterior wall and near the trigone.

Reference

Karcnik TJ, Simmons MZ, Abujudea HA: Ultrasound imaging of the adult urinary bladder. *Ultrasound Q* 1999;15:135–147

Cross-Reference

Genitourinary Radiology: THE REQUISITES, pp 197–204.

Comment

Bladder cancer is the 11th most common cancer in the world. It occurs in men three times more often than in women. At least 90% of bladder cancers are transitional cell cancers (TCC). Less than 5% are squamous cell, and an even lower percentage are adenocarcinomas, small cell carcinomas, and sarcomas. Smoking predisposes to TCC and contributes to approximately half of the cases seen in men. Certain occupational exposures also seem to predispose to bladder cancer, including the dye, rubber, and aluminum industries. Excessive exposure to diesel exhaust and excessive consumption of phenacetin and acetaminophen are also associated with TCC of the bladder.

The majority of patients with bladder cancer present with hematuria. Less commonly, they will have voiding symptoms such as urgency, dysuria, and frequency. Flank pain may develop in the setting of ureteral obstruction. Rarely, patients present with symptoms related to metastatic disease to the liver, lung, or bones.

Sonography is very good at identifying bladder cancers, with a sensitivity and specificity of approximately 90%. However, most of these patients have cystoscopy done as the primary means of finding and quantitating bladder cancer. Nevertheless, it is very important to look carefully at the bladder in patients with hematuria, since ultrasound may be the first study that documents a tumor. Sonography may also be useful in patients with bladder diverticulae, in whom it may be difficult to pass the cystoscope past the neck of the diverticulum.

In patients with hematuria, bladder cancer must be distinguished from solid clots in the bladder. This is usually easy, since clots move with changes in patient position. Color Doppler is also valuable, since tumors often have detectable internal vascularity and clots do not. In men, an enlarged prostate may produce a mass that indents the base of the bladder and simulates a primary bladder mass. This situation should be suspected whenever the mass is located in the midline adjacent to the prostate. Occasionally, perivesicular tumors or perivesicular inflammatory processes involve the bladder wall and simulate a bladder tumor. Therefore, careful correlation with clinical history and careful analysis of perivesicular structures is important.

Splenomegaly

1. Upper limit of normal for splenic length is 13 cm. Upper limit of normal for splenic thickness is 6 cm.

2. Flow in the splenic vein is reversed.

3. Reversal of splenic vein flow and splenomegaly are both due to portal hypertension.

4. The spleen normally does not extend below the left kidney.

Reference

Permutter GS: Ultrasound measurements of the spleen. In Goldberg BB, Kurtz AB (eds): *Atlas of Ultrasound Measurements.* Chicago, Year Book, 1990, pp 126–138.

Cross-Reference

Ultrasound: THE REQUISITES, p 146.

Comment

Detection of splenomegaly is usually accomplished via physical examination of the abdomen. However, in some patients, physical examination may be limited by factors such as obesity, pain, and marked ascites. It can also be difficult to distinguish an enlarged spleen from other left upper quadrant masses. In these patients, sonography can be very valuable. Not only can ultrasound evaluate the size of the spleen, but in some patients it can also determine the cause of an enlarged spleen and exclude other processes.

Because the spleen is a curved, disk-shaped organ, it is somewhat difficult to measure in standard planes. One measurement that is relatively easy to obtain and to reproduce is the maximum splenic length. For spleens that are not long but are thick, the short-axis thickness of the spleen is also a valuable measurement. The short axis needs to be measured perpendicular to the long axis of the spleen.

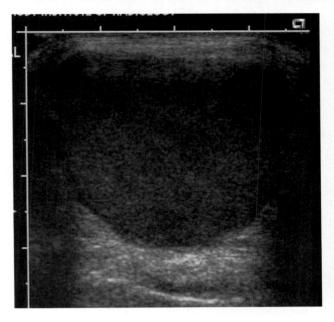 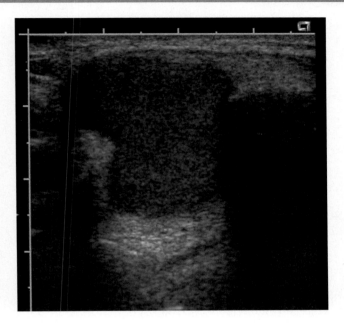

Transverse and longitudinal views of the neck between the thyroid cartilage and the hyoid bone.

1. Is it common to see internal echoes in these lesions?

2. Is this a common location for this abnormality?

3. Is this lesion usually unilocular or multilocular?

4. Is this lesion likely to be cured with percutaneous aspiration?

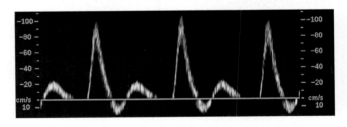 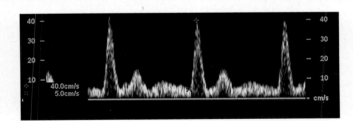

Pulsed Doppler waveforms from two arteries.

1. Would you characterize these waveforms as high or low resistance?

2. What arteries might display waveforms such as the ones shown in this case?

3. What causes the flow below base line on the waveform on the left?

4. What is the resistive index of these waveforms?

Thyroglossal Duct Cyst

1. Although thyroglossal duct cysts are filled with fluid, the fluid is usually complex-appearing on sonography, and internal echoes are common.

2. This is the classic location, between the thyroid cartilage and the hyoid bone.

3. Thyroglossal duct cysts are usually unilocular.

4. Aspiration will not cure a thyroglossal duct cyst. The cyst wall has to be completely resected, or else it will recur.

References

Koeller KK, Alamo L, Adair CF, Smirniotopoulos JG: From the archives of the AFIP: Congenital cystic masses of the neck: Radiologic-pathologic correlation. *Radiographics* 1999;19:121–146.

Wadsworth DT, Siegel MJ: Thyroglossal duct cysts: Variability of sonographic findings. *AJR Am J Roentgenol* 1994;163:1475–1477.

Cross-Reference

Neuroradiology: THE REQUISITES, p 438.

Comment

Thyroglossal duct cysts are the most common of the congenital cysts of the neck. They arise along the tract of the thyroglossal duct. This tract extends from the foramen cecum at the base of the tongue to the hyoid bone and finally to the thyroid isthmus or to a pyramidal lobe. Normally this tract involutes by the eighth week of fetal development. However, remnants of thyroid elements remain in approximately 5% of cases. These remnants can give rise to cysts, fistulae, or solid thyroid nodules. Histologically, the cyst wall is composed of squamous cell mucosa, although inflammatory changes may obscure this fact. Despite the pathogenesis, thyroid tissue is usually not detected on pathologic analysis of thyroglossal duct cysts. Thyroid cancer is even less common in these cysts (approximately 1%). When it occurs, it is usually papillary cancer.

Thyroglossal duct cysts typically manifest prior to age 10, although there is a second peak in the young adult years. They may be painful owing to hemorrhage or infection. However, many of these cysts are discovered as painless masses or as incidental findings on imaging studies done for other reasons. They are located in the midline, usually at the level of the hyoid bone (15%) or just below the level of the hyoid bone (65%). Only 20% are suprahyoid. Cysts that arise significantly below the hyoid bone tend to be farther from the midline.

Unlike cysts elsewhere, thyroglossal duct cysts are usually not anechoic. Low-level internal echoes, as seen in the case shown here, may be due to hemorrhage, infection, crystals, or proteinaceous material. Their usu-ally intimate relationship to the hyoid bone is best seen on longitudinal scans. Although they are usually in the midline, slight pressure applied with the transducer can sometimes push them to one side or the other.

High Resistance Waveforms

1. Both of these waveforms are high-resistance–type waveforms.

2. High-resistance waveforms can arise from arteries that supply nonparenchymal structures, such as the extremities and the bowel. The first waveform came from the superficial femoral artery, and the second came from the radial artery.

3. The short phase of early diastolic flow reversal is caused by elastic recoil of the artery.

4. The resistive index (RI) is calculated as the difference of peak systole and end diastole divided by peak systole. The RI equals 1.0 whenever the end diastolic flow is zero, as in the first image. In the second image the RI equals $(40 - 5)/40 = 0.88$.

Reference

Nelson TR, Pretorius DH: The Doppler signal: Where does it come from and what does it mean? *AJR Am J Roentgenol* 1988;151:439–447.

Cross-Reference

Ultrasound: THE REQUISITES, pp 464–465.

Comment

The waveforms shown in this case have very narrow and sharply pointed systolic peaks, rapid systolic deceleration into diastole, and little, if any, late diastolic flow. There is a short phase of early diastolic flow reversal seen on the first waveform. These are characteristics of a high-resistance waveform and typically come from vessels that supply nonparenchymal structures, such as the extremities. The first waveform is referred to as a triphasic pattern, since there is a phase above the base line, followed by a second phase below the base line, followed by a third phase above the base line. This is a classic appearance for an extremity artery. During systole, the vessel expands as the pressure increases. In early diastole, the elastic recoil properties of the vessel result in contraction of the lumen diameter. Resistance to forward flow is high enough that the majority of the blood filling the lumen is pushed backward during the period of elastic recoil, and this results in transient flow reversal. When the elastic recoil ceases, there is a short final phase of forward flow.

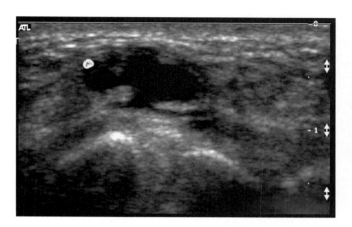 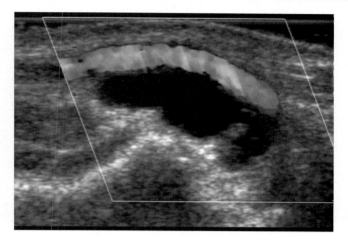

Transverse view of the dorsal surface of the wrist and longitudinal view of the volar surface of the wrist in two patients with the same abnormality.

1. What is the most common cause of cystic lesions in the wrist?
2. Where do these lesions most often occur?
3. What are these lesions composed of?
4. Are they usually firm or soft?

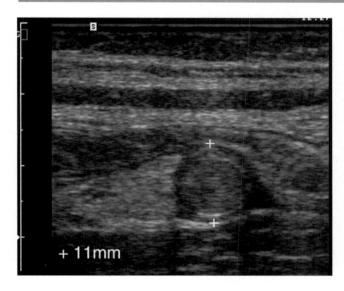 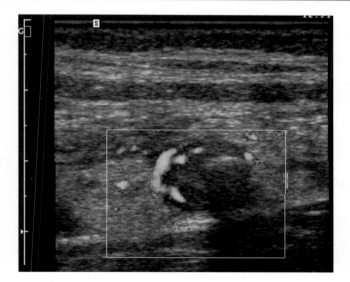

Transverse grey scale and color Doppler views of the right lower quadrant.

1. What is the sensitivity of ultrasound in making this diagnosis?
2. Is this diagnosis easier to make with ultrasound in children or in adults?
3. What are the sonographic criteria for this condition?
4. How do CT and ultrasound compare in evaluating patients suspected of having this condition?

Ganglion Cyst of the Wrist

1. Ganglion cysts are the most common cause of cysts in the wrist and hand.

2. The most common location is the dorsal wrist, superficial to the scapholunate joint. On the first image, the surface of the scaphoid and the lunate are seen as strong linear reflections deep to the cyst. The space between the two bones is the scapholunate joint.

3. Ganglion cysts are usually composed of very thick, gelatinous liquid.

4. Ganglion cysts are typically very firm and noncompressible on sonography.

Reference

Middleton WD, Teefey SA, Boyer MI: Hand and wrist sonography. *Ultrasound Q* 2001;17:21–36.

Cross-Reference

Musculoskeletal Imaging: THE REQUISITES, pp 241–243.

Comment

Ganglion cysts are the most common cause of palpable masses in the hand and wrist. They are most common in young women, although they can occur at any age and in both sexes. They manifest with either localized pain or a palpable mass.

There are four typical locations. Sixty percent to 70% occur over the dorsal wrist. Dorsal ganglia usually originate from the scapholunate joint. They may dissect proximally or distally. Twenty percent arise on the volar side of the wrist. Volar ganglia frequently extend around the flexor carpi radialis tendon or, as shown on the second image, the radial artery. They typically arise from one of the radiocarpal joints. The third most common location is along one of the flexor tendon sheaths. These cysts account for 10% of ganglia. Finally, ganglia can arise from the interphalangeal joints, usually due to underlying degenerative arthritis. These cysts have also been called mucous cysts.

The appearance of ganglia on ultrasound is predictable. Like other fluid-containing structures, ganglia are typically anechoic with well-defined walls. Through transmission is usually detectable unless the cyst is small. Due to slice thickness artifact, small ganglia may also have low-level internal echoes. In some cases, a neck may be seen leading toward the joint of origin. With large ganglia, there are often folds or septations, particularly near the neck of the cyst.

Detection of a wrist ganglion is limited by the size and depth of the cyst. Small and deep ganglia are the most difficult to detect. Ruptured ganglion cysts may appear as predominantly solid masses and can also lead to a confusing appearance. Nevertheless, ultrasound remains an excellent means of evaluating patients with a suspected ganglion cyst. Accuracy in skilled hands is similar to that of MRI.

Acute Appendicitis

1. The sensitivity of ultrasound for the diagnosis of appendicitis is 75% to 90%. Positive predictive value ranges from 91% to 94%, and negative predictive value ranges from 89% to 97%.

2. Children are usually easier to diagnose than adults because they typically have less abdominal wall fat.

3. The criteria for appendicitis are identification of a blind ending, noncompressible bowel loop that arises from the cecum and measures 6 mm or more in diameter. Identification of an appendicolith and inflamed periappendiceal fat are helpful secondary signs. Color Doppler demonstration of mural hypervascularity is also useful.

4. The success of CT and ultrasound in diagnosing appendicitis depends on institutional preference and local expertise. In general, radiologists probably do better with CT than with ultrasound. However, ultrasound is complementary to CT and is probably superior in thin patients.

Reference

Birnbaum BA, Wilson SR: Appendicitis at the millennium. *Radiology* 2000;215:337–348.

Cross-Reference

Ultrasound: THE REQUISITES, pp 457–458.

Comment

In the Western world, acute abdominal pain requiring surgery is more commonly due to appendicitis than to any other condition. The peak incidence of appendicitis is in the second decade of life. The most common etiology is obstruction from a fecalith. This obstruction results in increased luminal pressure and eventually in ischemia. Compromised mucosa subsequently becomes infected with luminal bacteria. Ongoing infection, ischemia, and infarction may lead to perforation.

Classic presentation is of vague lower abdominal pain, nausea, and vomiting, followed by more discrete right lower quadrant pain. Patients are usually afebrile or have a low-grade fever. Accuracy for clinical diagnosis of appendicitis is approximately 80%. Accuracy is lower in women of childbearing age owing to the clinical overlap of acute gynecologic disease and acute appendicitis.

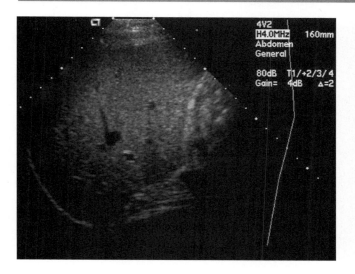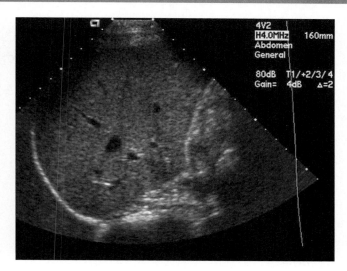

Two views of the liver.

1. Why is the deep aspect of the liver so hypoechoic on the first image?
2. What is the difference between gain and power?
3. Should image brightness be controlled first with gain or with power?
4. Are gain and power preprocessing or postprocessing controls?

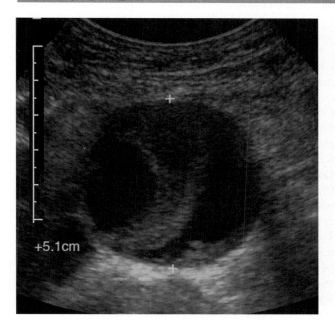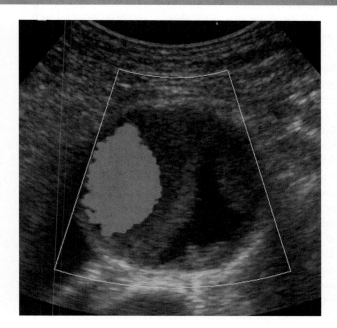

Transverse grey-scale and color Doppler view of the aorta.

1. Should surgery be considered in this patient?
2. What important information should be obtained when scanning a patient such as this one?
3. What is the significance of the hypoechoic crescent within the mural thrombus?
4. Is color Doppler necessary?

C A S E   2 6

Distance Gain Compensation Curve

1. The distance gain compensation curve is inappropriately adjusted on the first image. Increased gain settings were applied to the far field on the second image, and the liver appears normal throughout.

2. *Power* refers to the strength of the sound pulse that is transmitted by the transducer. *Gain* refers to the amount of electronic amplification of the signal that returns to the transducer.

3. Increasing the power and the gain both result in brighter images; however, increased power causes greater patient exposure and can cause artifacts. Therefore, it is best to increase power only when an optimal image cannot be obtained first with adjustment of gain.

4. *Preprocessing* refers to controls that must be adjusted in real-time while the patient is being scanned. *Postprocessing* refers to controls that can be adjusted on a frozen image. Gain and power are both preprocessing controls.

Reference

Zwiebel WJ: Image optimization, ultrasound artifacts, and safety considerations. In Zwiebel WJ, Sohaey R (eds): *Introduction to Ultrasound*. Philadelphia, WB Saunders, 1998, pp 18–30.

Comment

As sound travels through tissue, it undergoes a number of interactions. The interactions that allow an image to be created are reflection and scattering. In addition, sound is absorbed by the tissues. These interactions cause attenuation of the sound pulse as it passes through tissue. Since the transmitted pulse and the re-flected pulse both become weaker as they travel through the tissues, identical reflectors located in the near field and in the far field produce echoes of different strengths. To compensate for this, pulses that have trav-eled farther are electronically amplified after they return to the transducer. This process is called distance com-pensation, and it is displayed on the image as a curve, called the distance gain compensation (DGC) curve. On the images shown, the DGC curve appears as a line on the right side of the image that extends from the near field to the far field. On the second image, the curve slopes progressively to the right as it goes from the near to the far field. This indicates steady progressive amplification of the echoes returning from the far field. In the first image, the DGC curve tapers back to the left in the far field, indicating decreased amplification of the far field echoes.

For homogeneous structures like the liver that attenu-ate sound uniformly, the DGC curve should have a fairly constant up-slope. When fluid-filled structures such as the bladder are scanned, there is negligible attenuation, so the DGC curve does not need to provide compensa-tion until the solid structures deep to the bladder are encountered.

C A S E   2 7

Abdominal Aortic Aneurysm

1. Surgery should be considered when an aneurysm reaches 5 cm in diameter, since the cumulative risk of rupture over the next 8 years is 25%.

2. It is important to measure the diameter of the aneurysm and to determine where it starts and stops with respect to the renal arteries and the aortic bifurcation.

3. The crescent indicates liquefied clot. It does not indicate dissection, rupture, or impending rupture.

4. Color Doppler is rarely needed in the evaluation of an aortic aneurysm.

Reference

Nevitt MP, Ballard DJ, Hallett JW Jr: Prognosis of abdomi-nal aortic aneurysms: A population based study. *N Engl J Med* 1989;321:1009–1014.

Cross-Reference

Gastrointestinal Radiology: THE REQUISITES, p 102.

Comment

Abdominal aortic aneurysms are a common abnormality, especially in elderly men, with 95% occurring below the level of the renal arteries. They are strongly associ-ated with atherosclerosis. An aneurysm is present when there is a focal dilatation of the aorta that measures 3 cm or more in diameter. Different groups use different approaches to the measurement of aortic aneurysms. The most important issue is to use an approach that is reproducible, so that comparative measurements taken over time may accurately determine the stability of the aneurysm. In my practice, we measure from the outer wall to the outer wall. Anterior-to-posterior measure-ments are obtained from sagittal views, and transverse measurements are obtained from a left coronal view. I avoid measurements in the axial view, since it is not possible to determine whether such measurements are taken perpendicular to the long axis of the aorta, and the lateral borders of the aorta are not well seen. In addition, I believe that axial measurements are prone to significant interobserver and intraobserver variability.

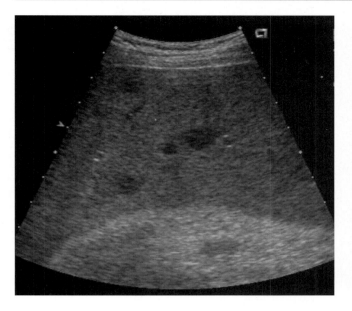
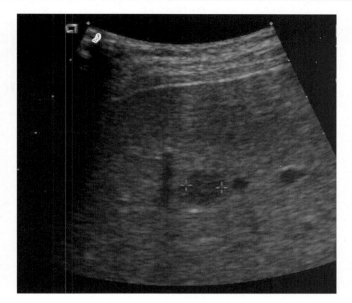

Two views of the liver in a patient with a history of lung cancer.

1. Are the lesions shown in this case most likely solid or cystic?

2. What is the most likely diagnosis?

3. What else should be considered?

4. How can the diagnosis be confirmed?

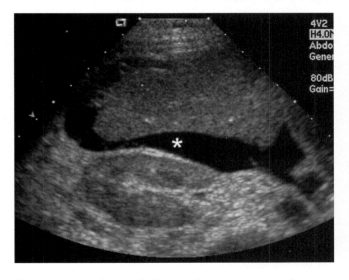
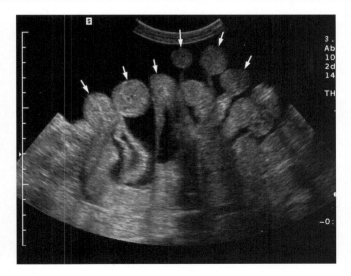

Transverse view of the right upper quadrant and the left lower quadrant in two patients.

1. What do these patients have in common?

2. To what are the arrows pointing?

3. In what anatomic location is the asterisk positioned?

4. What are the best places to look when searching for this abnormality?

CASE 28

Liver Metastases

1. The lesions shown in this case are homogeneous and hypoechoic. There is no detectable posterior enhancement, and the back wall is not sharply defined. These characteristics are most consistent with solid lesions. Cysts of this size in the liver should appear anechoic with readily detectable posterior enhancement. Occasionally, there is overlap in the grey-scale appearance of solid and fluid filled masses. In such cases, identification of internal vascularity on color Doppler will indicate that the lesion is solid.

2. The sonographic appearance is nonspecific. However, they are not simple cysts and do not have a typical appearance for hemangiomas. Given the patient's history of lung cancer, these lesions are most likely metastases.

3. Other possible causes of multiple solid lesions include lymphoma and multifocal hepatocellular cancer. Less likely considerations would be multiple focal nodular hyperplasia, sarcoidosis, multifocal adenomas, or abscesses. Hemangiomas are very common and can be multiple, so they should also be considered, although multiple hemangiomas that were all hypoechoic would be very atypical.

4. The diagnosis of metastases can be (and in this case was) confirmed with ultrasound-guided biopsy.

Reference

Marn CS, Bree RL, Silver TM: Ultrasonography of the liver. *Radiol Clin North Am* 1991;29:1151–1170.

Cross-Reference

Ultrasound: THE REQUISITES, pp 7–9.

Comment

Multiple solid hypoechoic masses in the liver are most likely to be metastases. In the majority of cases, patients with liver metastases have a prior history or current evidence of an extrahepatic malignancy. This patient had a history of lung cancer. If there were a history of lymphoma, then the most likely diagnosis would be lymphoma. If there were a history of fever and diverticulitis, liver abscesses would be a consideration. If there were a history of hepatitis C, then multifocal hepatocellular cancer would be most likely. In general, if there is no history to point toward another diagnosis, then metastatic disease is the leading possibility.

Further workup also depends on the patient's history. If there is a known primary malignancy and the presence of metastatic disease needs to be confirmed prior to chemotherapy, ultrasound-guided biopsy should be performed. In this situation, fine needle aspiration with cytologic evaluation is usually adequate. If there is no known primary malignancy, a standard evaluation for an unknown primary should be pursued. If the primary malignancy is not found, then a liver biopsy should be performed to establish the cell type that needs to be treated. In this situation, core biopsies are usually necessary to provide enough tissue so that immunohistochemical studies can be obtained to better define possible primaries. If the primary malignancy is found or if other sites of metastases are identified, then biopsy of the safest and most accessible site should be performed.

CASE 29

Ascites

1. Both demonstrate peritoneal fluid that is anechoic and conforms to the structures in the area. This is typical of ascites.

2. The arrows are pointing to loops of small bowel. Notice the mesentery surrounded by ascites.

3. The asterisk is in the hepatorenal fossa, also called Morrison's pouch.

4. The most common location for ascites is around the liver, in the pelvis, and in the pericolic gutters.

Reference

Nguyen KT, Sauerbrei EE, Nolan RL: The peritoneum and the diaphragm. In Rumack CM, Wilson SR, Charboneau JW (eds): *Diagnostic Ultrasound,* 2nd ed. St. Louis, Mosby, 1998, p 501–519.

Cross-Reference

Ultrasound: THE REQUISITES, p 50.

Comment

Ascites can be due to many underlying abnormalities, including congestive heart failure, hypoalbuminemia, portal hypertension, venous or lymphatic obstruction, infection or inflammation, and neoplasms. Because the peritoneal cavity is a continuum of multiple interconnecting spaces, ascites can localize in a variety of locations. Sonography is an excellent means of detecting ascites and is used routinely to localize an optimum site for paracentesis.

The best way to distinguish uncomplicated ascites and loculated peritoneal fluid collections is to look for the effect the fluid has on adjacent structures. Loculated collections such as abscesses, hematomas, and pseudocysts will displace and distort the structures around them. As shown in these images, simple ascites conforms to the shape of adjacent structures.

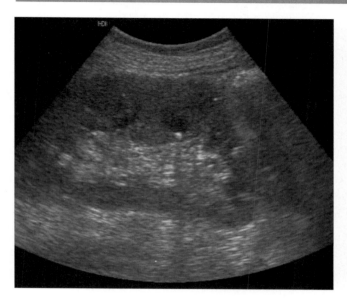
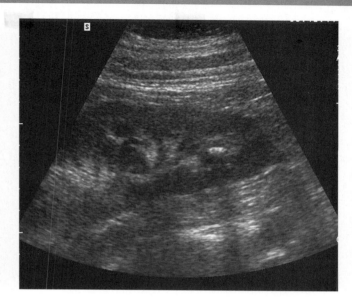

Longitudinal views of two patients with the same abnormality.

1. Describe the abnormality seen in both of these kidneys.
2. How good is ultrasound at making this diagnosis?
3. Is the abnormality seen in these kidneys likely to be seen on CT?
4. What are potential causes of shadowing in the kidney?

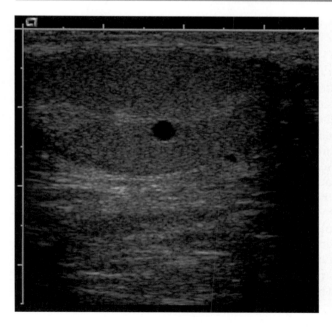
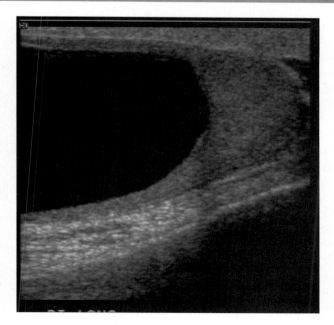

Longitudinal views of the testis in two patients.

1. Do these patients need further workup?
2. How common are these lesions?
3. Are they more common in young patients or in elderly patients?
4. With what condition are they sometimes associated?

Renal Stones

1. Both images show shadowing, echogenic structures in the kidney most consistent with renal stones.

2. Reports vary. Success is very dependent on stone size.

3. Yes. CT is more sensitive than ultrasound in detecting renal stones.

4. Stones, air, crystalline material in renal cysts, angiomyolipomas, calcified arteries, refraction from normal sinus structures, calcifications in tumors or cysts, catheters.

Reference

Middleton WD, Dodds WJ, Lawson TL, Foley WD: Renal calculi: Sensitivity for detection with US. *Radiology* 1988;167:234-244.

Cross-Reference

Ultrasound: THE REQUISITES, pp 103-104.

Comment

Renal stones are a common abnormality. They come in a variety of sizes, shapes, and compositions. Sonographically, they all look the same. Like gallstones, renal stones typically appear as hyperechoic reflectors with a posterior acoustic shadow. Unfortunately, renal stones are harder to visualize than gallstones. This is partially due to the fact that renal stones are usually surrounded by the hyperechoic renal sinus structures. This makes them less conspicuous than gallstones, which are usually surrounded by bile. In addition, the kidneys are deeper than the gallbladder; therefore, it is harder to get close to kidney stones, and resolution is often limited. Finally, the interface between kidney stones and the soft tissue around them produces less of an acoustic impedance mismatch than that caused by gallstones and bile. Therefore, the reflection from kidney stones is usually not as strong as from gallstones.

Reports on the sonographic sensitivity for detecting kidney stones vary. It is clear that the major factor that affects our ability to detect stones is the size of the stones. Stones that are larger than 5 mm are detected with a high sensitivity, while stones that are smaller are detected less reliably. It is important to realize that stones may be relatively easy to see from one approach and impossible to see from another approach. It should also be recognized that shadowing frequently occurs from the renal sinus structures due to refraction of the sound. This is not associated with a leading echogenic focus and should not be confused with renal stones.

Another limitation of ultrasound is accurate measurement of stone size. Therefore, it is difficult to document changes in stone size when patients are undergoing therapy. This is particularly true in patients who have had lithotripsy, because it is often impossible to distinguish a single large stone from a cluster of adjacent stone fragments.

Unlike gallstones, kidney stones are easier to detect with CT than with ultrasound. This is because kidney stones are mineralized enough to appear dense on CT. Even stones that are typically lucent on abdominal radiographs are detected as high attenuation structures with CT.

Testicular Cysts

1. Testicular cysts require no additional workup, provided they appear entirely simple on ultrasound.

2. Cysts are detected on approximately 10% of testicular sonograms.

3. Testicular cysts are more common in elderly men.

4. Testicular cysts are associated with tubular ectasia of the rete testis.

Reference

Gooding GA, Leonhardt W, Stein R: Testicular cysts: US findings. *Radiology* 1987;163:537-540.

Cross-Reference

Ultrasound: THE REQUISITES, pp 435-439.

Comment

Testicular cysts were once felt to be relatively rare lesions. However, widespread use of ultrasound to evaluate scrotal diseases has shown that they are actually common. Series have shown that intratesticular cysts are seen in approximately 10% of patients referred for scrotal sonograms. They often occur near the mediastinum. This is well demonstrated in the first image, where the small cyst is immediately adjacent to the linear, hyperechoic mediastinum. These cysts are often seen in patients with tubular ectasia of the rete testes, and both conditions may be caused by some degree of outflow obstruction of the seminal fluid. Testicular cysts range in size but are usually small. Even when they are large, testicular cysts are generally not palpable.

Like cysts elsewhere in the body, testicular cysts should be anechoic, have a strong back wall reflection, and demonstrate posterior acoustic enhancement. When an intratesticular lesion meets these classic criteria for a simple cyst, it requires no further evaluation. When there are any solid components or septations, the possibility of a cystic testicular neoplasm should be considered, particularly if the lesion is palpable.

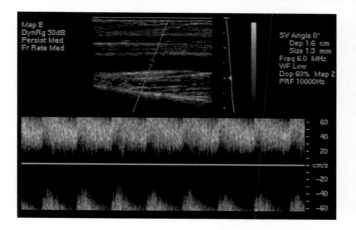 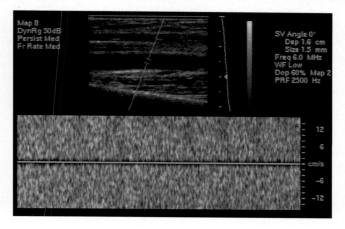

Pulsed Doppler waveforms from the common carotid artery.

1. What do these two waveforms have in common?
2. Will this finding be eliminated by proper adjustment of the Doppler gain?
3. Will this finding be eliminated by proper adjustment of the Doppler scale?
4. Will this finding be eliminated by changing to a higher frequency probe?

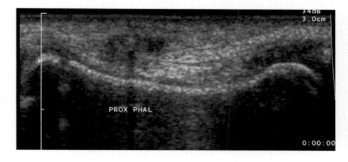 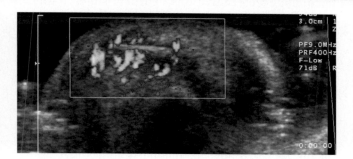

Longitudinal grey-scale view and transverse power Doppler view of the proximal fifth finger.

1. What are the pertinent findings?
2. What is the role of ultrasound in making this diagnosis?
3. What limits the ability of ultrasound to make this diagnosis?
4. How accurate is ultrasound in establishing this diagnosis in the hand and wrist?

Doppler Aliasing Artifact

1. Both of the waveforms show aliasing.

2. Doppler gain does not affect aliasing artifacts.

3. Increasing the Doppler scale can decrease or eliminate aliasing.

4. Lower frequency probes may eliminate aliasing, but higher frequency probes will make it worse.

Reference

Rubin JM: AAPM tutorial: Spectral Doppler US. *Radiographics* 1994;14:139–150.

Cross-Reference

Ultrasound: THE REQUISITES, p 474.

Comment

A number of artifacts can affect the Doppler waveform. One of the most common is the aliasing artifact. Aliasing artifacts arise owing to a basic principle of sampling theory that states that a periodic phenomenon must be sampled at twice its own frequency to be accurately reproduced. Sampling at less than twice the frequency will result in generation of artifactually low or negative frequency determinations. The classic example of aliasing artifact occurs when a rotating wheel on a movie appears to be rotating in the reverse direction. This happens because the frame rate of the movie is not twice the revolution rate of the wheel. The same phenomenon occurs with pulsed Doppler when the pulse repetition frequency is too low. This results in generation of artifactually negative frequency-shift information. On an arterial signal, the first effect is truncation of the systolic peaks with wrap-around of the peaks below the base line. As aliasing becomes increasingly severe, the result is multiple wrap-arounds, and, eventually, the Doppler signal overlaps itself and becomes completely non-arterial in appearance. As shown on the second image, this occurrence can simulate noise. Whenever this type of signal is encountered, the Doppler scale should be increased in order to determine if there is truly an arterial signal hidden within the waveform.

Since the frequency shift itself is proportional to the transmitted frequency, shifting to a lower frequency probe may assist in overcoming aliasing artifacts. Scanning at a larger Doppler angle also decreases the Doppler frequency shift and may assist in eliminating the aliasing artifact. When possible, scanning in another position so that the vessel is closer to the transducer allows the pulse repetition frequency to be increased, because the distance that the sound has to travel to reach the vessel and return to the transducer is decreased. Finally, some manufacturers have a function whereby pulse repetition frequency is increased by transmitting a sound pulse before the previous sound pulse returns to the transducer. This allows for larger Doppler scales but also creates one or more additional sample volumes that can result in some ambiguity as to the origin of the received Doppler signal.

Foreign Body

1. The grey-scale view shows a small echogenic structure in the soft tissue of the finger with a faint posterior shadow. The power Doppler view shows a linear echogenic structure with intense surrounding hyperemia.

2. Ultrasound is used to look for radiolucent foreign bodies. These include wood, glass, and plastic. Ultrasound is also used to localize foreign bodies for resection.

3. Size, depth, and composition of the foreign body limit the ability of ultrasound to make this diagnosis.

4. Very good. Sensitivity is about 95%.

Reference

Bray PW, Mahoney JL, Campbell JP: Sensitivity and specificity of ultrasound in the diagnosis of foreign bodies in the hand. *J Hand Surg* 1995;20(A):661–666.

Cross-Reference

Ultrasound: THE REQUISITES, p 455.

Comment

Foreign bodies retained after trauma can be a source of chronic pain or infection. Many foreign bodies are radio-opaque and can be detected and localized with radiographs. Those that are not radio-opaque can usually be seen with ultrasound. In the study of cadaveric hands and wrists referenced with this case, Bray and colleagues showed that sonographic detection of foreign bodies was excellent for objects between 1×4 mm and 2×5 mm. Visualization was 100% for all objects placed in the palm except for small glass particles. Visualization ranged from 79% to 100% for different types and sizes of foreign bodies placed in the fingers.

All foreign bodies appear as bright reflectors. They may or may not be associated with an adjacent hypoechoic inflammatory process or an adjacent abscess. Acoustic shadowing may be seen if the foreign body is large enough to block a significant amount of the ultrasound beam. Glass or metallic objects may show ringdown or comet-tail artifacts. If adjacent inflammation is present, color or power Doppler may demonstrate surrounding hyperemia, as seen in this case.

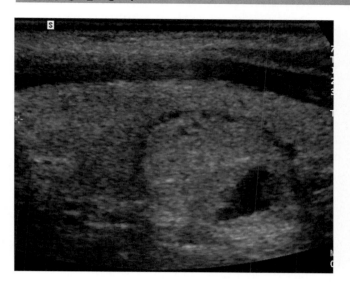
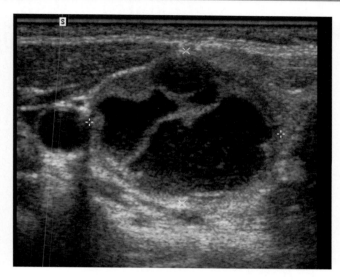

Longitudinal and transverse views of the thyroid in two patients.

1. Are the nodules shown in these patients most likely benign or malignant?
2. What is the incidence of thyroid nodules in the population?
3. What is the role of ultrasound in the evaluation of a thyroid nodule?
4. What gauge needle should be used for fine-needle aspiration of the thyroid?

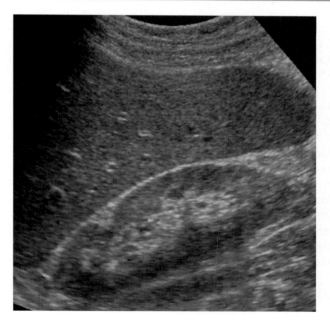
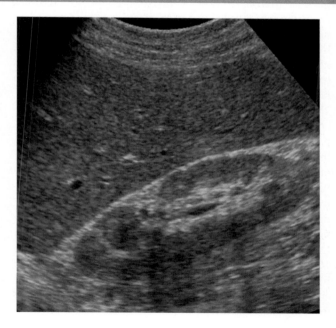

Longitudinal views of the right kidney.

1. What causes the anterior, triangular, echogenic defect at the junction of the upper and mid thirds of this kidney?
2. How often is this seen?
3. Is it more commonly visualized on the right or left kidney?
4. What further evaluation is needed?

Nodular Hyperplasia of the Thyroid

1. The nodule on the left is mostly solid and has a small cystic area and a uniform, thin, hypoechoic halo. The second nodule is mostly cystic and has thick, irregular septations. In thyroid nodules, all of these characteristics favor a benign etiology.

2. The incidence is roughtly equal to the age of the population that is studied.

3. The role of ultrasound in diagnosing thyroid nodules is: 1) to confirm that the nodule is in the thyroid; 2) to guide biopsy; 3) to monitor the response of the nodule to treatment; 4) to look for occult disease.

4. Usually a 25-gauge needle is used to perform fine-needle aspiration of thyroid nodules.

Reference

Solbiati L, Livraghi T, Ballarati E, et al: The Thyroid. In Solbiati L, Rizzatto G (eds): *Ultrasound of Superficial Structures*. Edinburgh, Churchill Livingstone, 1995, 49–86.

Cross-Reference

Ultrasound: THE REQUISITES, pp 448–451.

Comment

The most common indication for thyroid ultrasound is nodular thyroid disease. Approximately 80% of nodules are due to hyperplasia, which may be related to iodine deficiency, familial causes, or medications. An enlarged, hyperplastic gland is called a goiter. The male-to-female ratio is approximately 1:3. When hyperplasia progresses to nodule formation, the pathologic designation of the nodules may be hyperplastic, adenomatous, or colloid. These nodules have a wide range of sonographic appearances. They are often isoechoic or hyperechoic compared to the normal parenchyma. They may have a thin, uniform, hypoechoic halo due to compressed parenchyma or surrounding vessels. They very frequently have cystic components due to degeneration and hemorrhage. Bright foci, often with comet-tail artifacts, may be present and indicate inspissated colloid. Multiple internal septations and mural nodules can be seen.

Benign adenomas account for approximately 5% to 10% of thyroid nodules. A small minority may cause hyperthyroidism owing to autonomous function. They are usually solitary but may occur in a gland that has multiple nodules for other reasons. Follicular adenomas and follicular cancer can be distinguished only on the basis of vascular and capsular invasion. Therefore, fine-needle aspiration that indicates the presence of a follicular lesion should be followed by surgical resection.

Autopsy studies have shown that 50% of patients with a clinically normal thyroid have nodules. Sonography detects nodules in approximately 40% of patients who are scanned for other reasons. Despite the high prevalence of thyroid nodules, the percentage of thyroid malignancy is very low (2% to 4%). Therefore it is not practical to biopsy every nodule that is detected. This is especially true of incidentally detected nodules in patients being scanned for other reasons. Published indications for performing biopsies include: 1) nodules greater than 1.5 cm in size undergo biopsy regardless of the sonographic appearance; 2) nodules with malignant features on sonography, including microcalcifications, irregular margins, or thick halo, undergo biopsy regardless of size; 3) nodules less than 1.5 cm in size can be followed by regular physical examination, provided they do not have malignant sonographic features.

Junctional Parenchymal Defect

1. The defect is called the junctional parenchymal defect or the inter-renuncular junction.

2. It is visualized in approximately 20% of patients.

3. It is more commonly seen on the right side.

4. This requires no additional evaluation.

Reference

Carter AR, Horgan JG, Jennings TA, Rosenfield AT: The junctional parenchymal defect: A sonographic variant of renal anatomy. *Radiology* 1985;154:499–502.

Cross-Reference

Ultrasound: THE REQUISITES, p 73.

Comment

Longitudinal views of the right kidney frequently show a triangular-shaped defect along the anterior renal surface at the junction of the upper and middle third. Less commonly, the defect is seen on transverse scans. This is a normal variant located at the point of fusion of the embryologic upper and lower renunculus. It occurs equally often in both kidneys, but is sonographically seen less often on the left because acoustic access to the left kidney is more limited, and views from an anterior approach are seldom obtained.

The typical sonographic features of the junctional parenchymal defect are its triangular shape, its location at the upper to mid kidney, and its communication with the renal sinus fat. This communication is best visualized by following the defect medially on longitudinal views. In some cases, it is connected to the sinus by a thin, echogenic line. In other cases, the connection may be broader. This is demonstrated in the second image of this case. These characteristics should allow for a definitive distinction from other peripheral echogenic lesions, such as cortical scars or angiomyolipomas.

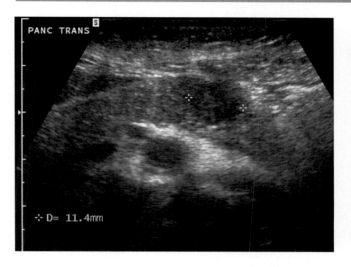
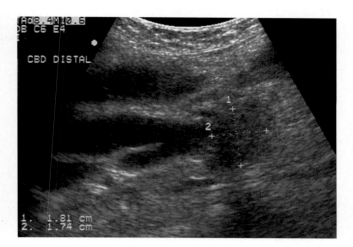

Transverse scan of the pancreas and longitudinal scan of the common bile duct in two patients.

1. What do these patients have in common?
2. Is this abnormality typically hypoechoic?
3. Would other imaging tests be useful?
4. What is the most common location of this lesion?

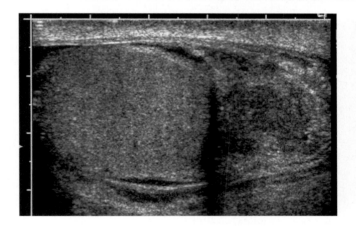
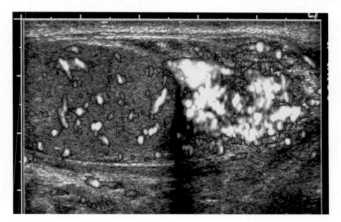

Transverse grey-scale and power Doppler views of the mid aspect of the left testis.

1. Describe the important findings in this case.
2. What are some of the potential complications of this condition?
3. What symptoms is this patient likely to have?
4. Is this condition usually diffuse or focal?

Adenocarcinoma of the Pancreas

1. Both patients have a focal pancreatic mass. The mass in the second image is located in the pancreatic head and is obstructing the bile duct.

2. Most abnormalities of the pancreas are hypoechoic, and pancreatic cancer is no exception.

3. CT would be useful to look for evidence of metastatic disease. ERCP would be useful to look at the pancreatic duct and potentially to establish a histologic diagnosis with brush biopsies.

4. Approximately 70% are located in the head, 20% in the body, and 5% in the tail of the pancreas. Diffuse involvement of the pancreas is also possible.

Reference

Karlson B-M, Ekbom A, Lindgren PG, et al: Abdominal US for diagnosis of pancreatic tumor: Prospective cohort analysis. *Radiology* 1999;213:107–111.

Cross-Reference

Ultrasound: THE REQUISITES, pp 133–136.

Comment

Pancreatic cancer is the fourth most common cause of cancer death in the United States. The prognosis is dismal, with a 1-year survival rate of approximately 10%. Only 15% of tumors are potentially resectable, and even in patients who undergo Whipple resection for cure, the 5-year survival rate is only 20%. Patients present most often with jaundice due to bile duct obstruction. Weight loss, pain, vomiting, unexplained venous thrombosis, and malabsorption are among the other possible symptoms. The vast majority of pancreatic adenocarcinomas arise from the ductal epithelium.

The typical sonographic appearance is of a poorly marginated hypoechoic mass. Most are homogeneous, but as they enlarge, they may become heterogeneous. Echogenic cancers are rare. The majority of pancreatic cancers arise in the head or uncinate process, and these lesions are often quite small, since they manifest early with bile duct obstruction and jaundice. Lesions in the body and tail tend to be larger. The average size of this tumor is 2 to 3 cm.

Although pancreatic cancer is by far the most common pancreatic tumor, other tumors should be considered when a focal hypoechoic solid mass is detected. Metastases to the pancreas and pancreatic lymphoma both appear as hypoechoic masses. These masses are often multiple, and the majority of these patients have a prior history of lymphoma or an extrapancreatic malignancy. Microcystic adenomas may appear solid on sonography, but they lack any evidence of metastases and appear cystic on CT. Focal pancreatitis can also produce a hypoechoic inflammatory mass in the pancreas that can simulate cancer. Fortunately a history of pancreatitis is usually present in these patients.

Epididymitis

1. There is marked enlargement of the body of the epididymis and intense hypervascularity of the epididymis when compared to the testis. This is typical of acute epididymitis.

2. Epididymitis can progress to cause an abscess, a pyocele, orchitis, or testicular ischemia.

3. Symptoms of epididymitis include primarily pain and swelling of the scrotum, possibly with fever and other signs of lower genitourinary tract infection.

4. Epididymitis can be either focal or diffuse. When focal, it is important to survey the entire epididymis from head to tail to make the diagnosis.

Reference

Horstman WG, Middleton WD, Melson GL: Scrotal inflammatory disease: Color Doppler ultrasonographic findings. *Radiology* 1991;179:55–59.

Cross-Reference

Ultrasound: THE REQUISITES, pp 445–446.

Comment

Epididymitis is the most common cause of scrotal pain and swelling in postpubertal men. It usually arises from an infection elsewhere in the lower urinary tract, such as prostatitis. Other etiologies include hematogenous spread and trauma. Common organisms are *Escherichia coli*, *Pseudomonas*, and *Aerobacter*. In younger men, *Gonococcus* and *Chlamydia* are also common.

On sonography, epididymitis produces an enlarged and hypervascular epididymis. The process may be diffuse or may be localized to just the head or the tail of the epididymis. Isolated involvement of the tail can be overlooked if careful scanning of the inferior scrotum is not performed. In most cases, the epididymis becomes hypoechoic. Occasionally, a mixed echogenic appearance develops, perhaps due to edema in the structures adjacent to the epididymis. It is important to realize that the hyperemia generally precedes the grey-scale changes. Therefore, color Doppler is more sensitive to epididymitis than grey-scale sonography. In addition to epididymitis, another common cause of an enlarged epididymis is post-vasectomy changes. This can be distinguished because it is bilateral and is not hyperemic.

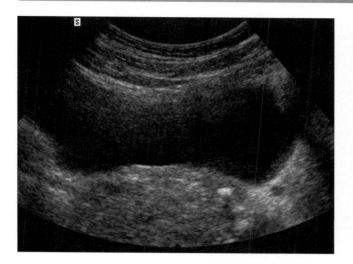 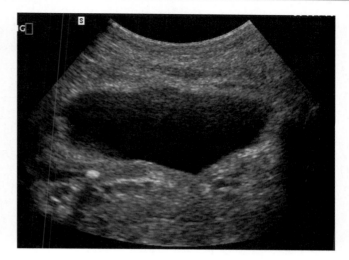

Transverse view of the pelvis just above the bladder trigone and longitudinal view of the pelvis just to the left of the midline in a patient who is 18 weeks pregnant.

1. Describe the abnormality shown in this patient.
2. What is the role of ultrasound in making this diagnosis?
3. When considering the diagnosis shown in this patient, where is the best place to look initially?
4. Is this abnormality easier to see in men or in women?

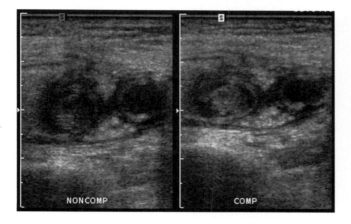 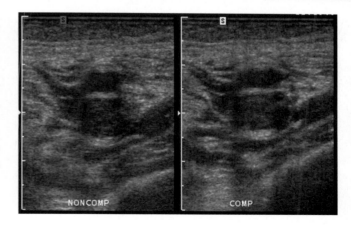

Transverse views of the groin and mid thigh.

1. How good is ultrasound at making this diagnosis in the thigh?
2. Is it possible to make this diagnosis reliably without color Doppler?
3. Does this condition most commonly produce unilateral or bilateral symptoms?
4. How important is luminal echogenicity in establishing the diagnosis?

Distal Ureteral Stone

1. The transverse view shows an echogenic shadowing structure in the left pelvis in the expected location of the distal ureter. The longitudinal view shows the same abnormality and confirms that it is located in the ureter.

2. Ultrasound is generally not used as a primary means of evaluating patients with suspected ureteral stones. The exception is when the patient is pregnant and radiation needs to be avoided.

3. The majority of ureteral stones impact in the distal ureter. Therefore, views through the urinary bladder give the highest yield for stone detection.

4. Stones in the distal ureter are seen with similar success in men and in women using transabdominal scanning through the fluid-filled bladder. In women, transvaginal scanning can be used to sort out difficult cases.

Reference

Ohnishi K, Watanabe H, Ohe H, Saitoh M: Ultrasound findings in urolithiasis in the lower ureter. *Ultrasound Med Biol* 1986;12:577–579.

Cross-Reference

Ultrasound: THE REQUISITES, pp 103–104.

Comment

Patients with renal colic can be imaged in a number of ways. Traditionally, intravenous urography was the method of choice. Currently, noncontrast CT is the recommended first test since it avoids the small risk of reactions to contrast media and provides information about structures other than the kidneys, ureters, and bladder. Ultrasound has a very limited role in the initial workup of patients with suspected renal colic. This is not to say that ultrasound is not capable of establishing the correct diagnosis in the majority of patients. It is simply easier and more effective to start with other tests. One legitimate role of ultrasound is in the pregnant patient in whom radiation needs to be avoided.

Most, but certainly not all, patients who are passing a kidney stone will have at least mild hydronephrosis. They may also have a small amount of perinephric fluid, usually best seen around the upper or lower pole. In the proper clinical setting, either of these findings is very specific for ureteral stones. Identification of the ureteral calculus itself is easiest when it is in the proximal ureter near the ureteropelvic junction (using the kidney as a window), and in the distal ureter near the ureterovesicle junction (using the fluid-filled bladder as a window). The most common place for stones to impact is in the distal ureter, so it is very important to carefully evaluate the distal ureters. In addition to a transabdominal approach using the bladder as a window, the distal ureters in women can be imaged quite well from a transvaginal approach. In men, a transrectal approach can be used, although it is not as successful as the transvaginal approach in women.

Lower Extremity Deep Vein Thrombosis

1. Ultrasound is very good at diagnosing deep vein thrombosis (DVT) in the femoral-popliteal system.

2. Color Doppler plays a minor role in diagnosing DVT. It is usually evaluated completely with grey-scale imaging.

3. Lower extremity DVT is usually unilateral.

4. The diagnosis of DVT is made based on lack of venous compressibility. Detection of intraluminal echoes is not a reliable way to diagnose DVT, and lack of intraluminal echoes is not a reliable way to exclude DVT.

Reference

Fraser JD, Anderson DR: Deep venous thrombosis: Recent advances and optimal investigation with US. *Radiology* 1999;211:9–24.

Cross Reference

Ultrasound: THE REQUISITES, pp 483–485.

Comment

Ultrasound has become the procedure of choice in the evaluation of suspected lower extremity DVT. In symptomatic patients, the sensitivity and specificity exceed 95% and 98%, respectively, in the femoral-popliteal system. Results in asymptomatic high-risk patients (predominantly post hip and knee surgery) and in the calf are more variable.

Normally, the deep veins should be completely compressible. The diagnosis of DVT is made when the veins fail to compress completely. Many normal veins will have low level internal echoes that are artifactual, and it is not uncommon for an intraluminal clot to be hypoechoic or anechoic. Therefore, analysis of echogenicity is not a primary focus of lower extremity venous examinations.

In patients with marked obesity or with severe edema, identification of the femoral and popliteal veins may be very difficult. In these situations, color Doppler may help to localize the vessels. Augmentation of proximal venous flow by compression of the calf or plantarflexion can accentuate the veins and further assist when color Doppler is required.

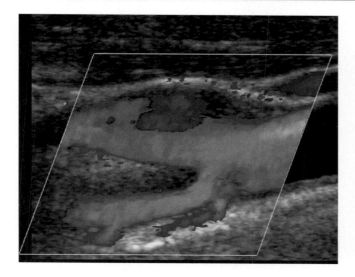

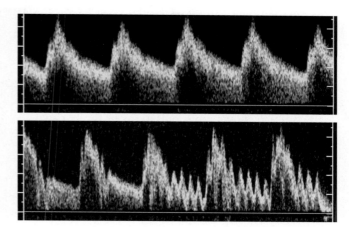

Longitudinal color Doppler view of the carotid bifurcation and pulsed Doppler waveforms from the internal and external carotid arteries. (See color plates.)

1. Identify the internal and the external carotid arteries on the color Doppler image.
2. Which vessel is typically located anterior and medial?
3. Which waveform is from the internal and which is from the external carotid artery?
4. On longitudinal views of the bifurcation, is the internal carotid artery located superficial or deep to the external carotid?

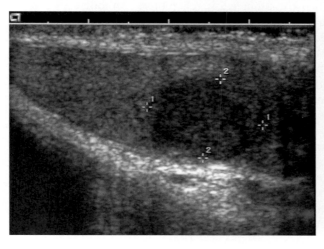

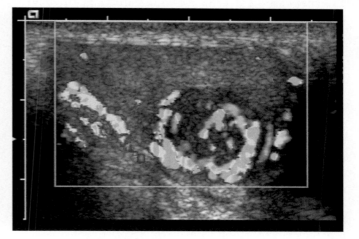

Longitudinal grey-scale and color Doppler images of the testis. (See color plates.)

1. Describe the abnormality.
2. What nonneoplastic conditions can appear as a focal hypoechoic mass in the testis?
3. Are testicular tumors most likely benign or malignant?
4. Does associated enlargement and hypervascularity of the epididymis favor a neoplastic or nonneoplastic condition?

Normal Carotid Bifurcation

1. Branches arise from the deep vessel, so that vessel is the external carotid artery. The larger vessel without branches is the internal carotid artery.

2. The external carotid artery is located anterior and medial to the internal carotid.

3. The top waveform shows a low resistance pattern typical of the internal carotid artery. The bottom waveform shows rapid pulsations in the last two cardiac cycles due to manual tapping on the superficial temporal artery. This is a way of identifying the external carotid.

4. When the transducer is positioned in the anterior and medial neck, the external carotid artery will be superficial. When the transducer is positioned in the posterior and lateral neck, the internal carotid will be superficial.

Reference

Cardoso T, Middleton WD: Duplex sonography and color Doppler of carotid artery disease. *Semin Interv Radiol* 1990;7:1–8.

Cross-Reference

Ultrasound: THE REQUISITES, pp 470–473.

Comment

Proper interpretation of carotid artery Doppler examinations requires reliable differentiation of the internal and external carotid arteries. Several features distinguish these vessels. Location, size, and branches are all useful. Realize, however, that although branches are always present on the external carotid artery, they are not always detectable on color Doppler. Therefore, branches are useful only when they are seen.

Doppler waveform analysis is also a valuable means of distinguishing the internal and external carotids. Since the internal carotid supplies a solid organ with a low vascular resistance, its waveform has a low resistance profile with broad systolic peaks, gradual systolic deceleration into early diastole, and well-maintained diastolic flow throughout the cardiac cycle. The external carotid supplies primarily muscle, bone, and cutaneous tissue, which has a high resistance to blood flow. Therefore the external carotid waveform has narrower systolic peaks, more abrupt transition between systole and diastole, and less end-diastolic flow. Another feature of the waveform that can be useful is transmission of fluctuations into the external carotid when the superficial temporal artery is tapped. This is called the temporal tap maneuver. Although the effects tend to be greatest and most frequent in the external carotid, occasionally some changes can be seen in the internal and in the common carotid.

Testicular Seminoma

1. The images show a homogeneous, hypoechoic, hypervascular mass. The most likely diagnosis is a testicular tumor, and the appearance is typical for a seminoma.

2. Infarcts, focal atrophy, focal orchitis, hematoma, abscess, sarcoid, and contusions can all appear as a hypoechoic lesion.

3. Testicular tumors are much more likely to be malignant than benign.

4. Involvement of the epididymis favors epididymo-orchitis.

Reference

Horstman WG, Melson GL, Middleton WD, Andriole GA: Color Doppler ultrasonography of testicular tumors. *Radiology* 1992;185:733–737.

Cross-Reference

Ultrasound: THE REQUISITES, pp 439–442.

Comment

Primary testicular tumors are the most common malignancy in young adult males. Germ cell tumors account for the vast majority of testicular tumors. Seminoma is the most common germ cell tumor, accounting for 40% to 50% of these malignancies. Seminomas frequently occur in a pure form as well as in mixed germ cell tumors. They tend to occur in a slightly older age group than the other germ cell tumors. Although 25% of patients with pure seminomas have metastases at the time of presentation, the 5-year survival rate is excellent. Most testicular tumors manifest as a painless, palpable mass. Approximately 10% will manifest with testicular pain and another 10% with symptoms related to metastatic disease (such as back pain due to retroperitoneal adenopathy).

On sonography, detection of an intratesticular lesion other than a simple cyst should always raise the possibility of a testicular tumor. Pure seminomas are typically homogeneous, hypoechoic, solid masses. When they are large, they tend to become more heterogeneous. Cystic components and calcification are distinctly uncommon in pure seminomas.

With modern color Doppler, most testicular tumors larger than 1 cm (and many that are less than 1 cm) are seen to have detectable internal blood flow. Detecting internal flow can be helpful in making a diagnosis, since many benign intratesticular lesions that can potentially be confused with tumors, such as hematomas, abscesses, and infarcts, do not have internal flow. In addition, many nonneoplastic lesions that are readily seen on ultrasound are not palpable, while the majority of testicular tumors are palpable.

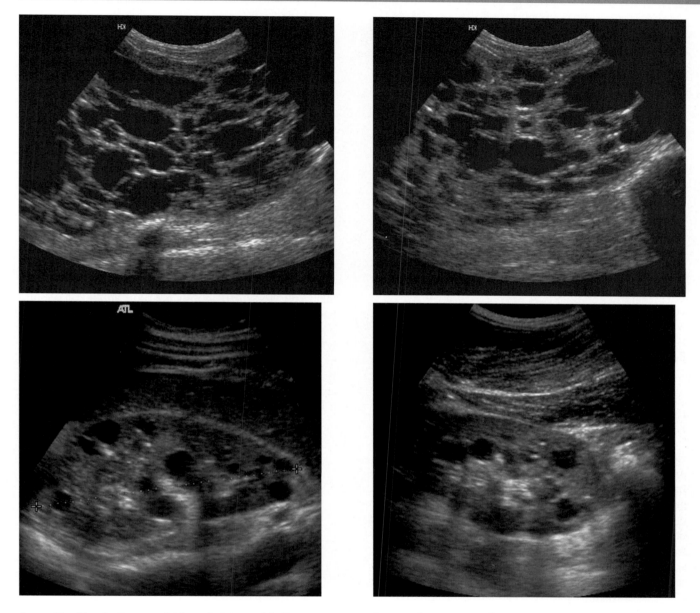

Longitudinal views of the right and left upper quadrants in two patients.

1. What are the major complications of the condition shown in this case?

2. What other associated findings are there?

3. Would your diagnosis be the same if there were no family history of renal disease?

4. Is there any effective therapy?

Autosomal Dominant Polycystic Kidney Disease

1. The most devastating complications of polycystic kidney disease (PKD) are renal failure and hypertension. Patients are also at increased risk for cyst hemorrhage, renal infection, and stone formation

2. Findings besides renal cysts include cysts in the liver (and rarely in the pancreas) and berry aneurysms.

3. Up to 50% of cases of PKD are due to spontaneous mutations and have no family history.

4. There is no proven therapy. Laparoscopic cyst decortication can help relieve symptoms and may improve renal function.

References

Levine E, Hartman DS, Meilstrup JW, et al: Current concepts and controversies in imaging of renal cystic diseases. *Urol Clin North Am* 1997;24:523–544.

Ravine D, Gibson RN, Walker RG, et al: Evaluation of ultrasonographic criteria for autosomal dominant polycystic kidney disease 1. *Lancet* 1994;343:824.

Cross-Reference

Ultrasound: THE REQUISITES, pp 86–87.

Comment

Autosomal dominant PKD is an inherited disorder that has 100% penetrance but is expressed to varying degrees. Patients generally present in the fourth or fifth decade with symptoms related to the mass effect of enlarged kidneys, hypertension, hematuria, or urinary tract infections. Renal failure develops on average in the sixth decade of life. Up to 10% of cases of end-stage renal disease in North America and Europe are due to PKD. If untreated, patients survive approximately 10 years from the onset of symptoms.

Two genetic defects cause PKD. Type 1 accounts for approximately 90% of families and is due to a defect on the short arm of chromosome 16. Type 2 is caused by a defect on the long arm of chromosome 4 and accounts for 10% of families. The major clinical difference in these two types is the lower age of onset of end-stage renal disease in type 1 than in type 2.

Although the kidneys are affected to a greater degree than any other organ, cysts can also develop in the liver (in up to 50% of patients), the pancreas (in up to 7% of patients), and the spleen (in less than 5% of patients). Cysts in these organs rarely cause clinical symptoms. In particular, the liver can be almost replaced by multiple cysts and still function normally. Approximately 10% of patients have intracranial aneurysms.

On sonography, the diagnosis is made by detecting multiple, bilateral renal cysts located in the renal cortex. In older patients the kidneys are almost always enlarged, sometimes to the point that they cannot be effectively measured with sonography. Hemorrhage into renal cysts is very common and may result in low level internal echoes, fluid-blood levels, or solid nodular internal structures. Cyst wall calcification and renal stones are also common.

In affected families, it is common to screen children to determine whether they inherited the disease. Criteria that have been established include the presence of at least two cysts in one kidney or one cyst in each kidney in an at-risk person under 30 years of age, the presence of at least two cysts in each kidney in an at-risk person between 30 and 59 years of age, and at least four cysts in each kidney for persons at risk aged 60 years and older. Most patients have many cysts present bilaterally, and the diagnosis is not in doubt. Ultrasound has a high sensitivity in making the diagnosis in patients with type 1 disease and in patients with type 2 disease who are over 30 years old. Ultrasound is less sensitive in patients with type 2 disease who are less than 30 years old. When ultrasound results are indeterminate or are confusing, DNA linkage analysis can be performed if it is available.

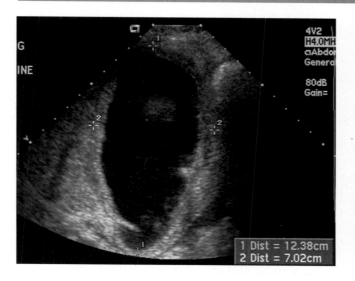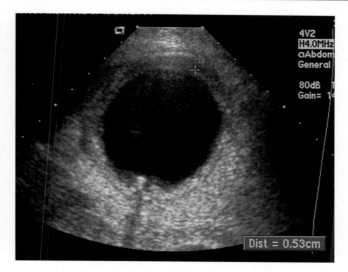

Longitudinal and transverse views of the gallbladder in a patient with fever.

1. What are the abnormalities in the images shown above?
2. What is the differential diagnosis?
3. What is the preferred way of establishing this diagnosis?
4. What is the treatment of choice?

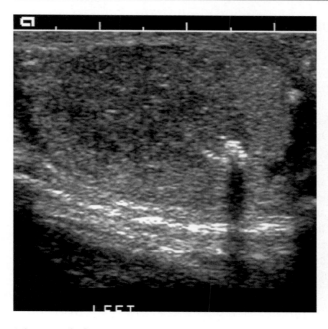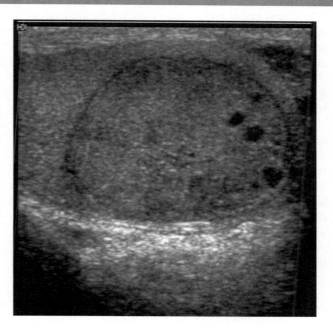

Views of the testis in two patients.

1. What is the significance of the shadowing shown in the first image?
2. In patients such as these, what else should be scanned in addition to the scrotum?
3. Is scrotal MRI useful in patients with sonographic findings such as these?
4. What conditions predispose to this abnormality?

Acute Cholecystitis

1. The gallbladder is enlarged (12 cm × 7 cm), has a thick wall (5 mm), and has an intraluminal stone.

2. The most likely diagnosis is acute cholecystitis. Many things can cause wall thickening, including edema-forming states, portal hypertension, hepatitis, adenomyomatosis, and gallbladder cancer. But the association of gallbladder enlargement, stones, and wall thickening in a febrile patient is strongly predictive of acute cholecystitis.

3. Ultrasound is the best initial test in patients with suspected acute cholecystitis. Scintigraphy is also very helpful in a problem-solving mode when the sonogram is confusing or indefinite.

4. Surgery. In some cases surgery will be postponed until the patient has been treated with antibiotics, and the acute inflammatory changes have resolved.

Reference
Middleton WD: Right upper quadrant pain. In Bluth EI, Benson C, Arger P, et al (eds): *The Practice of Ultrasonography.* New York, Thieme, 1999, pp 3-16.

Cross-Reference
Ultrasound: THE REQUISITES, pp 41-45.

Comment
Ultrasound is the procedure of choice in the evaluation of patients with suspected acute cholecystitis. In the majority of patients, by documenting a gallstone-free gallbladder, ultrasound can exclude the diagnosis rapidly and effectively. This is important, since most patients with suspected acute cholecystitis do not actually have that problem. Ultrasound has also been shown to be as effective at establishing the diagnosis of acute cholecystitis as any other noninvasive technique.

The signs of acute cholecystitis are gallstones, wall thickening (greater than 3 mm), gallbladder enlargement (greater than 4 cm transverse diameter), pericholecystic fluid, an impacted stone in the gallbladder neck or cystic duct, and a positive sonographic Murphy's sign. The combination of stones and either wall thickening or a positive sonographic Murphy's sign has a very high positive predictive value for acute cholecystitis.

Cholescintigraphy can also be used in patients with suspected acute cholecystitis. Accuracy is similar to ultrasound. However, there are several limitations to scintigraphy. Cholescintigraphy does not give morphologic information about the gallbladder (such as gallbladder size, wall thickness, pericholecystic abscess formation, or presence and size of stones), which is important prior to laparoscopic cholecystectomy. It also fails to provide information about other organs that might account for the patient's problem when the gallbladder is normal. Finally, it is more time-consuming and expensive than sonography. Because of these limitations, cholescintigraphy is generally not the initial examination in patients with suspected cholecystitis. Nevertheless, it is a very good way to evaluate patients who have equivocal or confusing findings on ultrasound.

Mixed Germ Cell Tumors

1. The shadowing indicates calcification, which is rare in pure seminomas but is common in mixed germ cell tumors.

2. In a patient with what appears to be a testicular tumor, it is helpful to scan the retroperitoneum to look for adenopathy.

3. Scrotal MRI is needed only rarely following scrotal ultrasound and would not add any valuable information in cases such as these.

4. Cryptorchidism, testicular atrophy, prior testicular tumor, and maybe microlithiasis predispose to testicular tumors.

References
Choyke PL. Dynamic contrast-enhanced MR imaging of the scrotum: Reality check. *Radiology* 2000;217: 14-15.

Horstman WG: Scrotal imaging. *Urol Clin North Am* 1997;24:653-671.

Cross-Reference
Ultrasound: THE REQUISITES, pp 439-440.

Comment
Of primary tumors of the testis, 95% are malignant germ cell neoplasms. These tumors are divided into seminomas and nonseminomas. Tumors that are composed of a mixture of seminomatous elements and nonseminomatous elements are grouped with the nonseminomas. Nonseminomatous tumors include teratoma, choriocarcinoma, embryonal cell carcinoma (also referred to as yolk sac tumors and endodermal sinus tumors in the pediatric age group), and any combination of these tumors. Teratocarcinoma refers to the relatively common combination of teratoma and embryonal cell carcinoma.

Unlike most seminomas, which are homogeneous and hypoechoic, nonseminomatous tumors are usually heterogeneous. This is at least partly due to the frequency of hemorrhage and necrosis. In addition, they often have cystic areas as well as calcifications. Cystic areas are most frequently seen in tumors that contain teratomatous elements.

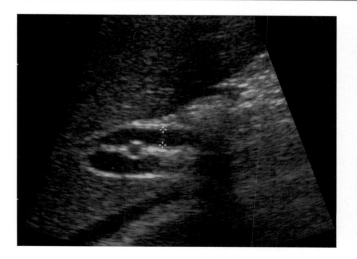
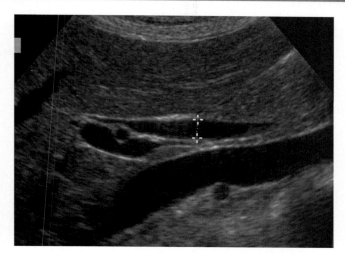

Longitudinal views of the porta hepatis in two patients. The first image is from a 21-year-old man and the second is from a 65-year-old woman.

1. Which of the patients shown in this case is more likely to have biliary obstruction?
2. Is the common duct frequently ectatic following a cholecystectomy?
3. How sensitive is ultrasound in determining the level and cause of biliary obstruction?
4. What is the theory behind giving patients a fatty meal when biliary obstruction is suspected?

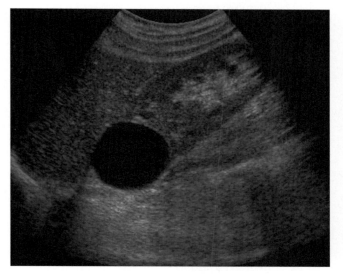
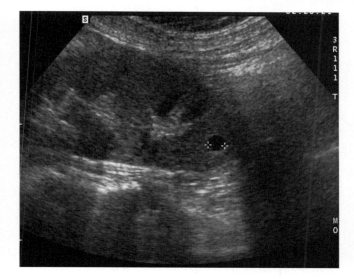

Longitudinal views of the kidney in two patients.
1. Is ultrasound a good means of characterizing lesions such as the ones shown here?
2. What are the three characteristics of this lesion?
3. What other lesions should be included in the differential diagnosis?
4. How common are these lesions?

Extrahepatic Biliary Dilation

1. Both images show dilated common bile ducts. In the second image, the duct is dilated in its mid portion, but it tapers to a normal caliber distally and proximally. In the first image overlying gas obscures the distal duct, but the proximal duct is dilated where it crosses over the right hepatic artery. Because of this, it is more likely to be obstructed. Additional images showed distal duct stones in the first patient and no abnormalities in the second patient.

2. The size of the extrahepatic duct increases with age and following a cholecystectomy. Therefore, an enlarged duct is less concerning in these patients.

3. Reports indicate that sensitivities up to 80% to 90% can be obtained with good technique.

4. A fatty meal stimulates bile production by the liver and contraction of the gallbladder. In patients with obstruction, this results in enlargement of the duct. Fatty meals also stimulate relaxation of the sphincter of Oddi, so that there is no change or reduction in the size of the duct in patients who do not have obstruction. Intrinsic variability in measurements of the bile duct diameter often limits the use of this technique.

Reference

Middleton WD: The bile ducts. In: Goldberg BB (ed): *Diagnostic Ultrasound.* Baltimore, Williams & Wilkins, 1993, pp 146–172.

Cross-Reference

Ultrasound: THE REQUISITES, pp 59–61.

Comment

Diagnosis of bile duct obstruction with sonography depends on detection of ductal dilatation. Different studies have proposed different measurements for the upper limits of normal for the extrahepatic ducts. Unfortunately, some obstructed ducts may not be dilated, and many things other than obstruction can cause dilated ducts. Therefore, rigid reliance on any single measurement value is dangerous. Important factors to realize when analyzing the common duct is that the duct normally enlarges with age (due to degeneration of the elastic fibers in the wall) and often enlarges following a cholecystectomy (this is controversial). Thus, borderline enlarged ductal measurements are more likely to indicate obstruction in young patients and in patients with their gallbladders than in older patients or patients who have had a cholecystectomy. In addition, it is not uncommon for the common duct to be ectatic in its mid portion between the liver and the head of the pancreas.

Therefore, if the duct is of normal caliber proximally where it crosses the right hepatic artery and distally within the head of the pancreas, then measurements slightly above the normal range in the mid segment are much less likely to indicate obstruction. With these caveats in mind, a reasonable value to use as the upper limits of normal for the maximum duct diameter is 6 mm. Some experts use 5 mm as the upper limits of normal and allow an additional 1 mm for each decade beyond age 50. In other words, a 5-mm duct is normal at age 50; a 6-mm duct is normal at age 60, and so forth.

Renal Cysts

1. As in other parts of the body, ultrasound is an excellent way to evaluate the characteristics of cystic renal lesions.

2. Characteristics of a simple cyst include lack of internal echoes, well-defined back wall, and posterior acoustic enhancement.

3. Lesions that can simulate a simple cyst include calyx diverticulum, aneurysm, pseudoaneurysm, lymphoma, or upper pole duplication.

4. Approximately 50% of patients over age 50 have at least one renal cyst.

Reference

Curry NS, Bissada NK: Radiologic evaluation of small and indeterminant renal masses. *Urol Clin North Am* 1997;24:493–505.

Cross-Reference

Ultrasound: THE REQUISITES, pp 81–84.

Comment

Renal cysts are extremely common. Provided they satisfy the classic sonographic criteria for cysts, renal cysts require no further evaluation. It is important to realize that all three of the criteria for cysts may not be seen on all images of the cyst. For instance, the image that shows increased through transmission may not demonstrate an anechoic lumen. As long as the three criteria can be shown on a group of images, then a confident diagnosis of a cyst can be made.

A common dilemma is a cyst that appears to contain internal echoes. Internal echoes may be real or may be artifacts created by the body wall. Imaging from multiple, different approaches varies the interactions from overlying tissues and often helps to clear out the internal artifacts. These types of artifacts can also be dramatically reduced or completely eliminated through the use of tissue harmonic imaging.

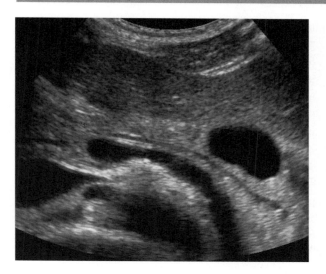 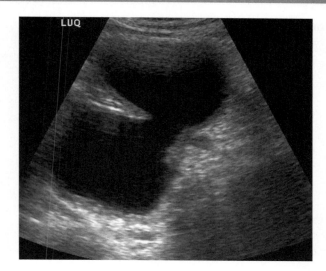

Transverse view of the pancreas and left upper quadrant in two patients with the same abnormality.

1. What question would you want to ask these patients?
2. How often do pancreatic adenocarcinomas have cystic components?
3. Does the differential diagnosis vary if the patient is a man or a woman?
4. Are pseudocysts more common in alcohol-induced or in gallstone-induced pancreatitis?

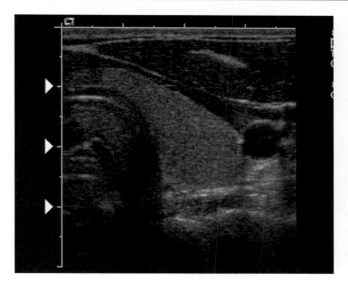 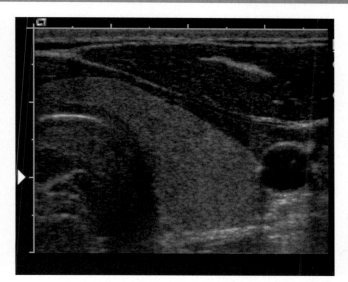

Two transverse views of the thyroid.

1. What do the arrowheads at the left side of the images indicate?
2. Which image would you expect to have the higher frame rate?
3. What can you do to improve the frame rate while performing real-time scans?
4. What can you do to improve the resolution while performing real-time scans?

Pancreatic Pseudocysts

1. In patients with cystic lesions of the pancreas, it is important to know whether they have a history of pancreatitis.

2. Cystic areas are rare in adenocarcinoma of the pancreas.

3. Women have a higher risk of cystic pancreatic neoplasms.

4. The large majority of pseudocysts are due to alcoholic pancreatitis.

Reference

Ros PR, Hamrick-Turner JE, Chiechi MV, et al: Cystic masses of the pancreas. *Radiographics* 1992;12:672–686.

Cross-Reference

Ultrasound: THE REQUISITES, pp 126–129.

Comment

Pancreatitis has a number of potential complications. The list of local complications potentially seen on sonography includes fluid collections, pseudocysts, abscesses, necrosis, pseudoaneurysms, venous thrombosis, and biliary obstruction. Fluid collections within or around the pancreas occur in 40% to 50% of patients with pancreatitis. The majority of fluid collections resolve spontaneously. If the collection organizes and forms a fibrous capsule, it is referred to as a pseudocyst. It takes approximately 6 weeks for a fluid collection to mature into a well-encapsulated pseudocyst. Approximately 2% to 10% of patients with acute pancreatitis ultimately develop a pseudocyst.

Pseudocysts can occur almost anywhere, but they are most commonly seen within or immediately adjacent to the pancreas. They appear as well-defined masses that are usually anechoic or hypoechoic. Pseudocysts may contain internal debris, hemorrhage, or septations. In such cases, the differential diagnosis often includes a cystic neoplasm such as a mucinous macrocystic neoplasm. The key to the correct diagnosis is the history of prior episodes of pancreatitis. Follow-up examinations are also useful, since the intraluminal echoes in a complex pseudocyst will usually clear over time. In some cases, aspiration is necessary to make the distinction, with increased levels of amylase expected in a pseudocyst and increased levels of carcinoembryonic antigen in mucinous cystic neoplasms. Endoscopic retrograde cholangiopancreatography can also be valuable, as it may demonstrate changes of pancreatitis that are not evident sonographically. It may also demonstrate communication between pseudocysts and the pancreatic duct in up to 70% of cases.

Frame Rate and Resolution

1. The arrowheads indicate the levels at which the image is focused.

2. Frame rate should be highest for the second image because the field of view is smaller, and there is only one focal zone.

3. Frame rate can be improved by decreasing the number of focal zones, decreasing the image depth, decreasing sector width, decreasing line density, and turning off Doppler modes.

4. Resolution can be improved by using a higher frequency transducer, increasing the number of focal zones, and increasing line density.

Reference

Kremkau FW: Multiple element transducers. *Radiographics* 1993;13:1163–1176.

Comment

Each ultrasound image is composed of multiple scan lines. The time required to create one frame of a real-time image is calculated by multiplying the speed of sound times the length of the scan lines times the number of lines per image times two. Multiplying by two is necessary because the sound has to make a round trip from the transducer to the target and back. The longer it takes to generate one frame, the lower the frame rate. Typical frame rates in diagnostic ultrasound range from approximately 5 to 40 frames per second. Increased frame rates can be obtained by decreasing the length of each scan line (less image depth) or decreasing the number of scan lines (less image width or narrower sector angles).

In many respects, frame rate and image resolution are competing parameters. As shown in this case, each scan line can be electronically focused at a certain depth. To focus at multiple depths requires multiple pulses for each scan line. In the first image shown in this case, pulses focused in the near field created the superficial aspect of the image, which was pasted to two different images obtained separately with mid- and far-field focusing. Therefore, the improved resolution throughout the field of view that comes with multiple focal zones results in a sacrifice in frame rate. It is also possible to improve resolution by moving the scan lines closer together. This is called increasing line density, and it also has an inverse relationship to frame rate.

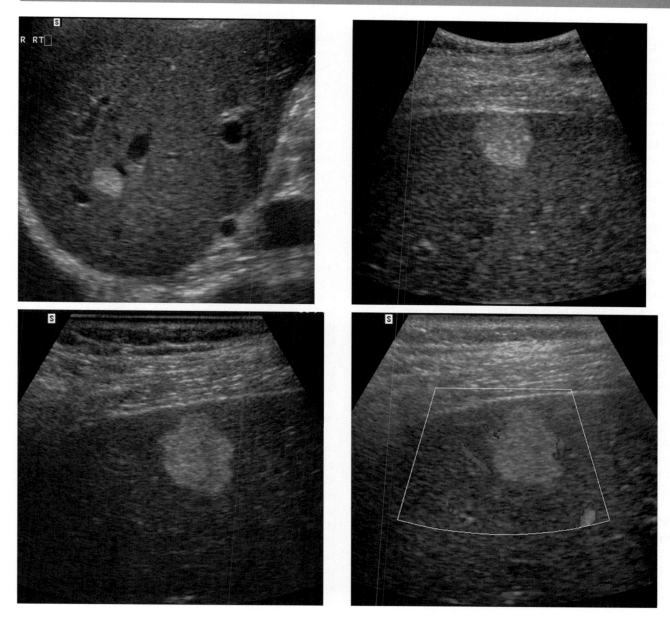

Magnified views of the liver in three patients. The bottom images are corresponding grey-scale and color Doppler views from the same patient. (See color plates.)

1. What is the differential diagnosis in these three patients with the same abnormality?
2. What factors determine the management of these patients?
3. Would the presence of increased through transmission affect your approach to this lesion?
4. Does the absence of detectable internal flow in the last image affect your differential diagnosis?

Hepatic Hemangioma

1. All images show a hyperechoic, homogeneous mass. Hemangioma is the most likely diagnosis. Metastasis, hyperechoic hepatocellular cancer, and nodular focal fat are other considerations. Focal nodular hyperplasia and hepatic adenoma are much less likely possibilities.

2. Management depends on the patient's risk factors for hepatic malignancy.

3. Hemangiomas occasionally have increased through transmission, but this can be seen with other solid lesions as well, so it should not affect your differential diagnosis significantly.

4. Usually hemangiomas have no detectable flow. Although some of the other lesions mentioned previously (hepatocellular cancer, hypervascular metastasis, focal nodular hyperplasia, and hepatic adenoma) might have detectable flow and may be hypervascular, in some cases it is not possible to detect flow in these other lesions also. Therefore, lack of detectable flow may make the diagnosis of hemangioma more likely, but it does not exclude the other possibilities.

Reference

Leifer DM, Middleton WD, Teefey SA, et al: Follow-up of patients at low risk for hepatic malignancy with a characteristic hemangioma at US. *Radiology* 2000; 214:167–172.

Cross-Reference

Ultrasound: THE REQUISITES, pp 9–12.

Comment

Hemangiomas are the most common solid, benign liver lesion, occurring in approximately 7% of adults. They are composed of multiple, small, blood-filled spaces that are separated by fibrous septations and lined by endothelial cells. They are most common in women. Approximately 10% are multiple. With the exception of cysts, they are the most common incidental lesion detected on hepatic sonography.

It is unusual for hemangiomas to cause symptoms. Giant hemangiomas may cause enough mass effect to be symptomatic, and rarely a hemangioma will bleed enough to cause symptoms. Platelet sequestration and destruction by hemangiomas has been reported as an extremely rare cause of thrombocytopenia (called Kasabach-Merritt syndrome).

The classic sonographic appearance, seen in approximately 60% to 70% of hemangiomas, is a well-marginated, homogeneous, hyperechoic mass. Hemangiomas are usually round (as shown on the first two images),

but they may have scalloped margins (as shown on the second two images). The majority are less than 3 cm in size. Atypical appearances tend to occur in larger lesions due to fibrosis, thrombosis, and necrosis. A significant percentage of atypical hemangiomas have a hyperechoic periphery and a hypoechoic center. This "atypical" appearance is actually fairly characteristic of hemangioma and is seen only rarely in malignant disease. Another finding occasionally seen in hemangioma is increased through transmission. A common misconception is that through transmission is an important characteristic necessary to make a confident diagnosis of hemangioma. This is certainly not true, since the majority of hemangiomas do not have through transmission, and many other tumors can have through transmission.

As expected for benign lesions, hemangiomas are usually stable over time. However, they will occasionally change in appearance over time. Typically they will convert from hyperechoic to hypoechoic. Rarely, they will change echogenicity over a matter of minutes or even seconds. No other hepatic mass has been observed to have this behavior.

The proper management of a homogeneous, hyperechoic hepatic mass depends on the patient's clinical history. In patients at increased risk for hepatic malignancy (prior history or current evidence of an extrahepatic malignancy or chronic liver disease), the presumed sonographic diagnosis of hemangioma should be confirmed with MRI or Tc^{99m}-tagged red blood cell scintigraphy. MRI is superior for small lesions (from less than 1 cm to 2 cm in size) and for larger lesions adjacent to the heart or to major hepatic vascular structures. For patients who are not at increased risk for hepatic malignancy, recommendations for the management of suspected hemangiomas are divergent. Some authorities have recommended no further evaluation. Others have recommended periodic sonographic follow-up. Still others have recommended confirmation with scintigraphy, MRI, or CT. We recently analyzed this group of patients at our own institution and found that the risk of malignancy in this group of patients is extremely low. Out of more than 200 patients, only one was subsequently found to have a malignant hepatic lesion. Therefore, we recommend no further evaluation of typical-appearing hemangiomas provided the patient has no prior history or current evidence of extrahepatic malignancy or chronic liver disease.

Occasionally, noninvasive tests do not establish the diagnosis of hemangioma, and it is necessary for the patient to have a biopsy. Biopsy can be performed safely; however, the needle should pass through normal parenchyma before entering the hemangioma in order to achieve some tamponade effect. Fine-needle aspirations generally obtain only blood and are not sufficient to make the diagnosis. Core biopsy needles can obtain sufficient tissue for diagnosis in the majority of cases.

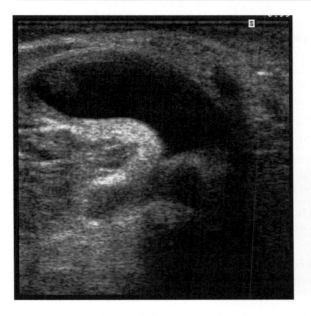
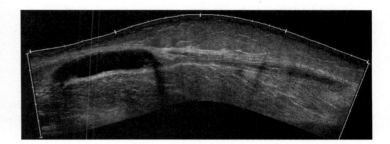

Transverse view of the posterior knee and extended-field-of-view scan of the posterior knee and calf.

1. Describe the abnormal findings.
2. Where does this condition occur?
3. How can this lesion be distinguished from other knee cysts?
4. Does this abnormality typically communicate with the joint space?

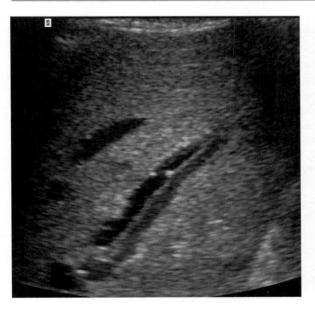
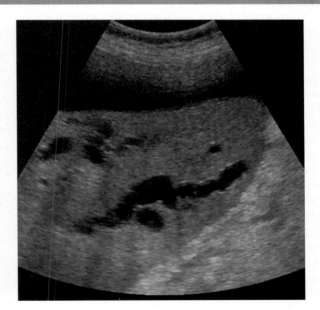

Views of the liver in two patients.

1. Is either of the images shown in this case abnormal?
2. Do the intrahepatic ducts run anterior or posterior to the portal veins?
3. What can simulate this abnormality in patients with cirrhosis?
4. Should a 3-mm intrahepatic duct be considered dilated?

Ruptured Baker's Cyst

1. The transverse view shows a cystic lesion with a curved beak-like extension heading toward the deep tissues. The longitudinal view shows the cystic lesion in the knee and a more complex appearing fluid collection extending into the calf. These features are typical of a Baker's cyst that has ruptured.

2. Baker's cysts occur in the medial aspect of the posterior knee. The cyst arises from fluid accumulation in the bursa between the medial head of the gastrocnemius and the semimembranosus tendon.

3. The location in the medial posterior knee and the beaked extension that wraps around the medial aspect of the medial head of the gastrocnemius muscle are the best confirmation that a knee cyst is a Baker's cyst.

4. Baker's cyst typically communicates with the joint.

Reference
Ptasznik R: Ultrasound in acute and chronic knee injury. *Radiol Clin North Am* 1999;37:797–830.

Cross-Reference
Musculoskeletal Imaging: THE REQUISITES, pp 28–29.

Comment
One of the earliest applications of musculoskeletal ultrasound was in the evaluation of patients with posterior knee pain and swelling due to a suspected Baker's cyst. Even prior to the advent of high-resolution linear array transducers, ultrasound was shown to be effective in identifying Baker's cysts and in distinguishing them from other posterior knee masses such as popliteal artery aneurysms.

Baker's cysts contain fluid distending the bursa between the medial head of the gastrocnemius and the semimembranosus tendon. They usually occur as a result of abnormalities that increase intra-articular fluid. They can also occur as a result of inflammatory conditions that affect the synovium of the joint and communicating bursae.

Baker's cysts may be filled with anechoic fluid and have thin, imperceptible walls. However, it is not uncommon to see internal septations; thick, irregular walls; nodular synovial proliferation; and loose bodies. The diagnostic feature that is most characteristic is the neck that extends between the medial gastrocnemius and the semimembranosus tendon. This usually appears as a beak when the knee is extended or as a channel when the knee is slightly flexed. Rupture of a Baker's cyst should be suspected whenever the inferior aspect of the cyst converts from a round to a pointed appearance, or when there is detectable fluid tracking from the inferior aspect of the cyst.

Intrahepatic Biliary Ductal Dilatation

1. Both images show dilated intrahepatic bile ducts. The first image shows the dilated bile duct running adjacent to the portal vein. The second image shows tortuous, dilated ducts with associated posterior enhancement.

2. The relationship of intrahepatic bile ducts and portal veins is variable.

3. Enlarged hepatic arteries can simulate dilated bile ducts on grey-scale imaging. This is particularly common in patients with cirrhosis.

4. The upper limit of normal for peripheral intrahepatic ducts is 2 mm.

Reference
Bressler EL, Rubin JM, McCracken S: Sonographic parallel channel sign: A reappraisal. *Radiology* 1987; 164:343-346.

Cross-Reference
Ultrasound: THE REQUISITES, pp 59–61.

Comment
The intrahepatic bile ducts travel in the portal triads adjacent to the portal veins and hepatic arteries. Although the extrahepatic ducts are located anterior to the portal vein and hepatic artery, the relationship of the intrahepatic ducts and the vessels is quite variable. Under normal circumstances, the portal vein is the largest vessel in the portal triads. A tubular structure adjacent to the portal vein may be either the hepatic artery or the bile duct. In the central aspect of the liver, it is usually possible to trace the arteries back to the proper hepatic artery and the bile ducts back to the common hepatic duct. When this is not possible, or when the peripheral aspect of the liver is being imaged, color Doppler can be used to distinguish the intrahepatic bile ducts from the intrahepatic arteries.

In the past, any time an intrahepatic duct was seen as a tubular structure running parallel to the portal vein, it was considered abnormal. This was called the parallel channel sign. However, the normal intrahepatic ducts can now be seen routinely with ultrasound. Therefore, current criteria used to diagnose intrahepatic dilatation are a duct that exceeds 40% of the diameter of the adjacent portal vein or a peripheral duct that is 3 mm or greater in diameter. With marked intrahepatic ductal dilatation, the ducts become tortuous, assume a stellate configuration centrally, and are associated with increased through transmission.

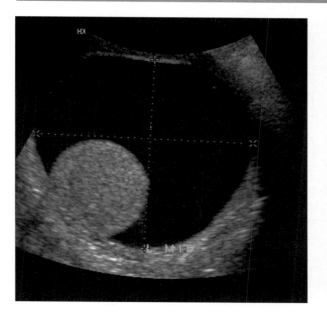
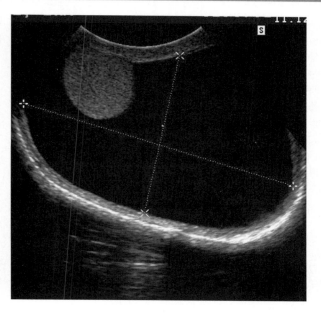

Transverse views of the scrotum in two patients with the same abnormality.

1. Is the location of the testis more typical in the first or in the second image?
2. What is the likely cause of this condition?
3. What would you expect to see at increased gain settings?
4. In what anatomic space is this abnormality located?

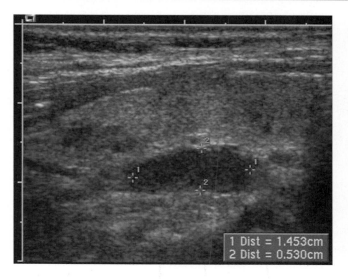
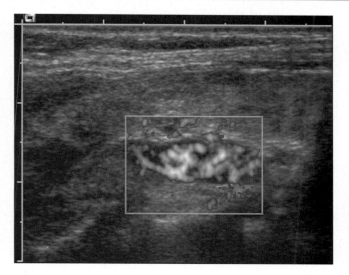

Longitudinal grey-scale and power Doppler views of the neck. (See color plates.)

1. Describe the abnormality.
2. What other test is useful in establishing this diagnosis?
3. Are these lesions usually hypervascular?
4. Are these lesions usually benign or malignant?

C A S E 5 2

Hydrocele

1. The testis is usually attached to the posterior aspect of the scrotal wall, as shown in the first image. However, this is variable, as shown in the second image.

2. Hydroceles of this size are usually idiopathic in origin.

3. Crystals often develop in chronic hydroceles and can be seen as low-level reflectors floating in the fluid when the gain is increased.

4. Hydrocele fluid is contained in the scrotal sac formed by the tunica vaginalis.

Reference

Feld R, Middleton WD: Recent advances in sonography of the testis and scrotum. *Radiol Clin North Am* 1992;30:1033–1051.

Cross-Reference

Ultrasound: THE REQUISITES, pp 446.

Comment

A hydrocele is a collection of increased fluid in the sac formed by the tunica vaginalis. A small amount of fluid around the testis is normal and is commonly seen on sonography. Collections that exceed approximately 1 cm in maximum dimension are less common. Hydroceles surround the testis over approximately 75% of their circumference on transverse views and over approximately 50% on longitudinal views. The remainder of the testis is adherent to the wall of the scrotum, so that hydrocele fluid cannot flow behind the entire testis. Although variable, hydroceles typically collect in the anterior aspect of the scrotum and displace the testis posteriorly. An unusual form of a hydrocele occurs when there is a fluid collection in a focally unobliterated portion of the processus vaginalis within the spermatic cord. This appears as a supratesticular cystic mass and is called a funiculocele or a hydrocele of the spermatic cord.

Causes of hydrocele include infections, torsion of the testis or one of its appendages, trauma, and testicular tumors. However, all of these conditions typically cause relatively small hydroceles. Large, simple-appearing hydroceles such as the ones shown in these patients are usually idiopathic.

In patients with large hydroceles, it is usually difficult to palpate the testis on physical examination. Therefore, one of the important roles of sonography is to image the testis and exclude testicular pathology. When the testis is displaced posteriorly, it can be difficult to get a good image of the testis from the typical anterior approach. Instead, a posterior approach brings the transducer closer to the testis and allows for a more detailed view.

C A S E 5 3

Parathyroid Adenoma

1. An oval-shaped, hypoechoic, hypervascular mass is located posterior to the thyroid.

2. The other valuable test for localization of a parathyroid adenoma is a sestamibi scan.

3. Parathyroid adenomas are usually hypervascular.

4. Parathyroid adenomas are benign. Parathyroid cancer is very rare.

Reference

Shawker TH, Avila NA, Premkumar A, et al: Ultrasound evaluation of primary hyperparathyroidism. *Ultrasound Q* 2000;16:73–87.

Cross-Reference

Ultrasound: THE REQUISITES, pp 452–454.

Comment

The most common cause of primary hyperparathyroidism is a solitary parathyroid adenoma. Approximately 15% of cases are caused by multiple enlarged glands (usually parathyroid hyperplasia and, less commonly, multiple adenomas). Parathyroid cancer is rare and causes less than 1% of cases of hyperparathyroidism. Primary hyperparathyroidism is more common in women.

Parathyroid adenomas are typically solid but very hypoechoic lesions. They are usually oval-shaped, with the long axis in the craniocaudal direction. On color Doppler imaging, many adenomas are hypervascular. The typical location for parathyroid adenomas arising from the superior gland is behind the mid aspect of the thyroid. Adenomas arising from the inferior glands are typically located close to the inferior aspect of the thyroid or a few centimeters below the thyroid.

Sensitivity of ultrasound for detecting parathyroid adenomas is approximately 80%, although both higher and lower values have been reported. False-negative examination results generally arise as a result of a small adenoma or an adenoma in an ectopic location, or in a patient with a large, multinodular thyroid gland. False-positive results are less of a problem but do occur. Lymph nodes can be misinterpreted as parathyroid adenomas. A useful clue is that parathyroid adenomas are essentially always located medial to the carotid arteries. Lymph nodes can be located in a variety of locations but are usually located lateral to the carotids. Posteriorly located thyroid nodules can also simulate parathyroid adenomas. Usually, there is a bright line that separates a parathyroid adenoma from the thyroid, while there is no such line between thyroid tissue and thyroid nodules.

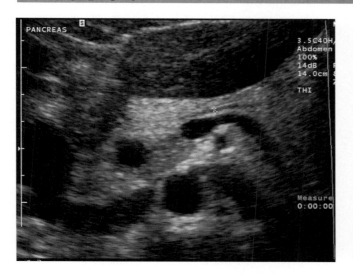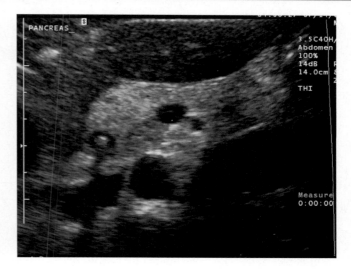

Magnified transverse views of the pancreatic head.

1. What are the two important findings on these scans?

2. Where is this abnormality usually located?

3. How good is ultrasound in visualizing this abnormality?

4. What is the treatment of this abnormality?

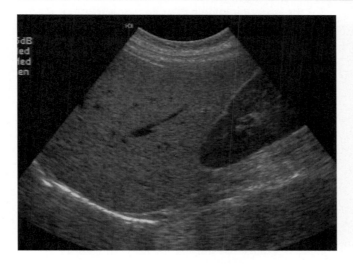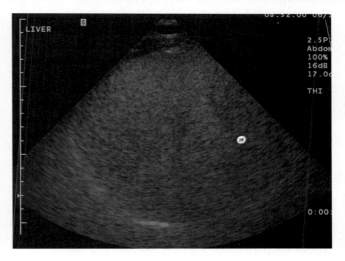

Longitudinal views of the right upper quadrant in two patients.

1. List the echogenicity of liver, kidney, spleen, and pancreas from most to least echogenic.

2. What is the most common cause of the abnormalities shown in these images?

3. In the first image, is the liver or the kidney more likely to be abnormal?

4. Why is the diaphragm so poorly seen in the second image?

Choledocholithiasis

1. The most important findings are a dilated bile duct, best seen on the first image, and a shadowing echogenic structure in the lumen of the duct on the second image.

2. Common bile duct stones are usually located in the distal, intrapancreatic portion of the duct.

3. In the best series, ultrasound has a sensitivity of 75% in identifying common duct stones.

4. Common duct stones are treated with endoscopic retrograde cholangiopancreatography (ERCP), balloon retrieval, and sphincterotomy.

Reference

Middleton WD: The bile ducts. In Goldberg BB (ed): *Diagnostic Ultrasound.* Baltimore, Williams & Wilkins, 1993, pp 146–172.

Cross-Reference

Ultrasound: THE REQUISITES, pp 61–63.

Comment

Choledocholithiasis is the most common cause of biliary obstruction. Approximately 85% of cases arise from gallstones that pass through the cystic duct and into the common bile duct. In fact, approximately 15% of patients with cholecystitis have choledocholithiasis. Pigmented stones can form de novo in the bile duct. Usually this is due to bile stasis or superimposed biliary infection. The majority of common duct stones are located in the distal, intrapancreatic portion of the duct. Only 10% are seen in the proximal portion of the common duct.

Ultrasound is frequently the initial imaging test used in patients with common duct stones. The primary finding that is usually observed is a dilated duct. This is typically the case in patients with jaundice due to choledocholithiasis. Unfortunately, a minority of patients with choledocholithiasis have an unobstructed or an intermittently obstructed duct, so that ductal diameter is normal. This is often the case in patients with cholecystitis or biliary colic who have also passed a stone into the bile duct. Therefore, the sensitivity of using dilated ducts to predict choledocholithiasis varies with the patient population being scanned.

Visualization of common duct stones is much more difficult than visualization of stones in the gallbladder. When ductal stones are seen, they appear as echogenic structures in the bile duct lumen. Although acoustic shadowing is usually present, it is seen less commonly than with stones in the gallbladder.

In the best of hands, the sensitivity of sonography in visualizing common duct stones is 70% to 80%. In many reported series, however, the sensitivity is less than 50%. The primary reason for this low sensitivity is that most common duct stones are located in the most distal aspect of the duct, and this segment is often not completely seen on sonograms. Using the gallbladder as a window, scanning through a fluid-filled stomach, and scanning the patient in an upright position are all techniques that can help to improve visualization of the distal duct.

Fatty Infiltration of the Liver

1. Pancreas → spleen → liver → kidney.

2. Fatty infiltration is by far the most common cause of hepatic hyperechogenicity.

3. Because fatty infiltration of the liver is so common, when there is a large discrepancy in the echogenicity of the liver and the kidney, it is much more likely that the liver is too echogenic than that the kidney is too echolucent.

4. Sound attenuation by the fatty liver limits visualization of the deeper structures, including the diaphragm.

References

Mergo PJ, Ros PR, Buetow PC, Buck JL: Diffuse disease of the liver: Radiologic-pathologic correlation. *Radiographics* 1994;14:1291–1307.

Zweibel WJ: Sonographic diagnosis of diffuse liver disease. *Semin US CT MRI* 1995;16:8–16.

Cross-Reference

Ultrasound: THE REQUISITES, pp 16–18

Comment

Normally the liver and the right kidney are either very similar in echogenicity or the liver is just slightly more echogenic than the kidney. In this case, the difference in echogenicity between the liver and the kidney is abnormal. In the majority of cases, this is due to fatty infiltration. A large number of processes can cause fatty infiltration of the liver, but the most common cause is obesity. Other common causes include alcohol abuse, total parenteral nutrition, diabetes, malnutrition, steroid use, hepatic toxins, and chemotherapy.

In addition to increased echogenicity, the fat-infiltrated liver appears to have a finer and more compact parenchymal echo pattern than normal liver. More severe fatty infiltration also causes sound attenuation, so that the deeper aspects of the liver are hard to penetrate. This may manifest as decreased echogenicity of the deep liver, poor definition of the diaphragm, or poor visualization of the hepatic vessels. These latter findings are seen in the second image.

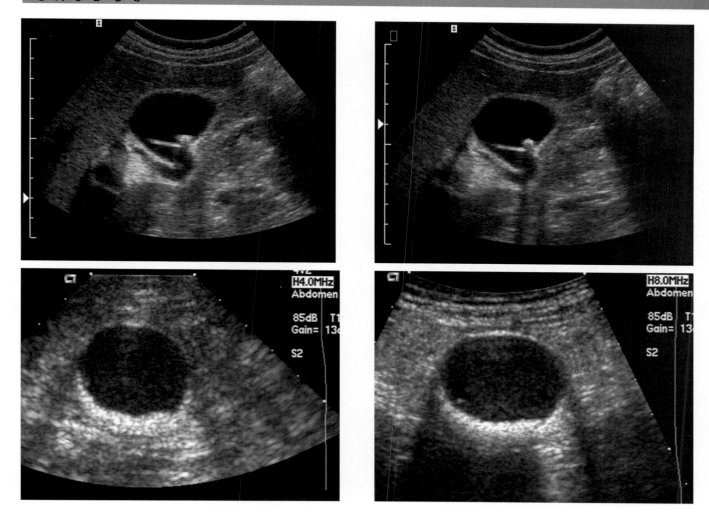

Paired longitudinal views of the gallbladder in one patient and paired transverse views of the gallbladder in another patient.

1. In each patient, which image is more diagnostic for gallstones?

2. What technical parameter causes the difference in the images of the first patient?

3. What technical parameter causes the difference in the images of the second patient?

4. Is there a significant difference between the sonographic appearance of calcified and noncalcified gallstones?

Technical Parameters Important in Producing Shadowing From Small Gallstones

1. In each patient, the second image is most diagnostic of gallstones because it shows shadowing.

2. In the first patient, the focal zone is properly positioned at the level of the stone in the second image. In the first image, the focal zone is located deep to the stone.

3. In the second patient, a higher frequency (8 MHz) probe has been used in the second image. A 4 MHz probe was used in the first image.

4. Calcified and noncalcified stones appear the same on sonography.

Reference

Middleton WD: Right upper quadrant pain. In Bluth EI, Benson C, Arger P, et al (eds): *The Practice of Ultrasonography.* New York, Thieme, 1999, pp 3–16.

Cross-Reference

Ultrasound: THE REQUISITES, pp 38–40.

Comment

The sonographic criteria for gallstones include: 1) echogenic structure in the gallbladder lumen; 2) mobility demonstrated by moving the patient into different positions; and 3) posterior acoustic shadowing. Sludge balls can appear as mobile, echogenic, intraluminal structures, but they do not shadow. Polyps can appear as echogenic, intraluminal structures, but they do not move and do not shadow. Rarely, gallstones are nonmobile because they are adherent to the gallbladder wall, are trapped behind a fold, or are embedded in a gallbladder full of viscous sludge.

Shadowing is related to sound attenuation, which in turn is related to reflection, refraction, scattering, and absorption of the sound. With gallstones, absorption of the sound is the key factor in producing shadowing. Shadowing is related to the size of the stone and is largely independent to the composition of the stone. In other words, noncalcified stones (approximately 85% of total stones) shadow just as much as calcified stones. Stones in the 3 mm or less size range may not shadow regardless of their composition.

In attempting to produce shadowing in small stones, it is important to optimize scanning technique. Focus the transducer at the level of the stone so that the beam profile is minimized and the stone blocks as much of the beam as possible. Also, use as high a probe frequency as possible because penetration through the stone will be minimized. Finally, if there are multiple, small, nonshadowing stones, change the patient position so that the stones are aggregated together and therefore act as a single larger stone.

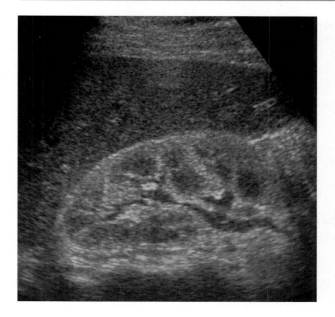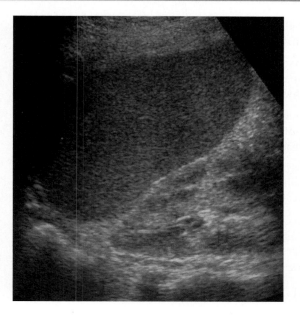

Longitudinal views of the right and left kidney.

1. What abnormality do both of these kidneys demonstrate?
2. What is the specificity of this abnormality?
3. What next test will help the most in establishing the diagnosis?
4. How well does normal renal echogenicity exclude renal dysfunction?

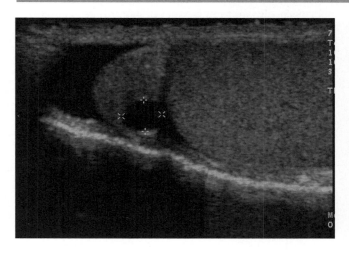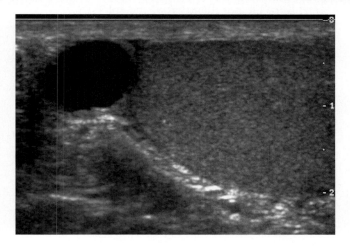

Longitudinal views of the scrotum in two patients.

1. Do these patients have anything in common?
2. Is this abnormality likely to be palpable?
3. Is this abnormality commonly or uncommonly seen on ultrasound?
4. What does this lesion contain?

Renal Parenchymal Disease

1. Both kidneys demonstrate increased echogenicity.

2. Increased renal echogenicity is relatively specific for renal parenchymal disease, but it does not predict the type of parenchymal disease.

3. The only effective way to distinguish the different types of parenchymal disease is to use clinical information or to do a biopsy.

4. Normal renal echogenicity does not exclude renal parenchymal disease.

Reference

Platt JF, Rubin JM, Bowerman RA, Marn CS: The inability to detect kidney disease on the basis of echogenicity. *AJR Am J Roentgenol* 1988;151:317-319.

Cross-Reference

Ultrasound: THE REQUISITES, pp 105-106.

Comment

Abnormalities of renal echogenicity can be detected by comparing the kidneys to the liver and the spleen. The right kidney is usually less echogenic than the liver, although it can be isoechoic to the liver and still be normal. If the right kidney is more echogenic than the liver, then it should be considered abnormal. Since the spleen is more echogenic than the liver, the left kidney should be considered abnormal if its echogenicity is equal to or greater than that of the spleen.

When comparing renal, hepatic, and splenic echogenicity, it is important to adjust the distance gain compensation (DGC) curve so that the hepatic and splenic echogenicity is uniform throughout. If this is not possible, then be sure to compare the kidney to regions of the liver and spleen that are at equivalent depths.

In some patients, it is not possible to directly compare the kidney to the liver and spleen. This might occur when the spleen is small, when there is abundant ascites separating the kidneys from the liver and spleen, or when the liver and spleen are not normal. In particular, in the setting of fatty infiltration of the liver, the kidney may be abnormally echogenic and still appear hypoechoic compared to the liver. In such cases, the renal cortex can be compared to the medullary pyramids. When the cortex is hyperechoic, the pyramids often appear unusually hypoechoic, and this can be used as a soft indicator of renal cortical disease.

Although increased renal echogenicity indicates renal parenchymal disease, it is extremely nonspecific. Many different processes produce the same appearance. Therefore, in a patient with renal dysfunction and echogenic kidneys, biopsy is frequently performed in order to determine the nature of the parenchymal disease.

Spermatocele

1. Both patients have simple-appearing extratesticular cysts located above the testis. In the first image, the cyst is clearly arising within the head of the epididymis. In the second image, the cyst obscures the epididymal head.

2. Spermatoceles are palpable unless they are very small.

3. Spermatoceles are very common.

4. The fluid in a spermatocele contains spermatozoa.

Reference

Feld R, Middleton WD: Recent advances in sonography of the testis and scrotum. *Radiol Clin North Am* 1992;30:1033-1051.

Cross-Reference

Ultrasound: THE REQUISITES, pp 435-437.

Comment

Cysts of the epididymis are extremely common. With improvements in resolution that have occurred since the mid 1990s, it is actually uncommon *not* to see a cyst in the epididymis. An epididymal cyst is the most common cause of a palpable mass in the scrotum. These cysts are called spermatoceles when they are filled with spermatozoa. They are called epididymal cysts when they contain serous fluid. In the majority of cases, spermatoceles and epididymal cysts both appear as simple cysts without internal echoes, so it is not possible to tell one from the other. Statistically, spermatoceles are more common. Spermatoceles most often occur in the head of the epididymis. They may contain internal septations, especially when they become large. It is uncommon to have symptoms related to a spermatocele, although they may become a cosmetic problem when they are large.

The differential diagnosis of a spermatocele is limited. Hydroceles are usually easily differentiated from spermatoceles because they surround the testis on all sides except for the bare area where the testis is anchored to the scrotal wall. Spermatoceles push the testis rather than surround the testis. An unusual form of hydrocele is called a funiculocele. This represents fluid that accumulates within a focally unobliterated portion of the processus vaginalis in the spermatic cord. Like a spermatocele, a funiculocele is located superior to the testis and may displace the testis inferiorly. If a normal epididymal head is visualized separate from the lesion, the cyst is very unlikely to be a spermatocele and much more likely to be a funiculocele.

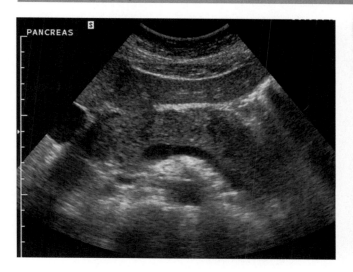
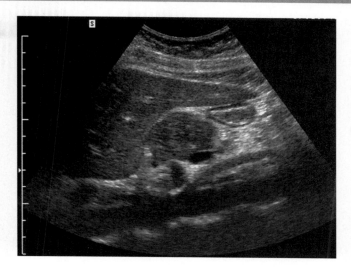

Transverse and longitudinal views of the pancreas.

1. What are the abnormal findings?
2. What are the two most common causes of this disorder?
3. What is the primary role of ultrasound in this disorder?
4. Are most abnormalities in the pancreas hypoechoic or hyperechoic?

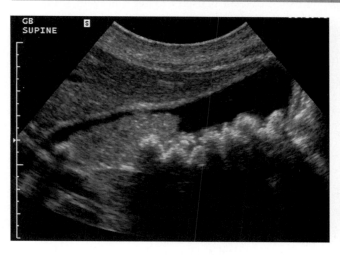
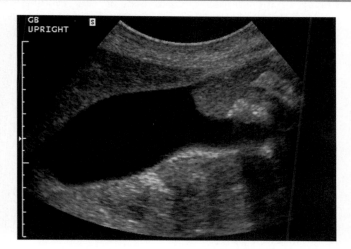

Longitudinal views of the gallbladder.

1. What is the differential diagnosis based only on the first image?
2. How does the second image help in establishing the diagnosis?
3. How can follow-up studies help?

Acute Pancreatitis

1. Both images show an enlarged and hypoechoic pancreas.

2. Gallstones and alcohol abuse are the most common causes of pancreatitis.

3. Ultrasound is used to look for gallstones or bile duct obstruction, and to help resolve questions raised by CT.

4. Most pancreatic pathology is hypoechoic.

Reference

Balthazar EJ, Freeny PC, vanSonnenberg E: Imaging and intervention in acute pancreatitis. *Radiology* 1994;193:297–306.

Cross-Reference

Ultrasound: THE REQUISITES, pp 126–129.

Comment

Either gallstones or alcohol abuse causes approximately 75% of cases of acute pancreatitis in the United States. Other, less common causes include drugs, hyperlipidemia, ischemia, viral infections, pancreas divisum, and trauma. Approximately 10% of cases are idiopathic. Many of the idiopathic cases may be due to biliary sludge. Obstruction of the pancreatic duct is believed to be responsible for increased intraductal pressure and release of pancreatic enzymes into the interstitial tissues. Alcohol causes precipitation of proteins that obstruct the ducts, and gallstones produce obstruction when they pass through the bile duct and lodge at the ampulla. The severity of pancreatitis ranges from the mildest interstitial (edematous) form, where there is edema isolated to the pancreas itself, to necrotizing pancreatitis, where there is extensive necrosis of the pancreatic parenchyma and adjacent tissues.

The role of sonography in patients with pancreatitis is primarily to evaluate the biliary tract for the presence of gallstones as a possible etiology and the bile duct for possible obstruction. Evaluation of the pancreas itself is certainly possible with ultrasound, but CT, especially contrast-enhanced CT, is superior in determining the severity and extent of pancreatitis.

Many patients with pancreatitis have a sonographically normal pancreas. When present, the sonographic signs of pancreatitis include increased size and decreased echogenicity of the pancreas, and slight enlargement of the pancreatic duct. Echogenicity is somewhat unreliable, since the base line echogenicity of the pancreas is variable, and since it is compared to the echogenicity of the liver, which varies depending on the presence and degree of fatty infiltration. The detection of pancreatic enlargement is also rather subjective. To further complicate the matter, the pancreas may be difficult to visualize owing to an associated ileus (which causes overlying gas-filled bowel loops) and pain (which precludes compression of the epigastrium). Therefore, it is important to look other places as well. Fortunately, edema and fluid collections frequently dissect into the anterior pararenal fascia, which is usually visible sonographically. In fact, detection of otherwise unexplained fluid around the kidney should always raise the suspicion of pancreatitis. Fluid may also dissect around the splenic hilum and the peripancreatic vessels. Tiny amounts of fluid may accumulate between the body of the pancreas and the portosplenic confluence. This is sometimes referred to as perivascular cloaking.

Tumefactive Sludge (Sludge ball)

1. In addition to gallstones, the first image shows well-formed, nonshadowing echogenic material. The differential diagnosis includes sludge, clotted blood, and neoplasm.

2. The second image excludes neoplasm because it documents mobility.

3. In some patients tumefactive sludge does not move. In such cases it is useful to get follow-up scans because the sludge usually changes over time.

Reference

Middleton WD: The gallbladder. In Goldberg BB (ed): *Diagnostic Ultrasound.* Baltimore, Williams & Wilkins, 1993, pp 116–142.

Cross-Reference

Ultrasound: THE REQUISITES, pp 40–42.

Comment

In most cases, sludge forms a layer of echogenic material along the dependent aspect of the gallbladder lumen. Occasionally, sludge forms a more mass-like aggregate referred to as a sludge ball or as tumefactive sludge. As is true with typical sludge, sludge balls are mobile and do not cast an acoustic shadow. The lack of shadowing helps to distinguish sludge balls from stones, and the mobility helps to distinguish sludge balls from tumors or polyps. Internal vascularity can be detected in many large polyps and polypoid cancers but is not present in sludge. Therefore, color Doppler can occasionally help in the differential diagnosis.

In some cases, tumefactive sludge forms in the presence of bile so viscous that it is impossible to document mobility. In such cases, a follow-up scan in several weeks can be useful, since sludge may resolve, regress, or change in some other way.

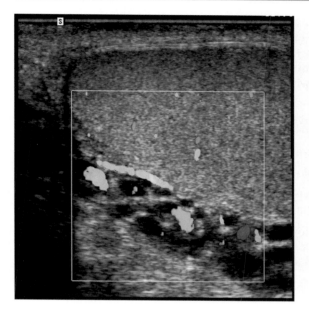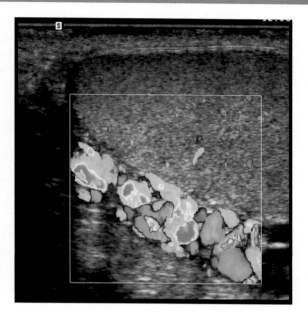

Longitudinal color Doppler views of the left scrotum. (See color plates).

1. What was the patient asked to do when the second color Doppler image was taken?
2. What is the etiology of this condition?
3. What is the significance of this lesion?
4. Are these lesions typically unilateral or bilateral?

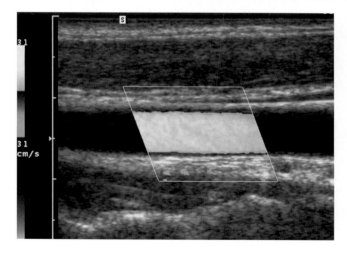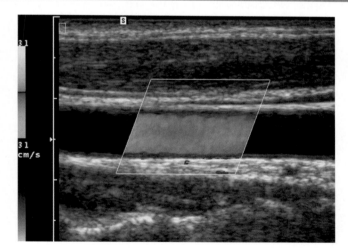

Two color Doppler images of the same vessel. (See color plates).

1. What is the direction of blood flow in the two images?
2. What is the significance of a positive Doppler frequency shift?
3. Would you usually expect it to be easier to determine flow direction at a Doppler angle of 5 degrees or of 85 degrees?
4. Under what circumstance would your answer to the preceding question be different?

C A S E 6 1

Varicocele

1. Flow is augmented and becomes detectable when the patient performs a Valsalva maneuver.

2. Incompetent valves in the spermatic vein cause varicoceles.

3. Varicoceles can potentially contribute to infertility. When large, they can cause pain.

4. Typically, 85% are unilateral on the left; 10% to 15% are bilateral. Unilateral right varicoceles are rare.

Reference

Feld R, Middleton WD: Recent advances in sonography of the testis and scrotum. *Radiol Clin North Am* 1992;30:1033-1051.

Cross-Reference

Ultrasound: THE REQUISITES, pp 446-449.

Comment

The veins of the pampiniform plexus enter the spermatic cord and drain into the internal spermatic veins. The left spermatic vein empties into the left renal vein, and the right empties into the inferior vena cava. Varicoceles are dilated veins of the pampiniform plexus. They are almost always caused by incompetent valves within the internal spermatic vein. Incompetent valves allow increased hydrostatic pressure when the patient is upright, which results in gradual enlargement of the veins. Varicoceles predominate on the left, because compression of the left renal vein as it passes between the superior mesenteric artery and the aorta causes higher pressure on the left side. In rare instances, varicoceles can be due to obstruction of the spermatic veins secondary to processes such as masses, retroperitoneal fibrosis, or venous tumor invasion.

Although controversial, most investigators believe that even small, subclinical varicoceles may contribute to abnormal semen analysis results, and that treatment of varicoceles may improve fertility. Therefore, the diagnosis of a varicocele is important, especially in the investigation of male infertility.

Varicoceles appear as an increased size, number, and tortuosity of the veins around the testis. When small, they are usually seen most prominently at the superior or lateral aspect of the testis. Large varicoceles extend to the posterior and inferior aspect of the scrotum. Reports indicate that normal peritesticular veins should be less than 2 or 3 mm in diameter. In my experience, they seldom exceed 2 mm. On color Doppler scanning, venous flow in varicoceles is generally too slow to be detected with the patient at rest. Sometimes, this slow flow is apparent on grey-scale imaging. With a Valsalva maneuver, there is augmented retrograde flow in the varicocele that is readily detectable on color Doppler imaging. This augmented flow usually lasts longer than one second. In a patient with infertility, if augmented flow is not seen when the patient is in the supine position, the patient should perform a Valsalva maneuver while being scanned in an upright position.

C A S E 6 2

Beam Steering and Color Assignment

1. Blood flow is from the right to the left.

2. A positive Doppler frequency shift indicates that the flow is toward the origin of the Doppler pulse.

3. Flow direction should be easiest to determine at a Doppler angle closest to 0 degrees and hardest to determine at an angle close to 90 degrees.

4. The preceding answer changes if there is extensive Doppler aliasing at the lower Doppler angles.

Reference

Middleton WD: Color Doppler image optimization and interpretation. *Ultrasound Q* 1998;14:194-208.

Cross-Reference

Ultrasound: THE REQUISITES, pp 464-470.

Comment

The most basic aspect of color Doppler image interpretation is the determination of flow direction. Blood flow going toward the origin of the Doppler pulse produces a positive frequency shift, while flow away from the Doppler pulse produces a negative frequency shift. Once the sign of the Doppler frequency shift is known, it is possible to determine which direction blood is flowing in a given vessel.

A color Doppler scale always indicates what color is assigned to different frequency shifts. This scale displays positive shifts on the top and negative shifts on the bottom. In general, red is assigned to positive shifts and blue to negative shifts. However, it is common to adjust the color assignment so that arterial flow is displayed in red even though it is directed away from the Doppler pulse. When the color assignment is inverted, the color scale displays red on the bottom and blue on the top. Another method of changing the color assignment in a vessel is to change the direction of the Doppler pulse. With linear array transducers, this can be done by electronically steering the beam, as was done in this case. With phased array sector or curved array probes, the Doppler pulse can be redirected by repositioning or reangling the probe. When a vessel is curved or tortuous, different segments may have different color assignments owing to variation in the direction of blood flow with respect to the transmitted Doppler pulse.

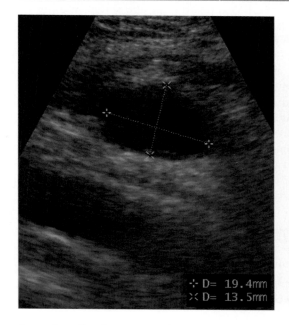
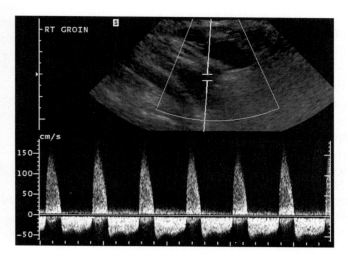

Longitudinal grey-scale view and pulsed Doppler waveform of the groin.

1. How does the waveform shown in this case differ from the normal triphasic waveform of extremity arteries?

2. What is the significance of this type of waveform?

3. How is the abnormality shown here treated?

4. What is the success of this treatment?

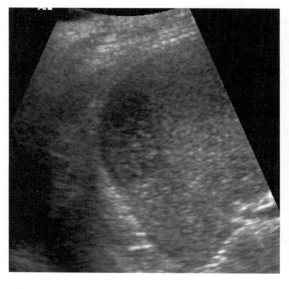
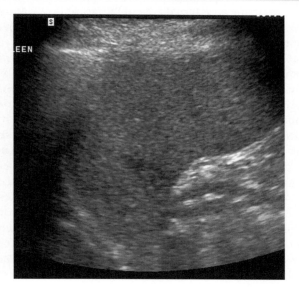

Views of the spleen in two patients.

1. Describe the abnormality seen in these patients.

2. Is this likely to be acute or chronic?

3. Would other tests be valuable in further characterization of this abnormality?

4. What are the common causes of this abnormality?

CASE 63

Post-Catheterization Pseudoaneurysm

1. The waveform exhibits pandiastolic flow reversal. The normal triphasic pattern has only a short period of flow reversal in early diastole.

2. It comes from the neck of a pseudoaneurysm and reflects flow into the aneurysm during systole and flow out of the aneurysm during diastole.

3. Treatment is with ultrasound-guided injection of thrombin or with compression repair.

4. The success rate of treatment with thrombin injection is 90% and is somewhat less with compression.

Reference

Paulson EK, Sheafor DH, Nelson RC, et al: Treatment of iatrogenic femoral arterial pseudoaneurysms: Comparison of US-guided thrombin injection with compression repair. *Radiology* 2000;215:403–408.

Cross-Reference

Ultrasound: THE REQUISITES, pp 479–481.

Comment

The frequency of post-catheterization pseudoaneurysm (PA) increased in the 1990s owing to the increased use of large-gauge catheters for vascular interventions as well as to the increased use of anticoagulation during and after these procedures. PA typically manifests with swelling and ecchymosis in the first day or two following the procedure. In this setting, a PA basically is a hematoma that maintains an internal area of extravascular blood flow via a patent neck that communicates with the femoral artery. With time, a fibrous capsule may develop around the PA.

On sonography, a PA appears as a collection of fluid adjacent to the injured artery. With grey-scale imaging, it is often possible to see the collection expand during systole and contract during diastole. Otherwise, it is not possible to distinguish a PA from a simple hematoma. A PA may or may not have a significant amount of clotted blood at the periphery. It is not uncommon to see several adjacent PAs connected to each other via thin tracts.

With color Doppler, it is possible to detect flowing blood in the lumen of a PA. Typically, blood flow into the PA concentrates along one wall, and flow out of the PA concentrates along the opposite wall. This produces the typical swirling, or "yin-yang," appearance, where one half of the lumen appears red and the other half appears blue. There are many variations on this pattern depending on the direction of the inflow jet into the aneurysm lumen. The key point is not the pattern of luminal flow but simply the presence of flow. Another frequently described characteristic of PAs is the "to and fro" pattern of flow in the neck. This refers to systolic flow (into the PA) appearing on one side of the pulsed Doppler base line and diastolic flow (out of the PA and back into the artery) appearing on the other side of the baseline.

Initial attempts at nonsurgical treatment of PAs concentrated on ultrasound-guided compression. Although this approach is reasonably effective, it is time-consuming, painful for the patient, and fatiguing for the doctor. Thrombin injection under ultrasound guidance is much faster, almost painless, and easy for the doctor. Also, thrombin injection is more successful and, unlike compression, does not require termination of anticoagulation.

CASE 64

Splenic Infarction

1. These lesions are peripherally located, hypoechoic, and wedge-shaped.

2. This is probably fairly acute, since infarcts tend to become more hyperechoic with age.

3. Contrast enhanced CT may be helpful, since the wedge shape may be more apparent and other infarcts may be seen.

4. Common causes of splenic infarction include emboli of cardiac or atherosclerotic origin, lymphoproliferative disease, arteritis, pancreatitis, sepsis, and sickle cell anemia.

Reference

Goerg C. Schwerk WB. Splenic infarction: Sonographic patterns, diagnosis, follow-up, and complications. *Radiology* 1990;174:803–807.

Cross-Reference

Ultrasound: THE REQUISITES, pp 147–148.

Comment

Infarcts are one of the most common causes of focal splenic lesions. When they are small, they usually produce no clinical symptoms or only minor symptoms. Therefore, it is not unusual to see them as incidental findings. Pain, fever, and diaphragmatic irritation can occur with large infarcts.

Classically, splenic infarctions appear as multiple or solitary wedge-shaped, peripherally located lesions, as shown in this case. They are usually hypoechoic but have also been reported as anechoic. They can also appear as spherical masses that are impossible to distinguish from neoplastic processes. In most cases, the clinical history will suggest the correct diagnosis. In some patients, imaging with CT may help in further characterization. If there is a contraindication to iodinated contrast, then MRI is an alternative approach.

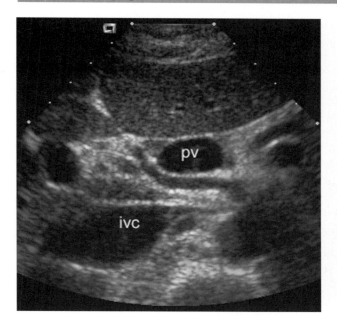 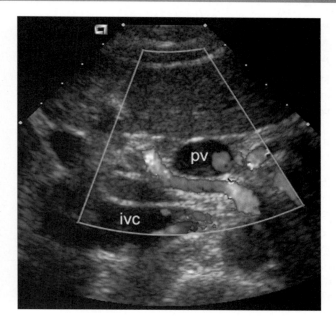

Transverse grey-scale and color Doppler view of the portal vein (pv) and inferior vena cava (ivc).

1. What type of Doppler signal would you expect from the vessel running between the PV and the IVC?
2. From where does this vessel usually arise?
3. How often is this vessel located in this location?
4. What is the normal course of this vessel?

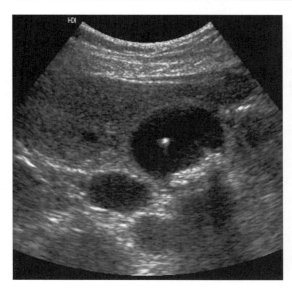 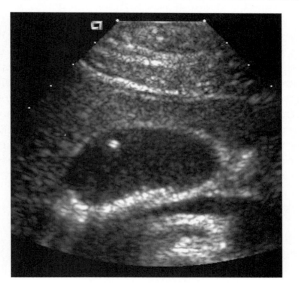

Views of the gallbladder in two patients.

1. What is unusual about both of these patients?
2. Is it possible to predict the composition of stones in these patients?
3. Is this a common finding?
4. Under what circumstance does this occur?

Replaced Right Hepatic Artery

1. A Doppler waveform would show an arterial signal with flow toward the liver.

2. Most of the time, an artery running between the PV and the IVC is an anomalous right hepatic artery coming from the superior mesenteric artery. Occasionally, a hepatic artery may arise normally from the celiac axis and then travel anomalously behind the PV prior to entering the liver.

3. Replaced or accessory right hepatic arteries occur in approximately 20% of the population.

4. Normally the hepatic artery runs anterior to the PV.

Reference

Lafortune M, Patriquin H: The hepatic artery: Studies using Doppler sonography. *Ultrasound Q* 1999; 15(1):9–26.

Comment

Normally, the celiac axis divides into the splenic artery, the left gastric artery, and the common hepatic artery. The first branch of the common hepatic artery is the gastroduodenal artery. Beyond the gastroduodenal, the name of the hepatic artery changes to proper hepatic artery. The proper hepatic artery then divides into the right and left hepatic artery. Some variation of this standard anatomy is present in just under half of the population.

An artery is called a *replaced* artery if the entire artery arises from an anomalous source. An artery is called an *accessory* artery if one of its portions originates from its usual origin and another branch arises from some other vessel. Replaced or accessory right hepatic arteries arising from the superior mesenteric artery are present in approximately 20% of patients. Unlike the normal hepatic artery, they travel behind the PV and then ascend to the liver in the hepatoduodenal ligament. After the replaced hepatic artery passes to the right behind the PV, it then wraps around the right side of the PV and eventually is located anterior to the PV and lateral to the common duct. This can produce a situation where there are three round structures anterior to the PV on transverse views, with the common duct placed between the normal left hepatic artery and the replaced right hepatic artery.

Floating Gallstones

1. In both cases, stones are seen layering in the dependent portion of the gallbladder, but a stone is also seen floating in the middle of the gallbladder.

2. Under most circumstances, it is not possible to predict gallstone composition. However, only cholesterol stones float, so in this case prediction is possible.

3. This is a very uncommon finding.

4. Gallstones float only when the specific gravity of the bile is greater than the specific gravity of the stone.

Reference

Yeh HC, Goodman J, Rabinowitz JG: Floating gallstones in bile without added contrast material. *AJR Am J Roentgenol* 1986;146:49–50.

Cross-Reference

Ultrasound: THE REQUISITES, pp 39–41.

Comment

In the age of oral cholecystography, it was not uncommon to see gallstones floating in the nondependent portion of the gallbladder. This was because the opacification of the bile caused by the medication also caused an increase in the specific gravity of the bile. If the specific gravity of the stones is less than that of the bile, then the stones will float.

Today, oral cholecystography is no longer performed, so it is very uncommon for the specific gravity of bile to exceed that of gallstones. One exception is when there is some degree of vicarious biliary excretion of iodinated intravenous contrast material. One of the patients shown in this case had a contrast enhanced CT prior to the ultrasound.

Regardless of the reason, when stones are seen to float in the nondependent portion of the gallbladder, it is safe to say that they are unusually buoyant, and therefore to predict that they are composed of cholesterol.

II Fair Game

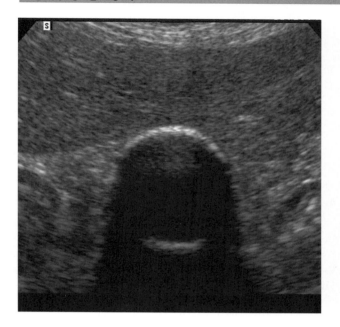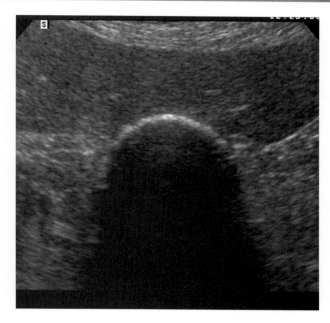

Transverse views of the gallbladder.

1. What two conditions are most likely to produce this sonographic appearance?
2. Does the nature of the shadowing help in favoring one of the two possibilities?
3. What other imaging examination could be used to confirm the diagnosis?
4. How can you exclude a gallbladder full of stones as a possible diagnosis?

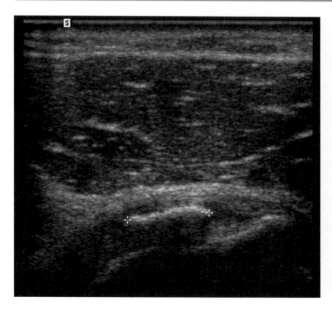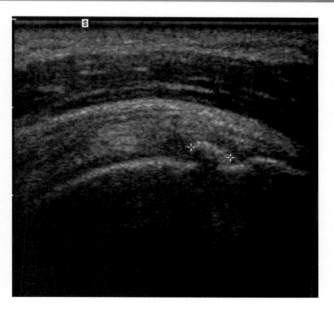

Long axis views of the rotator cuff in two patients.

1. What would you expect to see on these patients' shoulder radiographs?
2. What would you expect to see on these patients' MRI?
3. How good is ultrasound at making this diagnosis?
4. What type of transducer is used to scan the shoulder?

Porcelain Gallbladder

1. The primary considerations are a porcelain gallbladder and emphysematous cholecystitis.

2. A clean shadow favors porcelain gallbladder, and a dirty shadow favors emphysematous cholecystitis.

3. An abdominal radiograph or a CT scan could help to distinguish gallbladder wall calcification from gas.

4. It would not be possible to see the back wall of the gallbladder if the lumen were full of stones.

Reference
Middleton WD: The gallbladder. In Goldberg BB (ed): *Diagnostic Ultrasound*. Baltimore, Williams & Wilkins, 1993, pp 116-142.

Cross Reference
Ultrasound: THE REQUISITES, pp 50-52.

Comment
A porcelain gallbladder refers to calcification of the gallbladder wall. This occurs as a result of chronic inflammation and is almost always associated with gallstones. Patients with gallbladder wall calcification are at increased risk of gallbladder cancer. Although the exact risk is not uniformly agreed upon, most authorities agree that patients should undergo a prophylactic cholecystectomy unless there are contraindications to surgery.

The sonographic appearance of porcelain gallbladder depends on the distribution and thickness of the calcification. When the calcification is diffuse and thick, the superficial wall of the gallbladder is seen as a bright, curvilinear reflector with an associated shadow. Because of extensive attenuation of the sound pulse, the back wall is not visible when the calcification is thick. If the calcification is thin, enough sound may penetrate the superficial wall in order to image part of, or even the entire back wall. Such is the case in this patient. Ability to see the back wall is important because that excludes a gallbladder full of stones from the differential diagnosis.

The other consideration in this case is emphysematous cholecystitis. Both conditions can appear as a bright, curvilinear line with posterior shadowing. In general, gas appears brighter than calcification, and the shadowing from gas appears dirtier than shadowing from calcification. However, in an individual case these differences may be hard to rely on. Ring-down artifact, which appears as a bright line trailing deep to the gas, is only seen with gas and does not occur with calcification. In addition, if gas is confined to the lumen of the gallbladder, it is mobile. If there is difficulty in distinguishing gas from calcification based on the sonogram, an abdominal radiograph should be obtained. If it remains unclear after the abdominal radiograph, a CT scan should be obtained.

Calcific Tendinitis of the Rotator Cuff

1. Radiographs may show a focal area of soft tissue calcification in the region of the rotator cuff. The calcification may be difficult to see if it is projected over bone on all views.

2. MRI would show a signal void on all sequences. For this reason, calcific tendinitis is often missed on MRI.

3. Ultrasound is the best way to identify, quantitate, and localize calcific tendinitis of the rotator cuff.

4. As with other musculoskeletal examinations, shoulders should be scanned with a linear array transducer with a center frequency of 7 to 12 MHz.

Reference
Middleton WD, Teefey SA, Yamaguchi K: Sonography of the shoulder. *Semin Musculoskeletal Radiol* 1998; 2:211-221.

Cross Reference
Ultrasound: THE REQUISITES, pp 455-457.

Comment
Patients with chronic rotator cuff tendinitis may develop areas of calcification within the substance of the cuff. When the calcification is dense and well profiled, it can be seen on shoulder radiographs. However, it is much easier to see with sonography. In fact, sonography is the most accurate means of identifying, localizing, and quantifying rotator cuff calcification. In some centers, ultrasound guidance is used to aspirate soft areas of calcification. MRI is excellent at detecting most soft tissue abnormalities in the shoulder, but, as elsewhere in the body, it is poor at detecting calcification.

The sonographic appearance of calcific tendinitis is easy to understand. Like other forms of calcium deposition, calcium in the rotator cuff produces an area of increased echogenicity and in most cases an associated acoustic shadow. Extensive spur formation from the greater or lesser tuberosity rarely simulates calcium in the rotator cuff. However, with multiple views, it is usually possible to make this distinction.

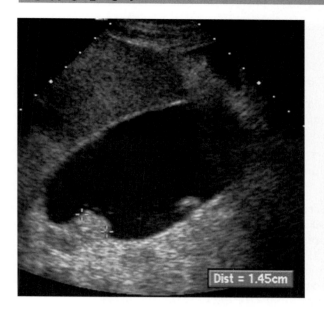
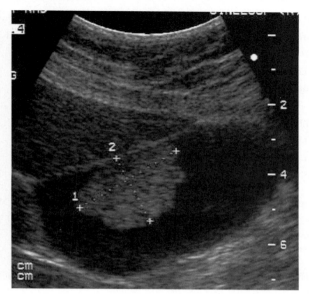

Views of the gallbladder in two patients.

1. What is the differential diagnosis?
2. How does color Doppler assist in the differential diagnosis?
3. What else helps in narrowing the differential diagnosis?
4. What is the treatment of this lesion?

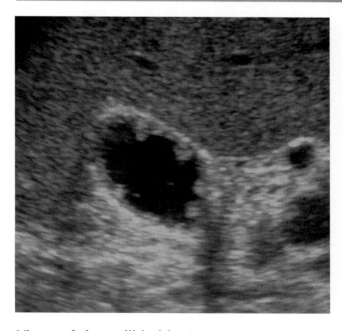
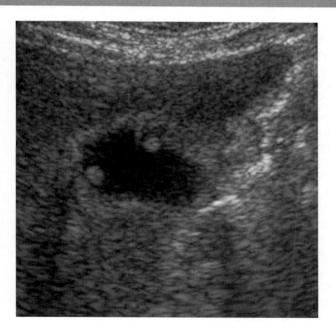

Views of the gallbladder in two patients.

1. Are these lesions typically sessile or pedunculated?
2. Is a cholecystectomy indicated?
3. Are these lesions usually solitary or multiple?
4. Is this abnormality associated with gallstones?

Adenomatous Polyps of the Gallbladder

1. The differential diagnosis includes polyp, tumefactive sludge, clotted blood, cancer.

2. Color Doppler may indicate that the lesion is vascularized and thus exclude the possibility of sludge and clotted blood.

3. Demonstration of mobility excludes the diagnosis of polyp or cancer.

4. Due to the possibility of malignancy, lesions of this size are usually treated with cholecystectomy.

Reference

Middleton WD: The gallbladder. In Goldberg BB (ed): *Diagnostic Ultrasound.* Baltimore, Williams & Wilkins, 1993, pp 116–142.

Cross Reference

Ultrasound: THE REQUISITES, pp 46–48.

Comment

Large polypoid-appearing lesions of the gallbladder may be true polyps or intraluminal material that simulates a polyp, such as tumefactive sludge. Sludge can be distinguished from a true polyp by noting mobility of the lesion. Clotted blood and pus behave like sludge and may simulate polyps but are much less common than sludge.

True gallbladder polyps, regardless of their histology, are all composed of viable soft tissue. Therefore, they all have internal blood flow. With current-generation scanners, it is often possible to detect this blood flow with color or power Doppler. Demonstration of flow eliminates sludge or clotted blood from the differential diagnosis. Inability to detect blood flow with Doppler does not help much with the differential diagnosis because some polyps may not have enough flow for it to be detectable.

Polypoid gallbladder neoplasms can arise from any of the elements of the gallbladder wall. Of the benign tumors, adenomatous polyps predominate, but leiomyomas, lipomas, neuromas, and fibromas have all been reported. Gallbladder cancer may also appear as an intraluminal polyp, but these lesions are very rarely seen when they are less than 1 cm in size. In general, the larger the size of the polyp, the more likely it is to be malignant. Polyps that are 5 mm or less in size can be ignored. Polyps between 5 and 10 mm in size can be followed to ensure stability. It is not clear when the risk of cancer exceeds the risk of cholecystectomy in patients with polyps. However, it is probably reasonable to remove polyps that are larger than 10 mm, unless there are contraindications to surgery. One should realize, however, that an 11-mm polyp is much less likely to be a cancer than is a 30-mm polyp.

Cholesterol Polyps of the Gallbladder

1. Cholesterol polyps are usually pedunculated.

2. These polyps are benign and do not cause symptoms, so a cholecystectomy is not indicated.

3. Polyps are usually multiple. However, it is not uncommon to see only the largest polyp on sonography.

4. There is no association between cholesterol polyps and gallstones.

Reference

Collett JA, Allan RB, Chisholm RJ, et al: Gallbladder polyps: A prospective study. *J Ultrasound Med* 1998;17:207–211.

Cross Reference

Ultrasound: THE REQUISITES, pp 46–48.

Comment

Nonshadowing, nonmobile, intraluminal defects are typical of gallbladder polyps. Small nonshadowing stones that are adherent to the gallbladder wall rarely produce a similar appearance. Tumefactive sludge can also occasionally be confused with a polyp.

The most common type of gallbladder polyp is a cholesterol polyp. These polyps are not true neoplasms but rather enlarged papillary fronds filled with lipid-laden macrophages. Cholesterol polyps represent one form of cholesterolosis of the gallbladder. The more common form is the planar variety, where there are smaller, but more diffuse accumulations of triglycerides, cholesterol precursors, and cholesterol esters in the lamina propria. The planar form of cholesterolosis is also known as the strawberry gallbladder. It is difficult to appreciate the subtle wall abnormality of planar cholesterolosis on sonography.

Cholesterol polyps are usually 5 mm or less in size and are attached to the gallbladder wall by a narrow stalk. They can occur in any portion of the gallbladder wall. Cholesterolosis occurs in equal numbers in men and women. Its etiology is unknown, but it is not associated with elevated levels of lipid in the blood. Likewise, it does not appear to be associated with an increased incidence of cholesterol gallstones.

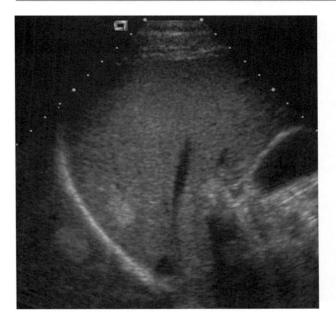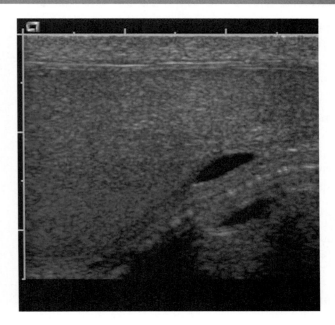

Longitudinal view of the liver and longitudinal view of the testis in different patients.

1. What artifact is demonstrated in the two images shown in this case?
2. What causes this artifact?
3. Where else is this type of artifact commonly seen?
4. Does this artifact produce lesions of similar size and shape?

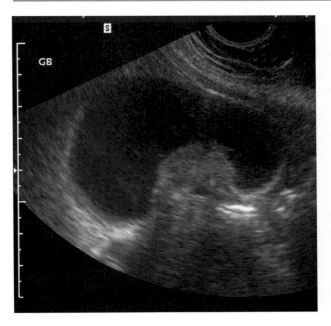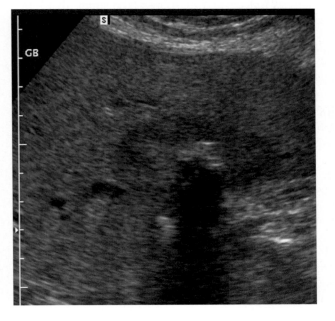

Views of the gallbladder in two patients.

1. Which image is more typical of this condition?
2. Is this abnormality more common in women or in men?
3. What predisposes to this condition?
4. Is this condition more commonly seen in elderly or in young patients?

Mirror Image Artifact

1. These images demonstrate mirror image artifact.

2. Air in the lung base and air around the scrotum acts as an acoustic mirror.

3. This artifact may be seen anywhere there is a large, smooth gas interface.

4. Usually lesions created as mirror images are similar in size and shape to the original lesion. However, if the mirror is curved, the mirror image may have a different size and shape.

Reference

Middleton WD: Ultrasound artifacts. In Siegel MJ, (ed): *Pediatric Sonography,* 2nd ed. New York, Raven Press, 1994, pp 13–28.

Comment

Acoustic mirrors can be compared to optical mirrors. With optical mirrors, a smooth, flat surface that reflects a large amount of light causes a visual duplication of structures. Surfaces that reflect more light (like a sil-vered piece of glass) act as better mirrors than surfaces that reflect less light (like a sheet of metal). Flat surfaces produce a mirror image that is identical in size and shape to the original object, but curved surfaces (like mirrors at the carnival) produce a distorted mirror image.

Since gas reflects almost 100% of the sound that hits it, gas is the best acoustic mirror in the body. This is particularly true where there are large, smooth gas interfaces—such as in the lung. Therefore, mirror images are very common on sonograms that include the interface between lung and adjacent soft tissues.

The base of the right lung serves as a mirror on right upper quadrant scans and produces a number of well-recognized mirror images. Although not always appreciated, the liver itself is duplicated above the diaphragm, and this accounts for the supradiaphragmatic echogenicity seen on right upper quadrant scans. The diaphragm is also commonly duplicated, and this becomes apparent in areas where the diaphragm is thick enough to be resolved sonographically. Focal hepatic lesions that contrast markedly with the normal liver parenchyma are also frequently duplicated above the diaphragm. However, because the diaphragm is curved, the mirror image may not be an exact reproduction of the actual lesion. In addition, the mirror image may arise from a lesion that is not in the plane of the image. This can produce an apparently isolated supradiaphragmatic lesion. The trachea is another structure with a large, smooth gas interface. It is therefore capable of acting as a mirror on scans of the neck.

Gallbladder Cancer

1. The second image, which shows a hypoechoic mass encasing a gallstone and invading the liver, is most typical of gallbladder cancer.

2. Gallbladder cancer is more common in women.

3. Gallstones, chronic wall inflammation, and gallbladder wall calcification predispose to gallbladder cancer.

4. Gallbladder cancer is a disease of the elderly.

Reference

Rooholamini SA, Tehrant NS, Razavi MK, et al: Imaging of gallbladder carcinoma. *Radiographics* 1994; 14:291–306.

Cross-Reference

Ultrasound: THE REQUISITES, pp 45–47.

Comment

Gallbladder cancer is strongly associated with gallstones and is likely related to chronic inflammation caused by the stones. It is usually extensive at the time of diagnosis, so the prognosis is very poor. Metastases are commonly present in regional lymph nodes, and direct invasion of the liver is also common. Spread to the peritoneum and direct invasion of adjacent bowel may also occur. Because of the association with gallstones, gallbladder cancer is more common in women than in men.

The most common sonographic appearance for gallbladder cancer is a large, soft-tissue mass that is centered in the gallbladder fossa. In many cases the mass completely obliterates the gallbladder so that there is no recognizable normal gallbladder. Because of this obliteration, it can be difficult to determine the origin of the mass. In such cases, identification of engulfed gallstones is very helpful because their presence makes it much more likely that the mass arose from the gallbladder.

Gallbladder cancer can also appear as diffuse or focal wall thickening. The wall thickening is usually irregular, eccentric, and solid in appearance. It is very unusual for gallbladder cancer to produce concentric, uniform thickening of the gallbladder wall.

The least common form of gallbladder cancer is a polypoid intraluminal mass. Polypoid cancers are usually much larger than benign gallbladder polyps and are attached to the wall of the gallbladder by a broad base rather than by a narrow stalk.

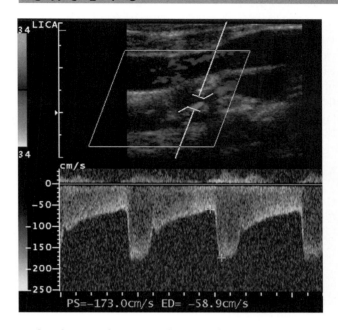 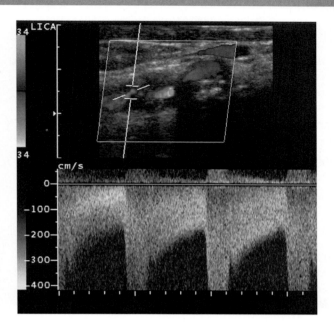

PS=-173.0cm/s ED= -58.9cm/s

Pulsed Doppler waveforms obtained from the internal carotid artery. (See color plates.)

1. What different parameters are used to grade carotid artery stenosis?
2. How severe is the stenosis shown in the figures in this case?
3. Which waveform and corresponding velocity is more indicative of the severity of this stenosis?
4. Can a severe stenosis ever be associated with a normal velocity?

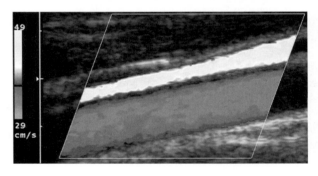 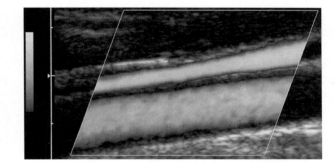

Longitudinal views of the carotid artery and the jugular vein. (See color plates.)

1. What different techniques were used to generate these two images?
2. What is the advantage of the technique shown on the left?
3. What is the advantage of the technique shown on the right?
4. Which technique is capable of determining the maximum flow velocity?

High-Grade Carotid Stenosis

1. Peak systolic velocity, end-diastolic velocity, the ratio of internal carotid artery (ICA) to common carotid artery (CCA) peak systolic velocity, and the ratio of ICA to CCA end-diastolic velocity are used to grade carotid artery stenosis.

2. This is a greater than 80% diameter stenosis.

3. The second waveform, which shows a velocity of greater than 400 cm/s, is more indicative of the high-grade stenosis.

4. A very tight stenosis may rarely be associated with normal velocities if the flow volume has dropped almost to zero.

Reference

Cardoso T, Middleton WD: Duplex sonography and color Doppler of carotid artery disease. *Semin Interv Radiol* 1990;7:1-8.

Cross-Reference

Ultrasound: THE REQUISITES, pp 470-474.

Comment

When an ICA stenosis reaches a value of approximately 50% diameter narrowing, velocities increase. The narrowing can be estimated based on the velocity. The easiest parameter to use is the peak systolic velocity. The end-diastolic velocity is also useful. Both are obtained at the site of the stenosis or in the region of the flow jet just slightly beyond the stenosis. As in this case, when the stenosis is long, the peak velocity may be isolated to a very small segment of the vessel, and it may not be detected with color Doppler. This can result in imprecise placement of the sample volume and velocities that are normal or only minimally elevated. Without careful sampling all along the course of the stenosis, the peak velocity may be missed.

A theoretical limitation of isolated velocity parameters occurs when base line velocities are higher or lower than normal. Low base line velocities may occur in the setting of decreased cardiac output, or if there is a second stenosis in the more proximal vessel or in the aortic valve. In such a situation, even if the velocity at the stenosis is increased compared with the base line values, the velocity may still underestimate the stenosis. High base line velocities may occur in the setting of a contralateral internal or common carotid artery occlusion when all of the flow to the head is through a single carotid artery. In such a case the velocity may overestimate the degree of stenosis.

To account for differences in base line velocity, one can compare the ICA velocity at the stenotic site to the velocity in a normal segment of the ipsilateral CCA. Doing this establishes the CCA velocity as a base line for each individual patient. Unfortunately, any velocity measurement has a moderate amount of variability, and when two measurements are combined in a ratio, the variability is multiplied. In addition, the CCA velocity varies along the length of the vessel, resulting in a range of ICA to CCA ratios for an individual patient. Therefore, despite the theoretical advantages, there is usually little additional accuracy gained by using the ICA to CCA ratio.

Comparison of Color Doppler with Power Doppler

1. The first image is color Doppler, and the second image is power Doppler.

2. The advantage of color Doppler is its capability to determine flow direction and its relative lack of sensitivity to tissue and transducer motion.

3. The advantage of power Doppler is its increased sensitivity to slow flow and decreased dependance on the Doppler angle.

4. Neither can determine maximum flow velocity. Pulsed Doppler waveforms are required to do this.

Reference

Desser TS, Jedrzejewicz T, Haller MI: Color and power Doppler sonography: Techniques, clinical applications, and trade-offs for image optimization. *Ultrasound Q* 1998;14(3):128-149.

Cross-Reference

Ultrasound: THE REQUISITES, pp 464-470.

Comment

Power Doppler encodes the returning Doppler signal based on the power of the signal rather than on the frequency shift. This is advantageous because there is less noise contained in the power information and therefore a better signal-to-noise ratio. This allows for higher gain settings without superimposed noise. Thus, power Doppler is somewhat more sensitive to low-velocity blood flow than is color Doppler. In addition, power Doppler is less dependent on the Doppler angle and is therefore slightly better at detecting flow when the vessel is close to perpendicular to the direction of the Doppler sound pulse.

The disadvantage of power Doppler is that it is very sensitive to tissue motion and therefore is prone to artifacts. In addition, power Doppler gives no directional information nor velocity information. Although power Doppler was initially met with great enthusiasm, with most modern equipment, its advantages are usually outweighed by its disadvantages.

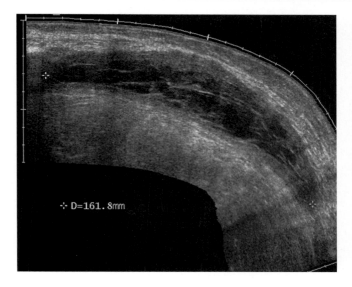

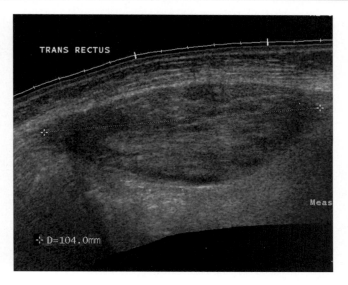

Transverse views of the abdominal wall in two patients.

1. Where is this lesion located?
2. Why do the two lesions appear different?
3. What is the most common cause for this abnormality?
4. Do these lesions cross the midline?

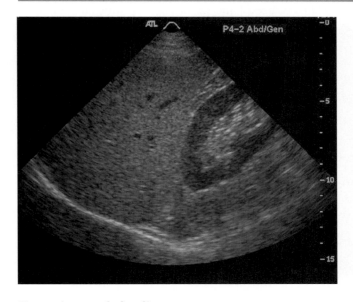

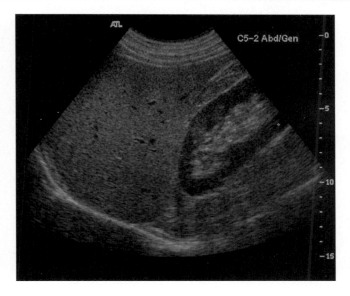

Two views of the liver.

1. What type of transducer was used to scan the liver in the first image?
2. What type of transducer was used to scan the liver in the second image?
3. What is the advantage of the first transducer?
4. What is the advantage of the second transducer?

Rectus Sheath Hematoma

1. The lenticular configuration suggests that this lesion is in the rectus muscle or sheath.

2. They appear different because the hematomas are of different ages. The more solid-appearing hematoma is more acute, and the more complex but liquefied hematoma is older.

3. Most rectus sheath hematomas are due to anticoagulation or to severe contraction of the rectus muscles from coughing, sneezing, defecation, and other activities.

4. When they extend below the arcuate line (located between the umbilicus and the pubis), they can cross the midline.

Reference

Fakuda T, Sakamoto I, Kohzaki S, et al: Spontaneous rectus sheath hematomas: Clinical and radiologic features. *Abdom Imaging* 1996;21:58–61.

Comment

In addition to anticoagulation, rectus sheath hematomas can also be caused by blunt or penetrating trauma or severe rectus muscle contraction. The hemorrhage can be either in the muscle itself or within the rectus sheath, but it is usually limited to one side by the linea alba. When large, rectus sheath hematomas may dissect inferior to the arcuate line, cross the midline, extend into the prevesicle space, and put significant mass effect on the bladder.

The sonographic appearance of a rectus sheath hematoma depends on when it is imaged. Like other hematomas, rectus hematomas are echogenic and solid-appearing in the acute phase. This is due to clotted blood in the hematoma. Over a matter of days, the clot begins to lyse, and the hematoma becomes complex, with cystic and solid components. With more time, the hematoma becomes progressively liquefactive and appears as a simple fluid collection. In some cases, a fluid level can be seen owing to a hematocrit effect.

Occasionally it can be difficult to tell whether a lesion is in the abdominal wall or within the peritoneal cavity. One maneuver that can help is to ask the patient to take deep breaths and observe the movement of the intraperitoneal contents (bowel and fat). Usually this localizes the depth of the parietal peritoneum and helps to determine whether the lesion is truly superficial to this level.

Comparison of Phased Array and Curved Array Transducers

1. The first image was obtained with a phased array transducer that has a frequency range of 4 to 2 MHz.

2. The second image was obtained with a curved array transducer that has a frequency range of 5 to 2 MHz.

3. Phased array transducers provide a large field of view of deeper structures. They are also small and can be easily used to scan between ribs and in other areas where acoustic access is limited.

4. Curved array transducers generally provide better resolution than phased array transducers, especially in the near field.

Reference

Kremkau FW: Multiple element transducers. *Radiographics* 1993;13:1163–1176.

Comment

Because of their ease of use, speed, and flexibility, most manufacturers have concentrated on multielement electronic array transducers and have abandoned mechanically driven transducers. The electronic probes consist of multiple small crystal elements arranged in an array at the surface of the probe. By adjusting the timing of activation of the different elements, an ultrasound pulse can be created that is steered in various directions and is focused at various depths. By changing the geometry of the probe, different advantages can be obtained.

Phased array transducers have a small, flat head and create a sound pulse from a composite of multiple pulses generated by all of the elements in the array. Curved array transducers have a broad, curved head and activate only a limited number of adjacent crystal elements to create a sound pulse. Phased arrays steer the beam electronically by adjusting the timing of activation of the different elements. Curved arrays steer the beam based on the shape of the probe. Most manufacturers identify a probe based on its type, frequency, and sometimes size. In the images shown in this case, the phased array is a P4-2. The curved array is a C5-2. Phased arrays can also be identified because the sector-shaped image comes to a pointed apex, whereas the image of a curved array has a curved apex that corresponds to the shape of the probe.

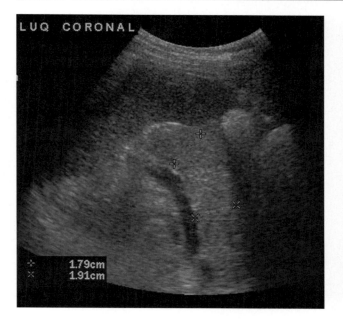
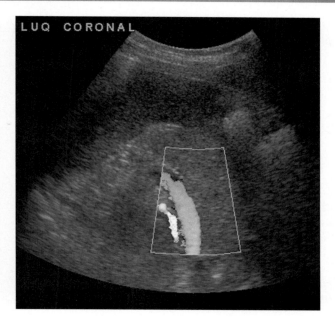

Longitudinal/coronal view of the left upper quadrant and pulsed Doppler waveform. (See color plates.)

1. What is the normal structure indicated by the cursors?
2. What is the normal relationship between this structure and the spleen?
3. What is the relationship of this structure and the splenic vein?
4. What is the relationship of this structure and the left kidney?

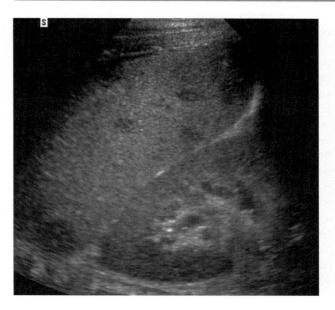
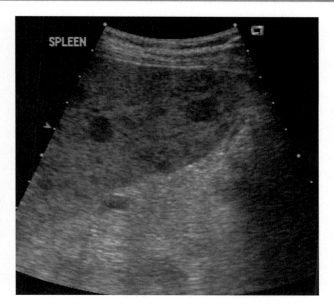

Views of the left upper quadrant in two patients.

1. Describe the abnormality.
2. What is the differential diagnosis?
3. Could these lesions be biopsied percutaneously with ultrasound guidance?
4. Would other imaging tests help in the workup of these patients?

Normal Relationship of Pancreatic Tail and Spleen

1. The cursors are placed on the tail of the pancreas.

2. The tail of the pancreas extends from the body of the pancreas toward the splenic hilum.

3. The pancreatic tail is positioned below the splenic vein as the splenic vein exits the splenic hilum.

4. The pancreatic tail is usually immediately anterior to the upper pole of the left kidney.

Reference

Paivansalo M, Suramo I: Ultrasonography of the pancreatic tail through the spleen and through the fluid-filled stomach. *Eur J Radiol* 1986;6:113–115.

Cross-Reference

Ultrasound: THE REQUISITES, pp 124–125.

Comment

Visualization of the pancreatic tail is a challenge with sonography. The challenge arises from its location high and deep in the left upper quadrant. When the standard anterior approach is used, shadowing from the gas-filled stomach and from the splenic flexure of the colon frequently obscures much, if not all, of the tail. Filling the stomach with fluid can displace the colon out of the left upper quadrant and can provide a suitable window for visualization of the pancreatic tail. However, results with this technique are variable, and in some patients visualization is actually diminished.

An alternative technique is to scan from a superior left lateral approach using the spleen as a window. The tail of the pancreas extends to the splenic hilum and is usually located immediately anterior to the upper pole of the kidney. To find it, start with a coronal, trans-splenic view of the left renal upper pole. The transducer should then be angled anteriorly until the kidney is no longer in view. The pancreas then appears as a band of tissue usually oriented directly at the transducer. In the splenic hilum, the splenic vein is located superior to the pancreatic tail and can thus serve as another landmark for identifying the tail. Even in situations where the tail of the pancreas cannot be seen as a discrete structure, the trans-splenic view often allows visualization of abnormalities related to the pancreatic tail, such as pseudocysts and tumors, that could not be seen from an anterior approach.

Focal Splenic Lesions

1. Both images show multifocal, solid, hypoechoic splenic lesions.

2. The differential diagnosis primarily includes metastasis, lymphoma, sarcoidosis, and abscess. Infarcts can also produce an appearance similar to this.

3. In general, it is preferable to avoid the spleen because it is very vascular. In most patients, other sites exist that can be biopsied with less risk of bleeding. However, when necessary, splenic lesions can be biopsied with ultrasound guidance. With the use of fine-needle aspiration (22- to 25-gauge needles) and cytologic analysis, the risk is very low.

4. CT could help to define a primary tumor or lymphadenopathy elsewhere in the chest or abdomen. With contrast enhancement, it might help to further characterize the splenic lesions.

Reference

Goerg C, Schwerk WB, Goerg K: Sonography of focal lesions in the spleen. *AJR Am J Roentgenol* 1991; 156:949–953.

Cross-Reference

Ultrasound: THE REQUISITES, pp 144–145.

Comment

The sonographic appearance of these splenic lesions indicates that they are not simple cysts, but it is otherwise relatively nonspecific. In situations such as this, it is very important to survey the rest of the abdomen for clues to the correct diagnosis. In some situations, either a primary abdominal tumor or adenopathy may be seen. If the adenopathy is extensive, then lymphoma and metastatic disease are the most likely possibilities. The first patient had extensive adenopathy, and subsequent biopsies showed lymphoma. If minimal adenopathy is seen, sarcoidosis should also be considered. If a primary tumor is identified elsewhere in the abdomen, then metastatic disease almost certainly explains the splenic lesions. In addition, clinical history will usually point in one direction or the other. The second patient had a history of lung cancer, and the splenic lesions were metastases. With the proper clinical history, splenic abscesses and infarcts should also be considered. If no other abnormalities are seen sonographically and the clinical history is not helpful, then CT should be considered for further evaluation.

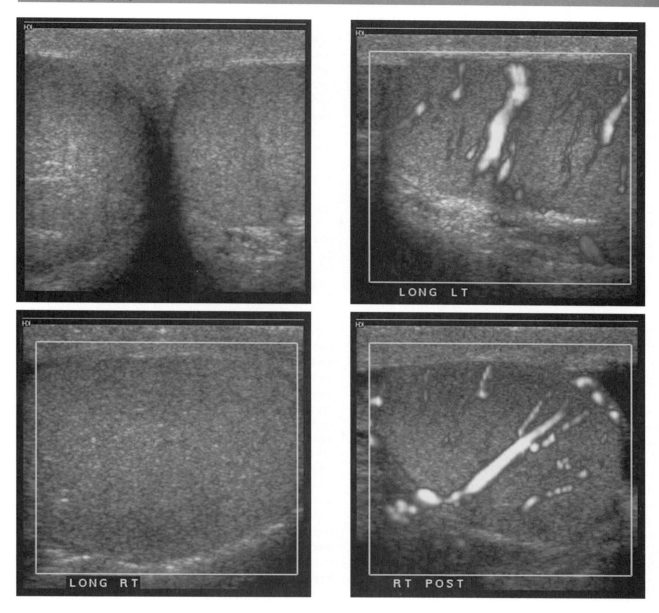

Images of the scrotum in a patient with right scrotal pain. The two images of the right testis shown here were taken approximately 3 minutes apart. (See color plates.)

1. Describe the abnormalities.

2. What congenital anomaly is this patient likely to have?

3. Is it likely that this patient has been symptomatic for less than 24 hours?

4. Explain the difference in appearance of the right testis in the lower left image compared with the lower right image.

Testicular Torsion

1. The grey-scale view shows testes that are symmetric in echogenicity and normal in appearance. The power Doppler view of the left testis shows normal distribution of flow in multiple intratesticular vessels. The first power Doppler view of the right testis shows no detectable blood flow. The second power Doppler view shows normal intratesticular flow. The first three views are typical of acute right testicular torsion. The lower right image was taken after manual detorsion.

2. The congenital anomaly that predisposes to testicular torsion is a "bell clapper" deformity.

3. The grey-scale appearance of the right testis is normal. This is very good evidence that the testis is still viable. Therefore, it is very likely that the patient has been symptomatic for less than 24 hours.

4. The patient was manually detorsed between the first and second power Doppler views of the right testis. The repeat view of the testis confirmed the success of the maneuver.

References

Cannon ML, Finger MJ, Bulas DI: Case Report: Manual testicular detorsion aided by color Doppler ultrasonography. *J Ultrasound Med* 1995;14:407–409.

Middleton WD, Siegel BA, Melson GL, et al: Prospective comparison of color Doppler ultrasonography and testicular scintigraphy in the evaluation of the acute scrotum. *Radiology* 1990;177:177–181.

Middleton WD, Middleton MA, Dierks M, et al: Sonographic prediction of viability in testicular torsion. *J Ultrasound Med* 1997;16:23–27.

Cross-Reference

Ultrasound: THE REQUISITES, pp 443–446.

Comment

Normally, the testis is anchored to the wall of the scrotum by a broad posterior attachment. This prevents the testis from significant degrees of rotation. The "bell clapper" deformity is a congenital anomaly in which this normal attachment is absent, so that the testis is suspended in the scrotal sac via its vascular pedicle, like a clapper in a bell. Patients with a bell clapper deformity are at significantly increased risk for torsion. It is believed that forceful contraction of the cremasteric muscles results in elevation and rotation of the testis and can be the precipitating event in testicular torsion.

Testicular torsion is a condition that most often affects boys in the peripubertal period or men during the young adult years. Patients often have previous episodes of torsion that spontaneously detorse before they arrive at their doctor's office or the emergency room with an episode of persistent torsion. Typical symptoms include pain and swelling of the scrotum. The pain may radiate into the groin and lower abdomen and is often associated with nausea and vomiting. On physical examination there is often marked tenderness, and the testis may be oriented in a transverse lie.

With prompt diagnosis and surgical detorsion, there is a good chance that the testis can be salvaged. In fact, if treated within 6 hours of onset, the majority of testes will maintain their viability. If surgery is delayed beyond 24 hours, ischemia causes permanent necrosis of the testis in the large majority of cases. Between 6 and 24 hours after onset, the chance of testicular salvage progressively diminishes.

The diagnosis of torsion is quite difficult to make based on grey-scale imaging alone. In some patients, the twisted cord can be seen as a heterogeneous mass superior to the testis. This is called the torsion knot. Unfortunately, it is possible to confuse the torsion knot with an enlarged epididymal head. In the early stages of torsion, the grey-scale appearance of the testis is normal. In fact, in the setting of torsion, it is possible to predict that the testis is still viable if it has a normal homogeneous echogenicity on grey-scale. On the other hand, if the testis appears heterogeneous or hypoechoic on grey-scale, then it is almost certainly nonviable. In addition to the changes in the testis, torsion also is frequently associated with a small reactive hydrocele and thickening of the scrotal skin.

The sonographic diagnosis of testicular torsion depends on detecting absent or, in some cases, diminished blood flow to the affected testis with color Doppler. It is important not to mistake color noise with true intratesticular blood flow. Color noise appears as very small, randomly positioned spots of red and blue color assignment that have no pulsed Doppler signal. True vessels appear as larger, better-formed areas of color assignment that can usually be elongated by various degrees of transducer rotation. In addition, true vessels should have a detectable pulsed Doppler signal. With prolonged torsion, an inflammatory reaction develops in the scrotal wall, and hyperemia can be detected in the tissues around the testis.

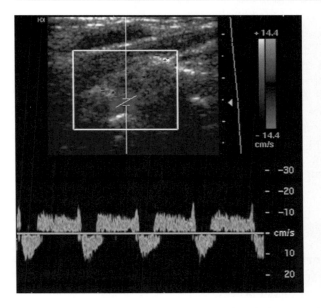
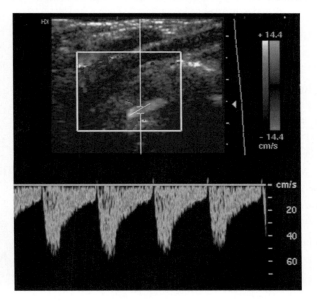

Pulsed Doppler waveforms of the left vertebral artery. Please note that both waveforms are inverted, with negative frequency shifts displayed above the base line.

1. What is the cause of this abnormality?

2. What was done to cause the difference in the two waveforms?

3. Is color Doppler alone adequate to make the diagnosis?

4. Is this abnormality more common on the right or on the left?

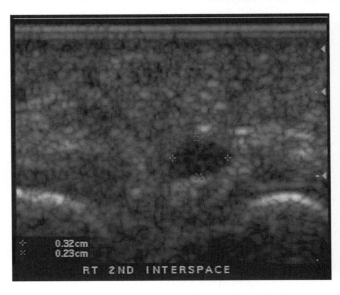
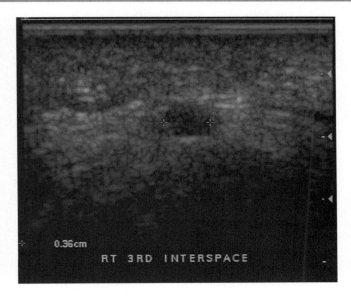

Transverse views of the second and third web space of the toes.

1. From what anatomic structure do these lesions arise?

2. What is the most common location of these lesions?

3. Are these lesions more common in men or in women?

4. Are they benign or malignant?

Subclavian Steal

1. This abnormality is caused by stenosis of the subclavian artery prior to the origin of the vertebral artery.

2. The first waveform was obtained at rest when there was a partial steal and retrograde flow only during peak systole. The second image was obtained after left arm exercise when there was complete steal and retrograde flow throughout the cardiac cycle.

3. A vertebral vein can be confused with an artery on color Doppler. Pulsed Doppler waveforms are needed to show that flow is arterial and not venous.

4. Subclavian steal is more common on the left.

Reference

Kliewer MA, Hertzberg BS, Kim DH, et al: Vertebral artery Doppler waveform changes indicating subclavian steal physiology. *AJR Am J Roentgenol* 2000;174:815–819.

Cross-Reference

Ultrasound: THE REQUISITES, pp 477–478.

Comment

The left subclavian artery arises in the superior mediastinum and is difficult to visualize with ultrasound. Therefore, abnormalities at its origin are typically diagnosed based on secondary criteria. Since the left vertebral artery arises from the left subclavian artery, the vertebral artery can potentially provide collateral flow to the arm when the subclavian artery is stenosed or occluded at its origin. When this occurs, flow in the left vertebral artery is at least partially directed toward the subclavian artery in a retrograde direction. Since the retrograde flow is being stolen from the internal carotid arteries and the right vertebral artery by crossover at the circle of Willis and the basilar artery, this is referred to as the subclavian steal phenomenon.

In most instances, the diagnosis is readily made by noting that flow in the left vertebral artery is going down toward the arm instead of up toward the head. When the subclavian artery is totally occluded, it makes sense that there is no way to establish effective antegrade vertebral flow, so all the flow that is seen in the vertebral artery is retrograde. In actuality, elastic recoil of the upper extremity arteries may result in some backflow from the arm and into the vertebral artery. This may be detected as a short phase of minimal antegrade diastolic vertebral flow despite the presence of complete subclavian artery occlusion.

When the subclavian artery is patent but stenosed, it is possible to have significant components of antegrade

flow in the vertebral artery. Since the arm is a high-resistance vascular bed, diastolic flow to the arm is ordinarily limited. Therefore, diastolic flow may proceed up the vertebral artery in an antegrade fashion, while systolic flow in the vertebral is reversed and supplying the arm. With less amounts of steal, antegrade systolic flow in the vertebral artery may be only partially affected. This can produce a dip in the systolic peak without resulting in actual flow reversal. Exercising the arm accentuates changes in the vertebral artery waveform and makes the diagnosis more certain.

Morton's Neuroma

1. Morton's neuromas arise from the plantar branch of the digital nerves.

2. They are most often located in the second and third web spaces of the foot at the level of the metacarpal heads.

3. They are more common in women.

4. They are benign.

Reference

Quinn TJ, Jacobson JA, Craig JG, van Holsbeeck MT: Sonography of Morton's neuromas. *AJR Am J Roentgenol* 2000;174:1723–1728.

Cross-Reference

Musculoskeletal Radiology: THE REQUISITES, p 455.

Comment

Morton's neuromas are benign masses of the plantar digital nerves of the foot. They are composed of perineural fibrosis and are likely due to repetitive trauma. The strong female predominance (80% occur in women) suggests a relationship with high-heeled shoes. The common symptoms are pain and paresthesias with walking and marked tenderness to direct palpation.

The interdigital nerves course in the space between the metatarsal heads. Under normal conditions, they are too small to be seen sonographically. Neuromas, on the other hand, can be seen with a reported sensitivity of approximately 95%. They appear as hypoechoic masses located in the interspaces of the toes, usually at or just proximal to the metatarsal heads. They may be associated with slight increased through transmission and occasionally are seen connecting to a swollen digital nerve. They occur most commonly in the third interspace and next most commonly in the second interspace. They may be multiple in approximately 25% of patients and bilateral in approximately 10% of patients.

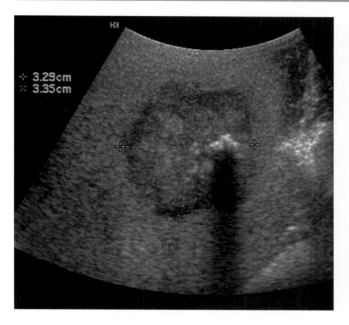 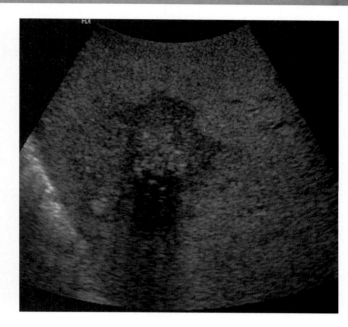

Views of the liver in two patients.

1. What are potential causes of shadowing in the liver?
2. Is the shadowing in the first case clean or dirty?
3. A liver tumor with calcification is most likely to be what?
4. Are calcifications frequently seen in focal nodular hyperplasia (FNH)?

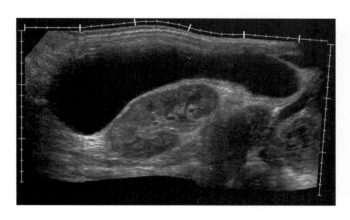 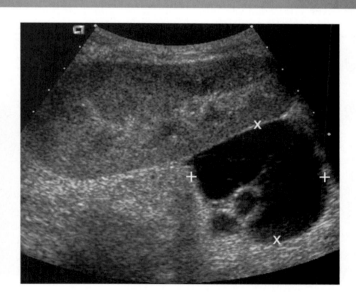

Views of renal transplants in two patients.

1. What is the abnormal finding?
2. What is the differential diagnosis?
3. How good is ultrasound at diagnosing transplant rejection?
4. Where do posttransplant urinomas usually occur?

Partially Calcified Liver Metastases

1. Shadowing in the liver is most often due to calcification, air, stones, and fat-containing lesions.

2. The shadowing in the first image is clean. This makes air an unlikely cause.

3. Metastases are the most common cause of a calcified liver tumor.

4. Focal nodular hyperplasia only rarely has calcification.

Reference

Stoupis C, Taylor HM, Paley MR, et al: The rocky liver: Radiologic-pathologic correlation of calcified hepatic masses. *Radiographics* 1998;18:675–685.

Cross Reference

Ultrasound: THE REQUISITES, pp 7–9.

Comment

Hepatic calcifications typically occur in inflammatory and neoplastic lesions. Inflammatory causes include granulomatous diseases, such as histoplasmosis and tuberculosis (small punctate calcifications) and echinococcus (peripheral curvilinear calcifications), or healed pyogenic or amebic abscesses (coarse calcification).

The most common cause of a calcified liver tumor is metastatic disease. Almost any metastatic tumor can potentially calcify, particularly during treatment. However, colorectal carcinoma is the most common primary to produce calcified liver metastases. Others that are also common are ovarian carcinoma, gastric carcinoma, and renal cell carcinoma. It is very uncommon for hemangioma, hepatocellular carcinoma, adenoma, or focal nodular hyperplasia to contain calcification. Fibrolamellar hepatocellular carcinoma more commonly contains calcification in the central scar.

On sonography, calcification is hyperechoic and is usually associated with shadowing. Gas is also hyperechoic and usually associated with shadowing. Typically, the shadow seen with gas contains medium- or low-level echoes and has fuzzy borders. This is referred to as dirty shadowing. The shadow associated with calcium contains fewer echoes and has sharper borders and is referred to as clean shadowing. Overlap exists between shadowing from calcification and from gas, and it is not always possible to distinguish between the two sonographically. When in doubt, radiographs or CT can help.

Fat attenuates sound more than normal liver parenchyma and can occasionally produce faint shadowing. This is sometimes seen in fat-containing tumors or in focal fatty infiltration.

Renal Transplant Lymphocele

1. Both images show a fluid collection adjacent to the renal transplant.

2. The differential diagnosis includes lymphocele, hematoma, seroma, urinoma, and abscess.

3. Like all other imaging tests, ultrasound is not good enough at diagnosing rejection to guide patient management. That is why biopsies are still necessary.

4. The leak usually occurs at the anastomosis of the ureter to the bladder. Therefore, the fluid collection usually is between the lower pole of the transplant and the bladder.

Reference

Brown ED, Chen MYM, Wolfman NT, et al: Complications of renal transplantation: Evaluation with US and radionuclide imaging. *Radiographics* 2000;20:607–622.

Cross-Reference

Ultrasound: THE REQUISITES, pp 116–118.

Comment

Peritransplant fluid collections are common following renal transplantation. In the immediate posttransplant period, hematomas are very common. They typically appear as complex collections adjacent to the transplant. Lymphoceles usually occur 1 to 2 months following transplant and are present in up to 15% of patients. They occur because of disruption of the renal lymphatics. Both hematomas and lymphoceles are usually asymptomatic. They may produce symptoms when they become large enough to compress the ureter or the renal parenchyma. The latter problem is particularly an issue with subcapsular hematomas. Urinomas are much less common and usually occur at the ureterovesicle anastomosis. They can also occur at other sites of the collecting system owing to ischemia. Abscesses can be a primary abnormality, or they can occur due to infection of another preexisting fluid collection.

The sonographic appearances of these various fluid collections overlap, so that it is usually necessary to rely on the clinical history, laboratory studies, and other imaging tests, such as radionuclide renography, to distinguish one from the other. In many instances, ultrasound guided aspiration is required to make a final diagnosis.

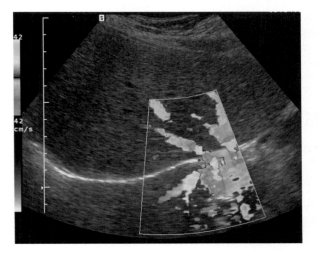
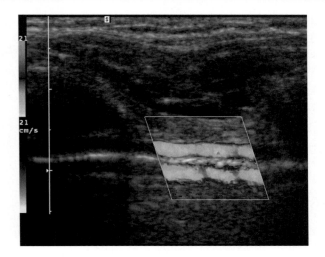

Transverse color Doppler view of the hepatic veins and longitudinal view of the internal mammary artery. (See color plates.)

1. What is unusual about both of these images?
2. Is this artifact more common on grey-scale images or on color Doppler images?
3. Where else is this type of Doppler artifact commonly seen?
4. How can pulsed Doppler help in confirming this artifact?

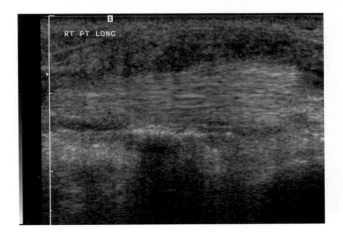
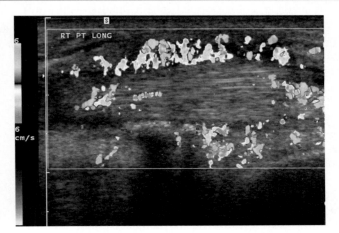

Longitudinal grey-scale image and color Doppler image of the posterior tibial tendon. (See color plates.)

1. What are the abnormal findings?
2. What is the most common cause of this condition?
3. Does the tendon appear intact?
4. Would you expect to see fluid in the tendon sheath?

Doppler Mirror Image Artifact

1. The first image shows what appears to be a vessel above the diaphragm, and the second shows a vessel deep to the internal mammary artery.

2. Mirror image artifacts are more common on color Doppler scans than on grey-scale scans.

3. Doppler mirror images can be seen anywhere that vessels course over the surface of the lung or other smooth gas interfaces. They are also seen deep to the common carotid artery and next to large, smooth, strong reflectors such as bone.

4. Pulsed Doppler can help by confirming that the signal arising from the artifact is similar to the signal in the real vessel.

Reference

Middleton WD: Ultrasound artifacts. In Siegel MJ (ed): *Pediatric Sonography,* 2nd ed. New York, Raven Press, 1994.

Comment

Because color Doppler creates images with marked contrast between vascular structures and soft tissues (i.e., color vs. grey scale), mirror image artifacts are particularly common on color Doppler scans. As with grey-scale imaging, color Doppler mirror images occur most frequently around the lung. However, the increased contrast also allows weaker acoustic interfaces to act as mirrors for color Doppler. For instance, bone can reflect enough sound to produce color Doppler mirror images. In fact, the back wall of the normal common carotid artery can act as a mirror and produce artifactual Doppler signals deep to these vessels. The artifactual arterial signal deep to the common carotid artery is referred to as the carotid ghost, and it can be detected on both color Doppler images and pulsed Doppler waveforms.

In some cases the etiology of the artifactual Doppler signal can be quite confusing. One helpful technique is to compare the Doppler waveform of the true vessel with the waveform of the mirror image. Since the artifactual signal is generated by blood flow in the real vessel (but is simply inappropriately localized), it should have the same size and shape as the signal from the true vessel. On the other hand, the intensity of the waveforms may differ. The Doppler signal from the true vessel arises from the strong, original sound pulse and appears as a strong signal. The artifactual signal arises from a sound pulse after it has reflected off the mirror. If 100% of the sound is reflected (as with a gas interface), then the mirror image signal will be almost as strong as the original signal. If some of the sound is transmitted through the mirror and only a portion of it is reflected, then the mirror image signal will be much weaker than the original signal. To decrease mirror image artifacts both on grey-scale and Doppler images, the power output and gain settings should be decreased. This produces a sound pulse that is too weak to reflect off the mirror and travel back to the transducer.

C A S E 8 5

Tenosynovitis

1. The images show thickening and increased vascularity of the tendon sheath around the tendon.

2. Tenosynovitis has many causes, but the most common is repetitive microtrauma from overuse.

3. The fibers of the tendon are well seen, and there are no defects identified. There is no evidence of tendon tear.

4. Usually tenosynovitis is associated with a tendon sheath effusion. Other images from this patient did show an effusion.

Reference

Martinoli C, Bianchi S, Derchi LE: Tendon and nerve sonography. *Radiol Clin North Am* 1999;37:691–711.

Cross-Reference

Ultrasound: THE REQUISITES, pp 455–456.

Comment

Sonography is particularly useful in evaluating disorders of the tendons. Tenosynovitis refers to inflammation of the tendon sheath and can be due to multiple etiologies. These include primary inflammatory processes (rheumatoid arthritis and other synovial-based arthritides), infection (either from penetrating trauma or blood borne), crystal-induced (gout), trauma (usually repetitive microtrauma), amyloidosis (chronic hemodialysis), or foreign bodies. Complications include tendon involvement and rupture, cellulitis, compressive neuropathies, abscess formation, and osteomyelitis.

Tenosynovitis can be diagnosed sonographically when there is fluid distending the tendon sheath and/or thickening of the tendon sheath. The fluid is usually anechoic, although complicated tenosynovitis (infectious or hemorrhagic) may have fluid with low-level echoes. Tendon sheath thickening may be diffuse and smooth or eccentric and nodular. With active inflammation, there is usually a detectable hypervascularity on color and power Doppler. In most cases, it is possible to determine the cause of the tenosynovitis based on the clinical history and associated laboratory findings. When necessary, ultrasound guided aspiration and biopsy can also be performed to establish the diagnosis.

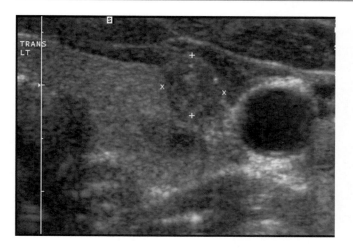 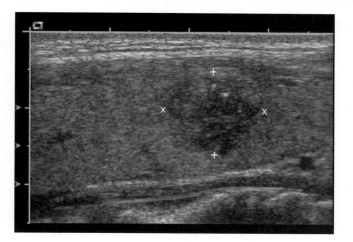

Transverse and longitudinal views of the thyroid in two patients.

1. What is the most important finding in the images shown here?
2. What is the echogenicity of most thyroid cancers?
3. What is the echogenicity of most benign thyroid lesions?
4. How often is thyroid cancer multifocal?

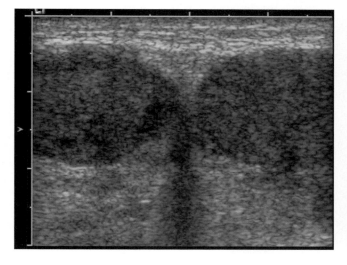 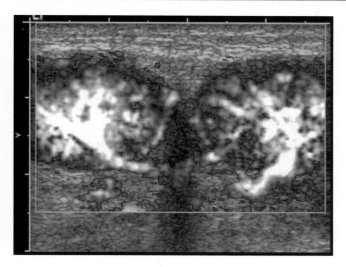

Transverse grey-scale and power Doppler views of the groin.

1. What is the most likely etiology for the lesion shown in this case?
2. Can ultrasound distinguish between a solid lesion and a complex cystic lesion?
3. Could this be due to a neoplastic process?
4. Could this be due to an inflammatory process?

Papillary Thyroid Cancer

1. Microcalcifications in a focal, solid, hypoechoic nodule are the most important finding here.

2. Most cancers are hypoechoic.

3. Echogenicity of benign nodules is variable.

4. Papillary cancer is multifocal in 20% of cases.

Reference

Ahuja AT, Metreweli C: Ultrasound of thyroid nodules. *Ultrasound Q* 2000;16:111-121.

Cross-Reference

Ultrasound: THE REQUISITES, pp 448-452.

Comment

Papillary cancer is the most common thyroid malignancy. It tends to occur in younger patients and is more common in women. As seen in this case, psammoma bodies (microcalcifications) are common. The prognosis is excellent, even when there are local lymph node metastases in the neck. Patients typically present with a painless palpable mass in the thyroid. It is not uncommon for these patients to present with palpable lymph node metastases and a nonpalpable tumor in the thyroid. Mortality at 20 years is approximately 5%. Papillary cancer often contains some follicular elements and is then referred to as mixed papillary/follicular or follicular variant. Mixed cancers behave like pure papillary cancers.

Follicular cancers account for approximately 10% of all thyroid malignancies. They may be minimally invasive or widely invasive. They metastasize via the hematogenous route rather than via the lymphatics. Common sites of metastases are lung, bone, liver, and brain. Mortality at 20 to 30 years is approximately 25%.

Medullary cancer accounts for 5% of thyroid cancers. These cancers arise from the parafollicular cells and frequently secrete calcitonin. Approximately 20% of these tumors are seen in patients with multiple endocrine neoplasia, type II (MEN-II) syndrome. The prognosis is slightly worse than for follicular cancer.

Thyroid lymphoma represents less than 5% of thyroid malignancies and can occur as either a manifestation of generalized lymphoma or as a primary abnormality. It is usually of the non-Hodgkin's variety. Women are affected more than men, and it tends to occur in the elderly. It generally manifests as a rapidly growing mass. On sonography, it is usually a large, hypoechoic mass that infiltrates much, if not all, of the thyroid.

Anaplastic cancer is the least common of the thyroid cancers. It occurs primarily in elderly patients. It is an extremely aggressive tumor, with a 5-year survival of only 5%. These tumors are locally invasive of the adjacent muscles, vessels, and nerves and are often not resectable at the time of diagnosis.

Distinguishing benign from malignant thyroid nodules is not possible with sonography. However, certain appearances should raise the suspicion for a malignancy. The most troublesome finding is microcalcifications. These typically appear as tiny, nonshadowing reflectors within the nodule. They are most often associated with papillary cancer but can also be seen with medullary cancer. Nodules that are entirely solid and hypoechoic are also more worrisome for cancer. If enlarged lymph nodes are seen in the neck, especially if they contain microcalcifications or areas of cystic degeneration, the chance of malignancy increases greatly.

Inguinal Adenopathy

1. Adenopathy.

2. There can be overlap in the grey-scale appearance of solid and complex cystic lesions. However, the vascularity shown on power Doppler would not be seen in a cystic lesion.

3. This could represent malignant lymphadenopathy.

4. This could also represent reactive lymphadenopathy.

Reference

Bruneton JN, Rubaltelli L, Solbiati L: Lymph nodes. In Solbiati L, Rizzatto G (eds): *Ultrasound of Superficial Structures.* Edinburgh, Churchill Livingstone, 1995, pp 279-302.

Comment

The differential diagnosis of a mass in the groin includes primarily hernia, enlarged lymph nodes, abscess, hematoma, and pseudoaneurysms. In most patients, the clinical history will point you in the right direction.

The images supplied show two adjacent hypoechoic masses with relatively intense hypervascularity. The vessels fan out into the periphery of the mass from a single site along the deep aspect of the mass. This pattern is typical of a lymph node. Inflammatory conditions with reactive lymphadenopathy can produce this degree of hypervascularity with a normal branching pattern, and, if the history were appropriate, that would be a consideration in this case. Neoplastic adenopathy can also produce hypervascularity. In metastatic disease, the normal vascular branching pattern is often disturbed and chaotic-appearing, and vessels are often predominantly peripheral. In lymphoma, the normal pattern is typically maintained. The diagnosis in this case was lymphoma, emphasizing that active lymphoma can be very vascular.

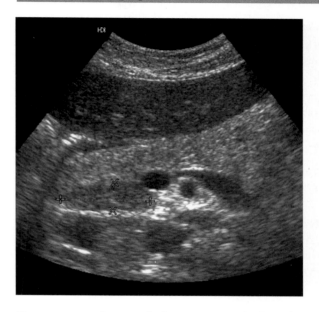
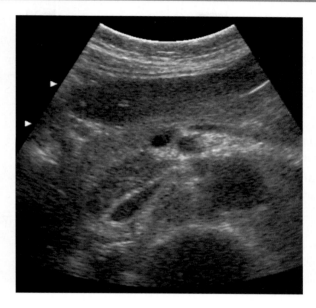

Transverse views of the pancreatic head in two patients.

1. What are the most common causes for focal areas of decreased pancreatic echogenicity?
2. What is the histologic explanation for this finding?
3. How can this condition be distinguished from the other possibilities?
4. How often is this seen?

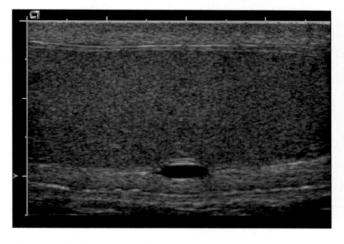
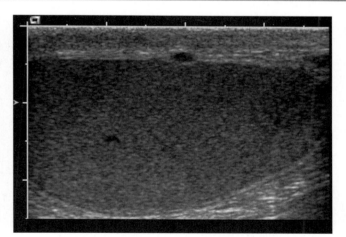

Views of the testis in two patients.

1. Is this lesion typically palpable?
2. How good is ultrasound at detecting this abnormality?
3. What is the typical size of this lesion?
4. How do these patients usually present?

Normal Variant Pancreatic Head

1. Pancreatitis and pancreatic tumors are probably the most widely described causes of decreased pancreatic echogenicity. However, the normal variant shown in these images is also a common cause.

2. Decreased fat in the posterior pancreatic head and uncinate process causes the difference in echogenicity.

3. The normal variant has a straight anterior border, produces no mass effect, and does not cause pancreatic or biliary ductal obstruction.

4. This is seen in 50% of autopsy specimens but in much less than 50% of cases seen in clinical practice.

References

Atri M, Nazarnia S, Mehio A, et al: Hypoechoic embryologic ventral aspect of the head and uncinate process of the pancreas: In vitro correlation of US with histopathologic findings. *Radiology* 1994;190:441–444.

Donald JJ, Shorvon PJ, Lees WR: Hypoechoic area within the head of the pancreas–A normal variant. *Clin Radiol* 1990;41:337.

Cross-Reference

Ultrasound: THE REQUISITES, pp 124–125.

Comment

The pancreas originates as two embryologic anlagen. The dorsal bud ultimately rotates into an anterior location and gives rise to the anterior aspect of the pancreatic head and to the pancreatic body and tail. The ventral bud rotates to a posterior location and gives rise to the posterior aspect of the pancreatic head and the uncinate process. Normally, the echogenicity of the pancreas is homogeneous throughout. However, in some patients an area of decreased echogenicity is seen in the portion of the pancreas corresponding in location to the ventral anlage. Studies have shown that this normal variant is due to decreased fatty deposition in the hypoechoic region.

This normal variant can be seen in approximately 20% of patients. It is seen more commonly in older patients and in patients in whom it is possible to get an unusually good look at the pancreatic head. Unlike pancreatic cancer and focal pancreatitis, this normal variant is well demarcated from the more echogenic pancreas, and the interface between the two areas is relatively straight. There is no mass effect on adjacent structures, and there is no obstruction of either the common bile duct or the pancreatic duct.

Tunica Albuginea Cyst

1. Unlike intratesticular cysts, tunica albuginea cysts are usually very firm and easily palpated.

2. Usually ultrasound is very good at detecting these cysts. However, the area of the palpable mass must be carefully scanned to avoid overlooking tunica albuginea cysts.

3. Cysts in the tunica albuginea are usually very small.

4. Patients usually present with a painless mass on physical examination.

Reference

Martinez-Berganza MT, Sarria L, Cozcolluela R: Cysts of the tunica albuginea: Sonographic appearance. *AJR Am J Roentgenol* 1998;170:183–185.

Cross-Reference

Ultrasound: THE REQUISITES, pp 435–439.

Comment

Cysts of the tunica albuginea are entities distinct from intratesticular cysts. Typically they are very firm on physical examination and often are first recognized by the patient himself. Since they arise from the tunica albuginea, they are always located at the periphery of the testis. Although they occur in a range of sizes, they are most often less than 5 mm in diameter. A fibrous plaque of the tunica albuginea is another lesion that can present as a firm, palpable nodule in the periphery of the testis. This lesion is usually the result of postinflammatory or posttraumatic scarring and is solid rather than cystic. Fibrous plaques of the tunica albuginea may calcify.

Because they are so small and they are not surrounded by testicular parenchyma, cysts of the tunica albuginea are occasionally difficult to find sonographically. This is true of other small peripheral masses as well. One technique that is useful is to place a finger over the lesion and then rotate the testis so that the palpable lesion is posterior. Then the transducer can be placed on the anterior aspect of the testis so that the palpating finger can be seen along the deep surface of the testis. Once the finger is located, the nature of the underlying palpable abnormality can usually be determined. In many cases, cysts of the tunica albuginea will satisfy all criteria for a simple cyst. However, the smaller lesions may contain artifactual internal echoes and may not demonstrate increased through transmission.

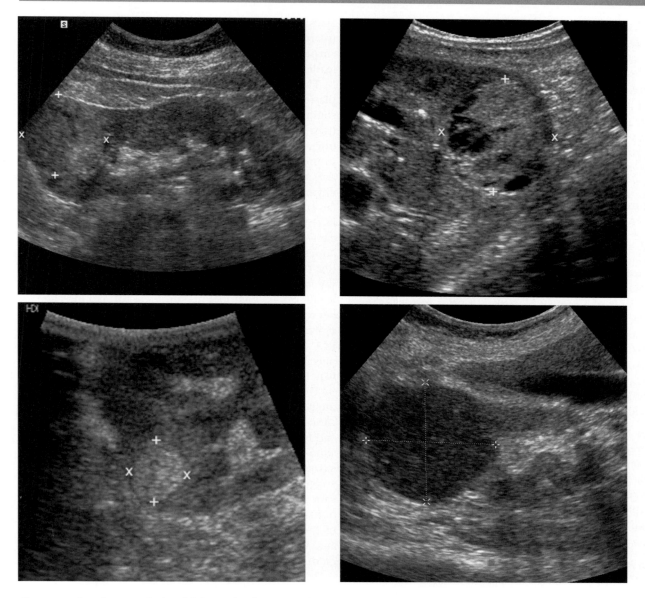

Grey-scale views of the kidney in four patients.

1. Describe the abnormalities shown in these images.
2. What is the differential diagnosis?
3. What is the role of percutaneous biopsy in lesions such as these?
4. Will CT or MRI assist in the differential diagnosis of these lesions?

Renal Cell Carcinoma

1. The first image shows an entirely solid-appearing mass in the upper pole of the kidney that is slightly hyperechoic to the renal parenchyma and produces a bulge in the external renal contour. The second image shows a predominantly solid mass in the lower pole of the kidney that is slightly hyperechoic and has several small, cystic components. The third image shows a small, homogeneous, hyperechoic mass. The fourth image shows a homogeneous, hypoechoic mass.

2. Cortical-based renal tumors such as renal cell cancer, angiomyolipoma, oncocytoma, lymphoma, or metastasis can all appear as a solid or predominantly solid mass.

3. The role of percutaneous biopsy is limited. Most lesions such as these will be resected regardless of the results of a biopsy. If there is a prior history of lymphoma or of another primary tumor likely to metastasize to the kidney, then biopsy would be useful, since a diagnosis of renal lymphoma or metastatic disease would not require surgery. Biopsy may also be necessary when it is not possible to distinguish neoplasm from infection on clinical and radiologic grounds.

4. CT or MRI would be helpful in evaluating the small, hyperechoic lesion because it could be an angiomyolipoma. It is unlikely that CT or MRI would help in further evaluating the other three solid renal lesions. However, CT and MRI provide valuable staging information, and one or the other should be performed prior to surgery.

Reference

Forman HP, Middleton WD, Melson GL, McClennan BL: Hyperechoic renal cell carcinomas: Increase in detection at US. *Radiology* 1993;188:431–434.

Cross-Reference

Ultrasound: THE REQUISITES, pp 89–93.

Comment

Renal cell carcinoma (RCC) is the most common solid renal neoplasm in the adult patient population. RCC is an adenocarcinoma arising from tubular cells. The most common histologic subtype is the clear cell type. Other types include papillary, granular cell, and sarcomatoid. In the past, the majority of RCCs were detected in patients with symptoms such as hematuria. Currently, approximately 50% of RCCs are discovered incidentally during sonograms or CTs done for other reasons. For this reason, RCCs are now being discovered at smaller sizes. Because surgical resection is the only effective treatment for RCC, detecting tumors when they are smaller and of lower stage has been one of the factors leading to improved survival.

The majority of renal cell cancers are solid neoplasms. They vary in echogenicity, but the majority are slightly hyperechoic to the adjacent renal parenchyma (first image). This is not hard to understand because the normal renal parenchyma is the most hypoechoic tissue in the upper abdomen. Approximately 10% of all RCCs are markedly hyperechoic compared to renal parenchyma and approximate the echogenicity of renal sinus fat (third image). Small renal cancers are even more likely to have this appearance. These are the types that can simulate an angiomyolipoma. A minority of RCCs appear either isoechoic or hypoechoic to the renal cortex (fourth image). Isoechoic RCC is detected only when it is large enough to distort the renal contour. Small cystic components or areas of hemorrhage or necrosis are common (second image). Color Doppler typically will identify internal vascularity in RCC, but RCC is usually less vascular than the adjacent renal parenchyma. Small tumors and hypovascular tumors may have no detectable flow on color Doppler.

The differential diagnosis of solid renal neoplasms includes other malignant tumors such as transitional cell cancer, medullary cancer, renal sarcoma, metastases, and lymphoma. Patients with metastases and lymphoma almost always have a history of prior lymphoma or extrarenal malignancy or have imaging evidence that suggests lymphoma or metastatic disease. Medullary cancer occurs in patients with sickle cell trait. Transitional cell cancer is typically based in the central aspect of the kidney, as opposed to the cortex, and is associated with typical abnormalities on an intravenous pyelogram.

Benign tumors are also a consideration and include renal adenoma and oncocytoma. It is not clear if there is a true distinction between renal adenoma and small, well-differentiated RCC. Oncocytoma is a variety of adenoma that has large cells with small, round nuclei and abundant eosinophilic cytoplasm and numerous mitochondria. In general, it is not possible to distinguish RCC from benign renal tumors with imaging tests. The exception is angiomyolipoma, which can be diagnosed by CT or MRI when fat is detected.

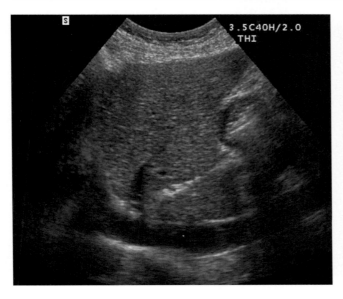
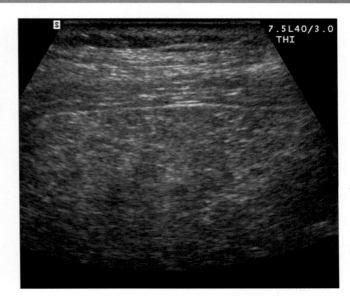

Two views of the liver.

1. What types of transducers have been used?
2. Which transducer shows the abnormality best?
3. What is the differential diagnosis?
4. Is there a role for Doppler sonography in establishing this diagnosis?

CASE 92

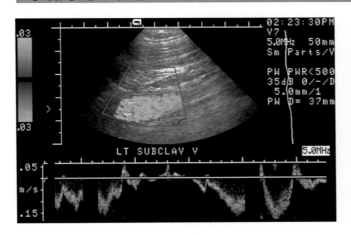
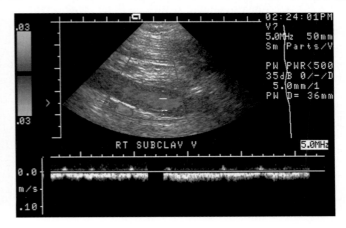

Pulsed Doppler waveforms from the left and right subclavian veins.

1. Which subclavian vein waveform is abnormal?
2. What does the abnormality indicate?
3. Is the superior vena cava likely to be normal in this patient?
4. What is the significance of reversed flow in the right and left internal mammary veins?

Cirrhosis

1. The first image was obtained with a 3.5 MHz curved array transducer. The second was obtained with a 7.5 MHz phased linear transducer.

2. The second image shows a coarsened and nodular-appearing liver parenchyma better than does the first image.

3. Cirrhosis is the most likely diagnosis. Metastatic disease, lymphoma, extensive hepatocellular cancer, and patchy fatty infiltration can also produce diffuse liver heterogeneity.

4. Doppler sonography can help in patients with suspected cirrhosis by finding portal systemic collaterals or other evidence of portal hypertension. This confirms the diagnosis of liver disease and helps to assess disease severity.

Reference

Mergo PJ, Ros PR, Buetow PC, Buck JL: Diffuse disease of the liver: Radiologic-pathologic correlation. *Radiographics* 1994;14:1291–1307.

Cross-Reference

Ultrasound: THE REQUISITES, pp 18–20.

Comment

Cirrhosis is a diffuse hepatic parenchymal process consisting of hepatocellular death, cellular regeneration, and fibrosis. It is divided into a micronodular form, when the regenerating nodules are less than 1 cm in size, and a macronodular form, when the nodules are greater than 1 cm in size. Sonographic signs of cirrhosis include a nodular liver surface, coarsening of the hepatic echotexture, multinodular hepatic echotexture, enlargement of the caudate and left lobe, atrophy of the right lobe, and signs of portal hypertension (ascites, splenomegaly, portosystemic collaterals). Evaluation of the liver surface is easiest when there is ascites. When there is no ascites, the liver surface is best visualized by using a high-frequency linear or curved array focused at the level of the liver surface. As shown in this case, high resolution transducers are also helpful for displaying the parenchymal nodularity of a cirrhotic liver.

It is important to realize that patients with early cirrhotic changes detected on sonography may have minimal, if any, clinical findings. Therefore, the diagnosis should not be excluded because of a low clinical suspicion if the sonographic findings are convincing. On the other hand, it is also important to know that patients with biopsy-proven cirrhosis may have a normal-appearing liver on sonography.

Subclavian Vein Obstruction

1. The left subclavian vein is normal. The right subclavian vein is abnormal.

2. The abnormality indicates some type of venous obstruction between the place where the sample was taken and the right atrium.

3. Since there is normal pulsatility in the left subclavian vein, the superior vena cava must be patent.

4. Reversed flow in the internal mammary veins indicates collateral flow owing to central venous obstruction, usually of the superior vena cava.

Reference

Patel MC, Berman LH, Moss HA, McPherson SJ: Subclavian and internal jugular veins at Doppler US: Abnormal cardiac pulsatility and respiratory phasicity as a predictor of complete central occlusion. *Radiology* 1999;211:579–583.

Cross-Reference

Ultrasound: THE REQUISITES, pp 486–487.

Comment

Doppler detection of subclavian vein thrombosis is more complicated than detection of lower extremity deep vein thrombosis because the thrombus frequently occurs in the central aspect of the vein, where the overlying bones (especially the clavicle) make compression impossible, and where visualization is in any case difficult or impossible. Therefore, the diagnosis often relies on secondary signs of obstruction. Since the subclavian vein is relatively close to the right atrium, the pressure fluctuations in the atrium are readily transmitted into the vein and produce a pulsatile waveform. When there is a venous obstruction between the heart and the site where the Doppler waveform is obtained, the normal pulsatility is blunted. The asymmetry in the right and left subclavian waveforms is well demonstrated in this case. It is also important to realize that many cases of subclavian vein thrombosis are associated with jugular vein thrombosis. Since the jugular vein is easy to evaluate with sonography, it should be a routine part of an upper extremity venous Doppler examination.

Although venous thrombosis is the most common cause of asymmetric waveforms, it should be realized that any obstructing process, such as venous stenosis or extrinsic compression, is a potential cause.

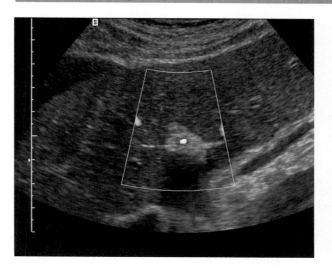 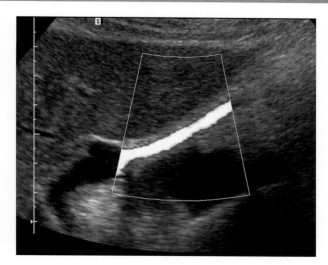

Transverse and longitudinal views of the left lobe of the liver.

1. What is the abnormality shown in this case?

2. In what direction is the blood flowing?

3. Where does this abnormality communicate with the portal venous system?

4. How does this blood flow return to the heart?

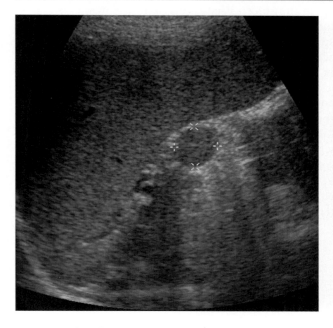 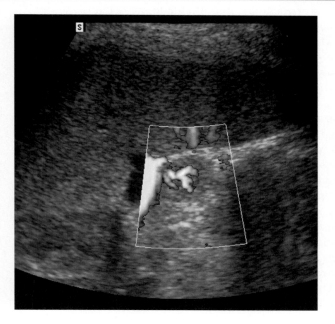

Longitudinal views of the left upper quadrant. (See color plates.)

1. Describe the abnormality that is being measured.

2. How common is this abnormality?

3. From where does the blood supply come?

4. What further evaluation is necessary?

Umbilical Vein Collateral

1. A vascular structure is seen in the ligamentum teres. This represents a recanalized umbilical vein.

2. Because the recanalized umbilical vein functions as a portosystemic shunt, blood flow is directed away from the liver (hepatofugal).

3. The umbilical vein communicates with the portal system at the anterior aspect of the terminal segment of the left portal vein. The ductus venosus communicates with the posterior aspect of this portion of the left portal vein. Therefore, in the fetus, this segment of the portal vein contains umbilical venous flow. That is why this segment of the left portal vein is called the umbilical segment.

4. The umbilical vein travels inferior to the liver along the deep aspect of the abdominal wall toward the umbilicus. It eventually connects to the inferior epigastric veins, which then drain into the femoral-iliac system. In some cases the umbilical vein turns superiorly to communicate with the superior epigastric veins and the internal mammary veins.

Reference

Gibson RN, Gibson PR, Donlan JD, Clunie DA: Identification of a patent paraumbilical vein by using Doppler sonography: importance in the diagnosis of portal hypertension. *AJR Am J Roentgenol* 1989;153: 513-516.

Cross-Reference

Ultrasound: THE REQUISITES, pp 19-22.

Comment

The umbilical vein is the portosystemic collateral that is the easiest to visualize sonographically. It has a constant relationship with the portal venous system; it always communicates with the umbilical segment of the left portal vein. Therefore, it can be seen between the medial and lateral segments of the left lobe within the ligamentum teres. In some normal individuals, the fibrous remnant of the obliterated umbilical vein can be seen as a hypoechoic band. However, this band should not exceed 3 mm and should not contain blood flow.

The umbilical vein normally exits the liver and travels along the anterior abdominal wall toward the umbilicus. The caput medusa sign refers to prominent visible superficial collaterals in the periumbilical region and represents an uncommon manifestation of umbilical vein collaterals. In patients with suspected portal hypertension, this is one of the potential collaterals that should be investigated to help confirm the diagnosis.

Splenule

1. The lesion being measured is a solid mass that is isoechoic to the spleen with detectable internal vascularity. This appearance is typical of a splenule.

2. Splenules are seen in up to 30% of autopsies.

3. Blood supply to splenules is from the splenic artery.

4. This is a common finding that requires no further evaluation.

Reference

Subramanyam BR, Balthazar EJ, Horii SC. Sonography of the accessory spleen. *AJR Am J Roentgenol* 1984; 143:47-49.

Cross-Reference

Ultrasound: THE REQUISITES, p 142.

Comment

Splenules are also referred to as splenunculi, accessory spleens, and supernumerary spleens. As indicated in the answer to question 2, they are very common and are frequently seen as incidental findings on imaging studies of the left upper quadrant. They are typically small lesions, measuring less than 3 cm in size. Small splenules may enlarge and become more readily evident when the spleen itself enlarges, or following a splenectomy. Although typically solitary, approximately 10% of splenules are multiple. In addition to the splenic hilum, accessory spleens can occur in the tail of the pancreas or in the suspensory ligaments of the spleen.

Under unusual circumstances, it may be necessary to confirm that a mass in the left upper quadrant with sonographic findings typical for a splenule is in fact functioning splenic tissue. For instance, in a patient with a suspected islet cell tumor of the pancreas, a splenule may cause diagnostic confusion. The best way to document that a lesion is a splenule is to perform either a sulfur colloid scan or a heat-damaged tagged red blood cell scan.

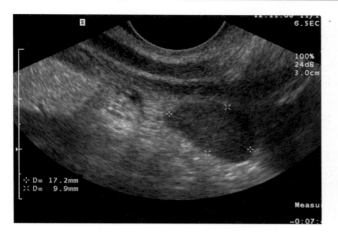
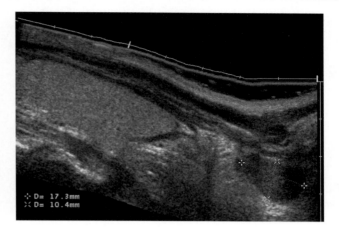

Longitudinal view and extended field of view scan of the neck in a patient with recurrent hyperparathyroidism following prior neck exploration.

1. Is imaging useful in patients such as this one?

2. Is a nodule lateral to the carotid artery more likely to be a lymph node or a parathyroid adenoma?

3. What is the sensitivity of ultrasound in detecting this abnormality in patients who have had prior neck dissection for hyperparathyroidism?

4. What is the incidence of this lesion?

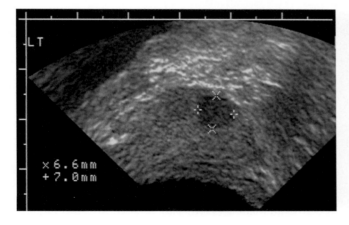
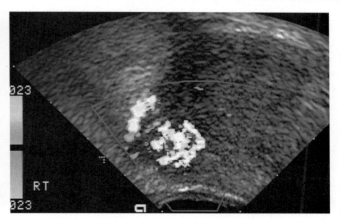

Sagittal grey-scale view of the lateral prostate and transverse color Doppler view of the right prostate in two patients.

1. Describe the abnormalities.

2. What is the most common location for prostate cancer?

3. Where is benign prostatic hypertrophy (BPH) located?

4. Is prostate cancer more often hypoechoic or hyperechoic?

Ectopic Parathyroid Adenoma

1. Imaging is most useful in localizing parathyroid adenoma following prior neck exploration.

2. Parathyroid adenomas are almost always medial to the carotid artery. A nodule seen lateral to the carotid is much more likely to be a lymph node.

3. The sensitivity is 60% to 80%.

4. The incidence of ectopic parathyroid nodules is approximately 10%.

Reference

DeFeo ML, Colagrande S, Bianini C, et al: Parathyroid glands: Combination of 99m Tc MIBI scintigraphy and US for demonstration of parathyroid glands and nodules. *Radiology* 2000;214:393–402.

Cross-Reference

Ultrasound: THE REQUISITES, pp 452–454.

Comment

One of the important reasons for a failed parathyroid operation is the presence of an ectopic adenoma. There are a number of potential ectopic locations. Behind the trachea or in the tracheoesophageal groove is a common ectopic location. These lesions can best be visualized by scanning from a lateral approach and having the patient turn his or her head away from the side being scanned. Other ectopic sites are low in the neck (as in this case) or in the mediastinum. Lesions in these sites can be a challenge to see, especially with a linear array transducer, which is usually used to scan the neck. Switching to a sector or curved array transducer can allow for better flexibility in the suprasternal area. In fact, a transvaginal probe is an excellent choice for looking into the superior mediastinum because it has a very small footprint. Intrathyroidal adenomas are rare but do occur. They have a similar appearance and orientation to other parathyroid adenomas and usually occur in the posterior aspect of the thyroid. Finally, ectopic adenomas can occur within the carotid sheath as high as the bifurcation.

Preoperative imaging of patients at their initial presentation with hyperparathyroidism is controversial. Experienced surgeons have a high success rate and a low complication rate without any preoperative localization. Less experienced surgeons can often benefit from preoperative imaging, since unilateral explorations can then be performed, and operative time can be diminished. On the other hand, even experienced neck surgeons benefit from the information provided by preoperative imaging in patients who have recurrent or persistent hyperparathyroidism after a previous neck exploration.

Other modalities used to identify parathyroid adenomas include scintigraphy, MRI, CT, angiography, and venous sampling. At my own institution, the combination of ultrasound and scintigraphy with technetium-99m sestamibi is the standard procedure for imaging patients with recurrent or persistent hyperparathyroidism.

Prostate Cancer

1. The abnormality on the grey-scale view is a hypoechoic nodule in the peripheral zone of the prostate. The abnormality on the color Doppler view is a hypervascular nodule in the peripheral zone. Although these findings are nonspecific, they are very typical of prostate cancer.

2. Seventy percent of prostate cancers occur in the peripheral zone.

3. Benign hypertrophy occurs in the central gland.

4. Prostate cancer is usually hypoechoic.

Reference

Choyke PL: Imaging of prostate cancer. *Abdom Imaging* 1995;20:505–515.

Cross-Reference

Ultrasound: THE REQUISITES, pp 458–460.

Comment

Prostate cancer is the most common malignancy in men. Ten percent of American men will be diagnosed with prostate cancer. Autopsy studies show that 20% of men between the ages of 40 and 60 and 60% older than age 80 have prostate cancer. Therefore, as screening for prostate cancer becomes more universal, the number of newly diagnosed patients will increase. Although the risk of dying from prostate cancer is only 2% to 3%, the tumor is so common that it is still the second leading cause of cancer death in men.

Men are screened for prostate cancer using digital rectal examination (DRE) and prostate-specific antigen (PSA) screening. Transrectal ultrasonography (TRUS) is used primarily to guide the biopsy of lesions felt on DRE, of lesions that are visible on TRUS, or of random areas of the prostate. TRUS is also used to measure the prostate so that volume-adjusted PSA (PSA density or PSAD) can be determined. TRUS is no longer used to screen for cancer.

Most prostate cancers are hypoechoic, but only 20% of hypoechoic lesions are cancer. Isoechoic cancer is also common, so ultrasound guided biopsies should be directed at random sites (usually the upper, mid, and lower third of the gland bilaterally) as well as at any visible lesion.

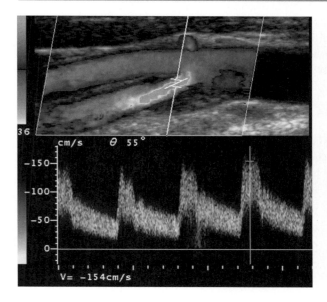
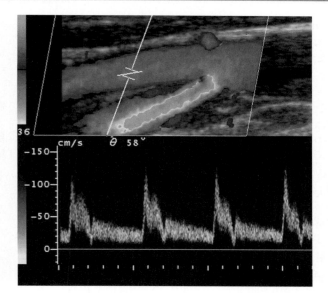

Longitudinal color Doppler views and pulsed Doppler waveforms from the carotid bifurcation. (See color plates.)

1. Identify the internal and external carotid arteries.

2. Do both vessels appear normal?

3. If this patient had a history of transient ischemic attacks, would he benefit from a carotid endarterectomy?

4. What is the most common site for carotid plaque formation?

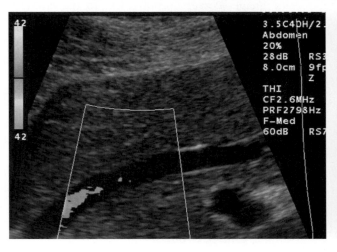
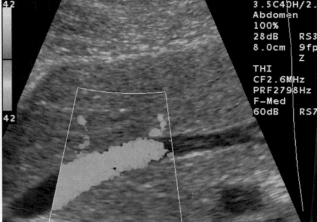

Longitudinal color Doppler views of the left hepatic vein. (See color plates.)

1. Why is blood flow seen better on the second image?

2. Why does the liver appear brighter on the second image?

3. Besides the technical control responsible for improved Doppler sensitivity in the second image, what two other controls are most important in increasing Doppler sensitivity?

4. If all other things are equal, what technical parameter should be adjusted first when attempting to improve Doppler sensitivity?

Low-Grade Internal Carotid Stenosis

1. In these images, the deep vessel is the internal and the superficial vessel is the external carotid artery. The internal waveform has a broader systolic peak with a more gradual deceleration into diastole. The external waveform has less diastolic flow.

2. The external carotid artery appears normal. Hypoechoic plaque is present at the origin of the internal carotid artery.

3. The peak flow velocity in the internal carotid artery is 154 cm/sec. This is elevated and would predict a stenosis of 40% to 60% of the arterial diameter. Endarterectomy is indicated for symptomatic patients when the stenosis exceeds 70%.

4. The location of plaque in this patient is the most common site, at the junction of the carotid bulb and the internal artery origin opposite the flow divider.

Reference

North American Symptomatic Carotid Endarterectomy Trial Collaborators: Beneficial effect of carotid endarterectomy in symptomatic patients with high-grade stenosis. *N Engl J Med* 1991;325:445–453.

Cross-Reference

Ultrasound: THE REQUISITES, pp 470–477.

Comment

Carotid Doppler imaging is used as a noninvasive way to detect atherosclerotic plaque and to estimate the degree of stenosis caused by the plaque. Early plaque formation is detected on grey-scale imaging as minimal thickening of the vessel wall. With progressive changes, the resulting luminal narrowing can be seen with both grey-scale and color Doppler imaging. Velocity increases begin to occur when the stenosis exceeds 40% to 50% of the diameter of the artery. Based on the results of the North American Symptomatic Carotid Endarterectomy Trial study, patients with neurologic symptoms benefit from carotid endarterectomy if the diameter stenosis (determined from a carotid arteriogram) is 70% or greater. In measuring the lesion, it is important to calculate the percentage of stenosis based on comparison of the lumen diameter at the stenotic site with that at a distal site where the diameter is normal.

The criteria for categorizing carotid stenosis are not uniformly agreed upon. In general, the higher the velocity, the greater the stenosis. Color Doppler is usually very useful in identifying the site of peak velocity, so placement of the pulsed Doppler sample volume can be precise. In this case, an area of aliasing is seen in the internal carotid origin indicating the site of the high velocity flow jet. The angle corrected pulsed Doppler waveform from this site shows that the peak systolic velocity is 154 cm/sec. The cutoff velocity used to indicate a stenosis of greater than 70% diameter narrowing is usually 200 cm/sec or higher.

Effect of Power Output on Color Doppler Images

1. The power output was increased in the second image.

2. For the same reason. The power output affects both the color image and the grey-scale image.

3. Doppler gain and Doppler scale are two basic controls that affect color sensitivity.

4. Doppler gain, because this does not affect patient exposure and does not increase the chance of aliasing.

Reference

Middleton WD: Color Doppler image optimization and interpretation. *Ultrasound Q* 1998;14:194–208.

Cross-Reference

Ultrasound: THE REQUISITES, pp 464–470.

Comment

Power output is one of several controls that will affect the color image. Power output refers to the strength of the transmitted ultrasound pulse. Stronger or more powerful sound pulses will produce stronger reflections that are more easily detected. Power output affects both the grey-scale and color Doppler image. In general, increasing the power output improves color Doppler sensitivity. This can be very important in deep abdominal applications, where tissue attenuation significantly weakens the Doppler signal. However, increasing the power output also causes increased patient exposure and can lead to a number of artifacts. Therefore, power levels should be kept as low as is reasonably achievable in order to obtain the desired information.

The two other basic controls that affect Doppler sensitivity are the Doppler gain and the Doppler scale. The Doppler gain electronically amplifies the Doppler signals received by the transducer. It also amplifies electronic noise. Therefore, it can be increased until image-degrading color-noise artifact is produced. Color Doppler sensitivity can also be improved by decreasing the color Doppler scale. The sacrifice is that aliasing artifacts may develop at low scales. With power, color gain, and color Doppler scale, it is worth realizing that attempts at improving sensitivity can have a paradoxical effect when they are adjusted to extreme levels.

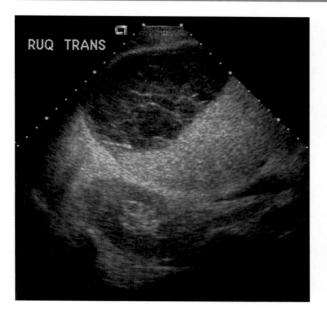
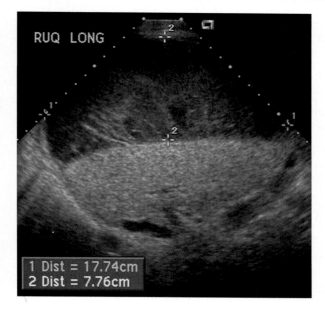

RUQ TRANS

RUQ LONG

1 Dist = 17.74cm
2 Dist = 7.76cm

Transverse and longitudinal views of the liver.
1. Describe the abnormality.
2. What is the differential diagnosis?
3. Given the compression of the liver, where is this lesion likely located?
4. What would the diagnosis be if this lesion contained bright reflectors with ring-down artifacts?

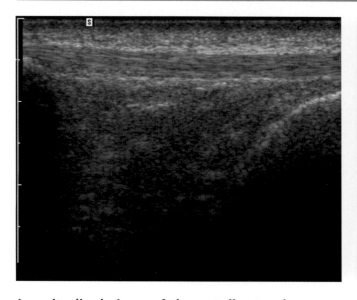
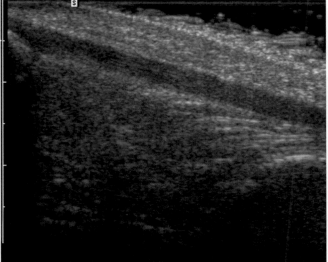

Longitudinal views of the patellar tendon.
1. Which view shows a normal patellar tendon?
2. What is the differential diagnosis for a hypoechoic tendon?
3. Are nerves more or less echogenic than tendons?
4. Does ultrasound demonstrate the internal fibers of tendons as well as MRI?

Hepatic Subcapsular Hematoma

1. The lesion is a complex fluid collection with low-level echoes and multiple internal septations.

2. The most likely diagnosis is hematoma. Other considerations include abscess and biloma.

3. Compression of the liver parenchyma suggests that this hematoma is subcapsular.

4. Distinguishing an abscess or an infected hematoma from a simple hematoma is very difficult. Ring-down artifacts usually indicate gas, and the presence of gas is a clue that there are gas-forming organisms present and thus allows for a diagnosis of infection. In the absence of gas, aspiration of the fluid is necessary if there is clinical concern about infection.

Reference

VanSonnenberg E, Simeone JF, Mueller PR, et al: Sonographic appearance of hematoma in liver, spleen and kidney: A clinical, pathologic and animal study. *Radiology* 1983;147:507–510.

Cross-Reference

Ultrasound: THE REQUISITES, pp 106–109.

Comment

Hematomas have a range of sonographic appearances depending primarily on their age. In the acute stage, they usually appear as a complex collection with solid and cystic components. If the proportion of clot predominates over the proportion of serum, then a hematoma may simulate a solid mass. With time, the clotted portion of the hematoma lyses, and the collection becomes more liquefactive. In this stage, sonography shows a complex fluid collection, usually with some combination of septations, internal fibrinous membranes, and fluid/fluid levels. Eventually, most hematomas liquefy completely and appear entirely cystic on sonography. The time of evolution of these sonographic changes varies greatly from one patient to the next. It typically takes a matter of weeks. In this case, the hematoma was in the subcapsular space and was caused by a liver biopsy. Trauma is the other most common cause of subcapsular hematoma.

Hematomas should always be considered when a complex fluid collection is identified sonographically. An abscess should also be included in the differential diagnosis. Other fluid collections should be considered, depending on the organ involved. In the case of the liver, a biloma is another consideration. If this collection were adjacent to the kidney, a urinoma would be a possibility.

Normal Tendon Anisotropy

1. The patellar tendon is normal in both views. In fact, it is the same tendon imaged once with the long axis parallel to the transducer and again with the long axis at an angle to the transducer.

2. Decreased echogenicity in a tendon may indicate tendinitis or a partial tear, or it may be due to anisotropy.

3. When imaged at 90 degrees, tendons are more echogenic than nerves.

4. Ultrasound displays the internal fibers of tendons better than MRI.

Reference

Martinoli C, Bianchi S, Derchi LE: Tendon and nerve sonography. *Radiol Clin North Am* 1999;37:691–711.

Cross-Reference

Ultrasound: THE REQUISITES, p 455.

Comment

Sonography displays the internal architecture of tendons better than any other modality. When imaged so that the sound reflects off the tendon at 90 degrees, the interfaces between tendon collagen and internal endotendineum septa produce strong specular reflections. This results in an appearance of bright, closely spaced, parallel, linear reflections within the substance of the tendon. When tendons are imaged at less than 90 degrees, the internal reflectors no longer act as specular reflectors, and the tendon becomes hypoechoic, and the internal fibrillar pattern is no longer seen. This effect (variable echogenicity depending on the relative orientation of the transducer and the tendon) is referred to as anisotropy. Anisotropy is present in many parts of the body but is particularly prominent in tendons.

Under most circumstances, tendons should be imaged at 90 degrees so that the internal fibrillar pattern is visible. However, when tendons are surrounded by echogenic tissue such as fat, it may be helpful to purposely angle the transducer so that the tendon appears hypoechoic and the contrast between tendon and peritendinous tissues is increased. In addition, echogenic lesions and abnormal intratendinous interfaces are occasionally best seen when the tendon itself is purposely made to appear hypoechoic by imaging at less than 90 degrees.

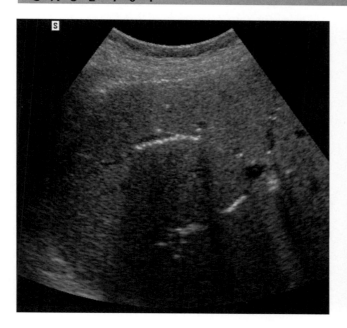 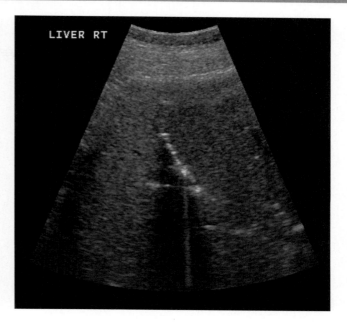

Two views of the liver.

1. Describe the abnormality.
2. What is the most common cause of this abnormality?
3. What would you consider if this finding were associated with dilated loops of small bowel?
4. Is this abnormality seen most often in the right or left lobe?

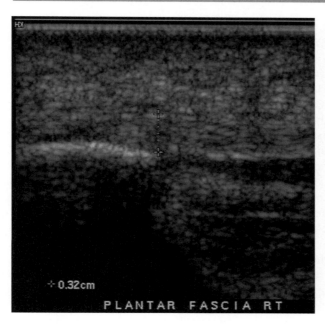 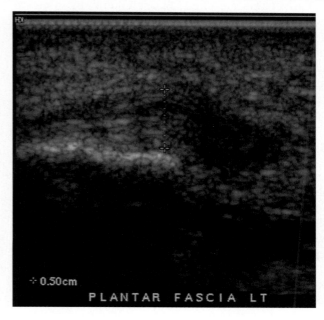

Longitudinal view of the plantar fascia of both feet.

1. Which side is abnormal?
2. What symptoms is this patient likely to have?
3. Is imaging required to make this diagnosis?
4. What is the etiology?

Intrabiliary Air

1. Both images show very bright, linear, branching structures in the liver. The second image shows a faint ring-down artifact arising from one of these structures.

2. Biliary air is most often caused by stents and surgical anastomosis between bile duct and bowel.

3. Biliary air and a small-bowel obstruction should raise the possibility of gallstone ileus.

4. Biliary air tends to move to the nondependent areas of the liver. Therefore, it is seen in the left lobe when patients are supine and in the right lobe when patients are in a left lateral decubitus position. This rule is frequently broken because free movement of the air is limited.

Reference

Middleton WD: The bile ducts. In Goldberg BB (ed): *Diagnostic Ultrasound.* Baltimore, Williams & Wilkins, 1993, pp 146–172.

Cross-Reference

Ultrasound: THE REQUISITES, pp 61–63.

Comment

Biliary gas is a common finding following various manipulations of the bile ducts. Biliary enteric anastomoses and biliary stents are probably the most common source of biliary gas. Endoscopic sphincterotomy is another common cause. Biliary enteric fistulas can also cause biliary gas but are much less common. Erosion of a gallstone through the gallbladder (or, less often, through the bile duct) into the bowel (usually the duodenum) is the most common cause for a biliary enteric fistula. Erosion of a duodenal or pyloric ulcer into the bile duct or gallbladder is another cause of a fistula.

On sonography, biliary air appears as a bright reflection in the lumen of the bile ducts. As with gas elsewhere, it often causes a ring-down artifact. It is generally most prominent in the nondependent portions of the biliary tree. Gas can be seen in the common duct, but this phenomenon is less common than in the intrahepatic ducts.

The differential diagnosis of pneumobilia includes intrahepatic bile duct stones, portal venous gas, and calcified hepatic arteries. Intrahepatic stones are usually less echogenic than air and do not produce ring-down artifacts. In addition, intrahepatic ductal stones are generally nonmobile and do not predominate in the nondependent portion of the liver. Portal venous gas can be confused with biliary air when it is confined to the peripheral intrahepatic portal veins. In such cases, careful grey-scale scanning of the more central portal veins often shows mobile bubbles flowing in the venous lumen. Pulse Doppler waveform analysis may also show characteristic spikes in the venous waveform that are indicative of portal vein gas. Hepatic arterial calcification can be as bright as air but is not mobile, does not produce ring-down artifacts, and does not predominate in the nondependent portion of the liver. When there is still confusion, abdominal radiographs can assist in differentiating biliary gas from the other entities mentioned here.

Plantar Fasciitis

1. The second image, showing the thicker plantar fascia, is abnormal.

2. The common symptoms are inferior heel pain and tenderness that worsens with prolonged activity.

3. Generally the diagnosis is made based on clinical evaluation, and imaging is not required.

4. The etiology is repetitive microtrauma.

Reference

Cardinal E, Chhem RK, Beauregard CG, et al: Plantar fasciitis: Sonographic evaluation. *Radiology* 1996; 201:257–259.

Cross-Reference

Ultrasound: THE REQUISITES, pp 455–456.

Comment

Plantar fasciitis is the most common cause of inferior heel pain. It occurs most commonly as a result of repetitive microtrauma in athletes engaged in activities such as running, dancing, tennis, and basketball. It may affect up to 10% of running athletes but can also occur in nonathletes. It can be exacerbated by prolonged weight-bearing and obesity. Rheumatologic conditions such as rheumatoid arthritis, systemic lupus erythematosus, Reiter's disease, and ankylosing spondylitis may also cause plantar fasciitis.

In most cases the diagnosis can be made based on the clinical history and physical examination. In atypical cases, sonography can be very helpful. The sonographic findings are thickening and, in some cases, decreased echogenicity of the fascia. In almost all instances, the fascia is thickest proximally at the site of attachment to the calcaneus. When the symptoms are unilateral, the asymptomatic side should be used as a base line for comparison of the thickness and echogenicity of the plantar fascia. When symptoms are bilateral, studies have shown that 4 mm is a reasonable upper limit of normal for plantar fascia thickness.

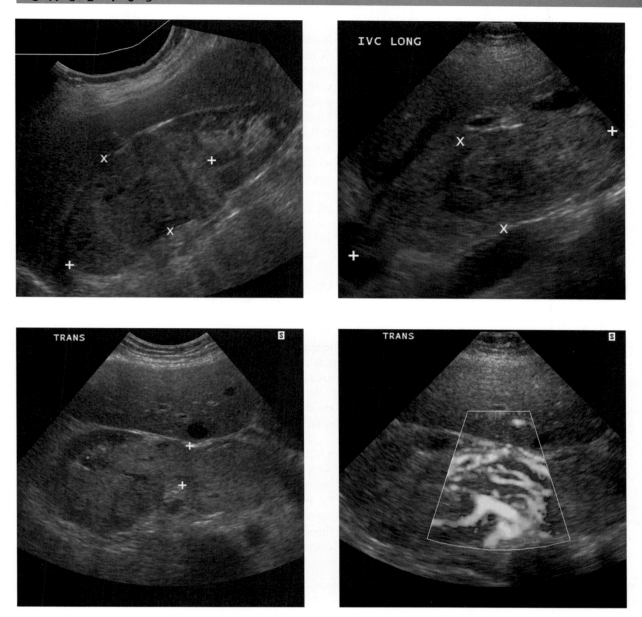

Grey-scale views of the right kidney, inferior vena cava, and right renal vein, and power Doppler view of the right renal vein.

1. Describe the abnormalities.

2. What is the most likely etiology of the abnormalities?

3. How common is this?

4. Is ultrasound a good way of evaluating this condition?

Tumor Thrombus of the Renal Vein and Inferior Vena Cava

1. A soft tissue mass is replacing the entire upper pole of the right kidney. Soft tissue extends from the right kidney into the markedly distended renal vein and inferior vena cava (IVC). Detection of internal vascularity on Doppler confirms that this is tumor thrombus.

2. Renal cell carcinoma (RCC) is almost always the cause of renal vein tumor thrombus.

3. Traditional estimates indicate that renal vein invasion occurs in up to 20% of patients with RCC, and IVC invasion occurs in up to 10% of patients. However, most renal cell cancers are now detected as incidental masses in patients undergoing CT or ultrasound for other reasons, and venous invasion is much less common in this group of patients.

4. Ultrasound is probably similar to CT and MRI in detecting clinically significant tumor thrombus and determining the extent in patients with RCC.

References

Bechtold RE, Zagoria RJ: Imaging approach to staging of renal cell carcinoma. *Urol Clin North Am* 1997;24:507–522.

Schwerk WB, Schwerk WN, Rodeck G: Venous renal tumor extension: A prospective US evaluation. *Radiology* 1985;156:491–495.

Cross-Reference

Ultrasound: THE REQUISITES, p 92.

Comment

RCC is the most common renal neoplasm. Survival is directly related to the stage and grade of the tumor. Chemotherapy and radiation therapy have little effect on RCC, so surgery is the only effective therapy at present. Imaging is critical in the preoperative evaluation of patients with RCC because it determines the surgical approach and the prognosis for patients who are not surgical candidates. The most common staging system used for RCC is the Robson system. In this system, stage I disease is tumor confined to the renal capsule. Stage II is tumor that has invaded the perinephric fat. Invasion of the renal vein or IVC indicates stage IIIA disease. Stage IIIB disease includes regional lymph node metastases. Stage IIIC disease has combined nodal and venous metastases. Direct invasion of adjacent organs indicates stage IVA, and distant metastases are stage IVB.

This case demonstrates stage IIIA disease, with invasion of the renal vein and the IVC. It is very uncommon for tumors smaller than 4 cm to invade the veins. In the majority of cases, tumor simply grows into the lumen of the vessel but does not invade the wall of the vessel. Interestingly, the prognosis is similar for stage IIIA disease and for tumor confined to the kidney. In fact, the prognosis is largely independent of the extent of IVC involvement. However, it is very important to detect and quantitate venous involvement because this dictates the surgical approach. If tumor extends into the supradiaphragmatic cava, then a combined thoracoabdominal approach is necessary, and cardiopulmonary bypass should be available. The relationship of the tumor to the hepatic veins is also important because the IVC can be clamped below the level of the hepatic veins, provided there is no tumor thrombus at that level.

In most patients, ultrasound is very good at detecting thrombus in the IVC and at identifying the superior extent. Detection of renal vein involvement is also usually possible, with the sensitivity depending on the extent of venous involvement. CT or MRI are almost always used to stage patients with RCC, and both tests are complementary to ultrasound in evaluating the status of the renal veins and IVC. In some patients, flow-related artifacts and other problems can make interpretation of venous and IVC invasion difficult on CT or MRI. In these situations, ultrasound is an excellent problem-solving tool.

In many cases, including the one shown here, the vascularity of the tumor thrombus can be documented with color or power Doppler. This distinguishes tumor thrombus from bland thrombus. Realize that the inability to detect intratumoral flow does not exclude the possibility of tumor thrombus. Also realize that venous thrombus in the setting of RCC is almost always tumor thrombus.

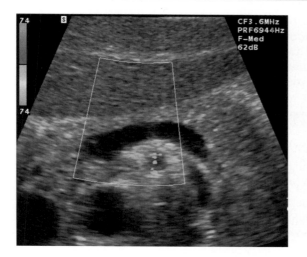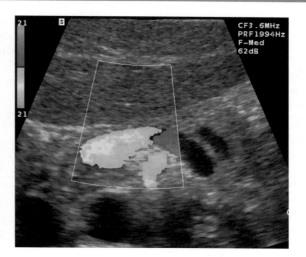

Transverse color Doppler views of the portosplenic confluence and the superior mesenteric artery. (See color plates.)

1. Why is blood flow not demonstrated in the vessels in the first image?

2. What does PRF stand for?

3. Is the PRF dependent on the Doppler gain?

4. Is the PRF dependent on the image depth?

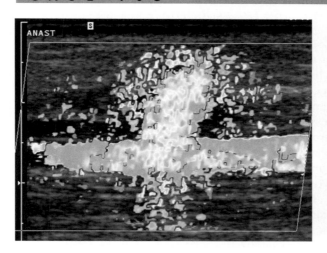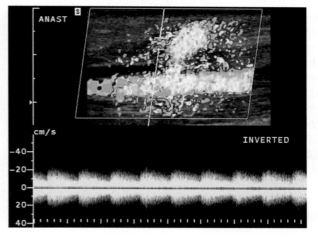

Color Doppler image and pulsed Doppler waveform obtained in the region of anastomosis of a hemodialysis arteriovenous fistula. (See color plates.)

1. Describe the abnormality shown on the color Doppler image.

2. Describe the abnormality shown on the Doppler waveform.

3. What is the explanation for these findings?

4. What pathologic processes can produce these findings?

Effect of Doppler Scale on Doppler Sensitivity

1. Blood flow is poorly seen on the first image because the Doppler scale is too high (± 74 cm/sec). The scale has been readjusted in the second image to a more appropriate level (± 21 cm/sec).

2. PRF stands for *pulse repetition frequency*. The PRF determines the Doppler scale.

3. The PRF is independent of the Doppler gain.

4. Deeper fields of view require a longer time delay between sound pulses because each pulse must travel farther. Therefore the PRF drops as the field of view deepens.

Reference

Middleton WD: Color Doppler image optimization and interpretation. *Ultrasound Q* 1998;14:194-208.

Cross-Reference

Ultrasound: THE REQUISITES, pp 464-470.

Comment

A number of user-adjustable parameters are available to optimize color Doppler images. The most basic is the color gain. This is simply a receiver end amplification of the color signal. In most situations, the color gain should be increased to a maximum value just prior to the point where random color noise begins to appear in nonvascular spaces. The color gain affects only the color portion of the image and does not affect the grey-scale background or the pulsed Doppler waveform.

The PRF refers to the number of sound pulses transmitted per second. The PRF determines the magnitude of the Doppler scale. Higher scales are produced by higher PRFs, while lower scales are produced by lower PRFs. The advantage of a low PRF (low scale) is improved sensitivity to low-velocity blood flow. The advantage of a high PRF (high scale) is display of high-velocity flow without aliasing. On most equipment there is a control labeled *Doppler scale* that varies the PRF and thus adjusts the Doppler scale. The PRF is usually displayed with the rest of the technical information on the image. On these images, the PRF is 6944 and 1994 pulses per second.

Another means of improving the sensitivity is to increase the number of sound pulses used to generate each individual line of color Doppler information. This control has been referred to as the "dwell time" or the "ensemble length" or "color sensitivity." If more pulses are used for each line in the color Doppler image, then it will take longer to generate each individual color Doppler frame. Thus, the trade-off is a lowered frame rate. In some situations where background motion is limited (such as neck or extremity examinations), a low frame rate is acceptable. However, in other situations, background motion requires a higher frame rate (cardiac, abdominal, and obstetrical scans) and thus there is a practical limit to the number of pulses that can be used to generate each color Doppler line.

Tissue Vibration

1. The color Doppler image shows focal, random color assignment in the tissues around the vessel.

2. The Doppler waveform shows strong but low-frequency Doppler signal symmetrically displayed above and below the base line.

3. Both findings are typical of soft tissue vibration.

4. Vibration of the soft tissues is caused by turbulent flow in the vessels. Usually it is associated with a stenosis, aneurysm, or arteriovenous fistula.

Reference

Middleton WD, Erickson S, Melson GL: Perivascular color artifact: Pathologic significance and appearance on color Doppler US imaging. *Radiology* 1989; 171:647-652.

Cross-Reference

Ultrasound: THE REQUISITES, pp 64-65.

Comment

In situations where flow velocity is extremely high or where flow is extremely disordered, turbulence may occur. Turbulence causes pressure fluctuations in the lumen of the vessel. The pressure fluctuations cause the vessel wall to vibrate. If the vessel wall vibration is strong enough, the vibrations are transmitted into the adjacent soft tissue. This perivascular soft tissue vibration may be auscultated with a stethoscope as a bruit. When it is severe, it can be palpated as a thrill.

Tissue vibrations can also be detected on Doppler scans. Since motion produces a Doppler frequency shift, the back-and-forth vibratory motion of soft tissue reflectors is recognized as a Doppler signal and displayed as random scattered red and blue color assignment centered around the abnormal vessel. The peak effect is during systole, when the velocities are the greatest. During diastole, the perivascular artifact recedes significantly. On a pulsed Doppler waveform, the signal from vibrating soft tissues is symmetric above and below the base line because the soft tissue reflections are going back and forth. In addition, the signal is strong because reflections from soft tissue interfaces are stronger than the reflections from red blood cells. On the other hand, since the speed of the vibrational motion is slow, the size of the pulsed Doppler signal is low.

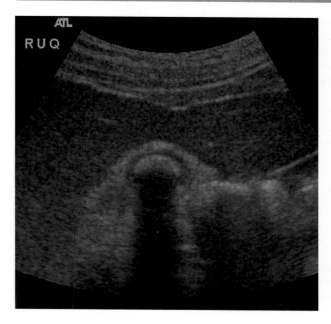 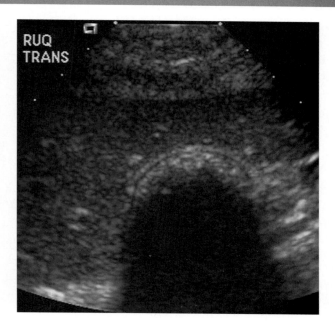

Transverse views of two gallbladders.

1. Describe the abnormal finding on these images.
2. What is the diagnosis?
3. How likely is this to be detected with CT?
4. How likely is this to be detected on an abdominal radiograph?

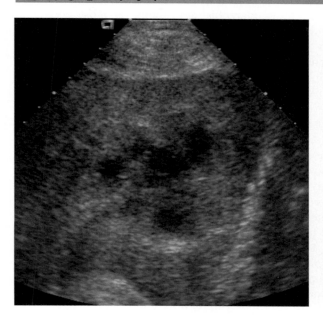 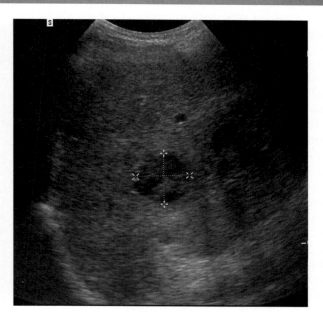

Views of the liver in two patients.

1. Describe the abnormality in these two patients.
2. What should be included in the differential diagnosis?
3. Is this lesion easier to diagnose with CT or with ultrasound?
4. What fluid-filled hepatic lesion often looks solid on sonography?

Wall-Echo-Shadow Complex

1. The finding is a bright curvilinear reflector with a dense posterior shadow (the echo and shadow) and a more superficial hypoechoic layer (the wall).

2. This finding indicates a gallbladder that is contracted and filled with stones.

3. The sensitivity of CT in detecting gallstones is less than 80%.

4. The sensitivity of radiography in detecting gallstones is 15%.

Reference

Ryubicki FJ: The WES sign. *Radiology* 2000;214:881–882.

Cross-Reference

Ultrasound: THE REQUISITES, pp 38–40.

Comment

Ultrasound is used in many situations because it is cheaper, more readily available, or safer than alternative imaging modalities. When it comes to gallstone detection, ultrasound is used simply because it is better than alternative modalities. However, in order to maintain a high sensitivity it is important to detect stones other than those that appear as the classic mobile, shadowing, echogenic structure in the lumen of a bile-filled gallbladder. One situation where stones do not have the classic appearance is when they completely fill the gallbladder lumen. In this situation, the gallbladder no longer appears as a fluid-filled (i.e., bile-filled) structure, and thus it is much more difficult to identify. Instead, a stone-filled gallbladder appears as an echogenic structure with posterior shadowing. The problem then becomes distinguishing the echogenic, shadowing, stone-filled gallbladder from the multiple echogenic, shadowing, gas-filled loops of bowel.

One means of distinguishing these entities is the wall-echo-shadow (WES) complex that is demonstrated in this case. The WES sign consists of a hypoechoic layer (the gallbladder wall), a hyperechoic layer (the leading edge of the stones), and a shadow. The WES complex is seen in many, but not all, gallbladders that are filled with stones. However, it is very unusual to see a WES complex in gas-filled bowel loops. Another factor that aids in this distinction is the nature of the shadow. Stones typically produce a well-defined, clean shadow. Gas, on the other hand, produces a less well-defined, dirty shadow. Finally, the location is also helpful, because the gallbladder is almost always located adjacent to the interlobar fissure, between the left and right lobe of the liver.

Hepatic Abscess

1. Both images show hypoechoic lesions with posterior acoustic enhancement.

2. The differential diagnosis is broad. The posterior enhancement suggests that the lesions are fluid-filled, and this makes abscess and hematoma possibilities. Solid lesions can also be associated with some degree of posterior enhancement, so metastatic disease and hepatocellular cancer are also considerations.

3. Liver abscesses often appear more characteristic on CT than on ultrasound.

4. Abscesses can appear solid on ultrasound.

Reference

Singh, Y, Winic AB, Tabbara SO: Residents' teaching files: Multiloculated cystic liver lesions: Radiologic-pathologic differential diagnosis. *Radiographics* 1997;17:219–224.

Cross-Reference

Ultrasound: THE REQUISITES, pp 14–16.

Comment

The lesions shown in this case are heterogeneous but predominantly hypoechoic. The increased through transmission suggests that the lesion is composed of fluid. Its sonographic appearance is most consistent with a complex fluid collection such as a hematoma or an abscess. It is not possible to distinguish these two abnormalities with ultrasound. In a case like this, the clinical history is critical. These patients had fever and leukocytosis, and both were subsequently proven to have an abscess when the fluid was drained percutaneously.

Gram-negative bacilli are the most common cause of pyogenic hepatic abscesses. *Escherichia coli* is cultured most often. Up to 50% of abscesses are anaerobic or mixed aerobic and anaerobic. They usually occur in the setting of infectious or inflammatory disease of the intestines, biliary tract, or adjacent organs, or are due to truma or septicemia.

Liver metastases usually appear as solid masses and typically have a target appearance or are hypoechoic. Some metastases can have cystic components and could therefore simulate a hematoma or an abscess. If patients in this case had a history of a prior malignancy, then metastatic disease to the liver would be a consideration. Hepatocellular cancer is usually entirely solid, but it may demonstrate increased through transmission and in the proper clinical setting would also be a consideration.

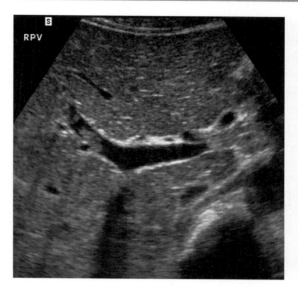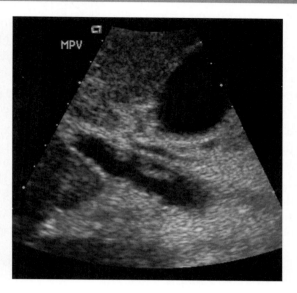

Views of the right lobe of the liver and of the porta hepatis in two patients.

1. Describe the abnormal findings.

2. What is the normal blood flow velocity in the portal vein?

3. What is the sensitivity of color Doppler in detecting the abnormality shown in this case?

4. What sorts of conditions predispose patients to this abnormality?

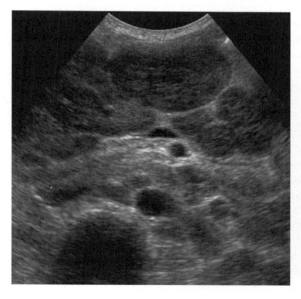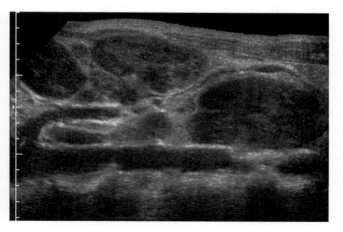

Transverse view and longitudinal extended-field-of-view scan of the mid abdomen.

1. What abnormality is demonstrated in this patient?

2. What two conditions are most likely?

3. If you were performing a biopsy on this patient, in what should the specimen be stored?

4. Would the presence of central liquefaction affect your interpretation?

Portal Vein Thrombosis

1. Both images show localized material in the lumen of the portal vein that is typical of nonobstructive thrombosis.

2. Normal portal vein flow velocity is approximately 20 cm/sec.

3. Ultrasound with color Doppler is very sensitive to portal vein thrombosis and is an appropriate initial study in patients suspected of having this diagnosis.

4. Hypercoagulable states of any sort, metastatic disease, abdominal infections or inflammatory conditions, trauma, and pregnancy predispose patients to portal vein thrombosis.

Reference

Tessler FN, Gehring BJ, Gomes AS, et al: Diagnosis of portal vein thrombosis: Value of color Doppler imaging. *AJR Am J Roentgenol* 1991;157:293–296.

Cross-Reference

Ultrasound: THE REQUISITES, pp 23–25.

Comment

Portal vein thrombosis may appear hyperechoic, iso-echoic, hypoechoic, or anechoic. When the thrombus is clearly seen on grey-scale sonography, the diagnosis is easy. However, hypoechoic or anechoic thrombus can be difficult to distinguish from low-level artifactual echoes that are often seen in the portal vein. In such cases, color Doppler is important in establishing the diagnosis. With occlusive thrombus, no flow is detectable in the affected segment of the portal vein. With nonocclusive thrombus, a flow void is present in the affected segment.

One limitation of color Doppler is that a patent portal vein may have very slow flow that cannot be detected with color Doppler. Therefore, whenever the diagnosis of portal vein thrombosis is being entertained based on lack of detectable flow, but thrombus is not confirmed on grey-scale imaging, the possibility of slow flow should also be considered. Careful attention should be paid to technical parameters that affect Doppler sensitivity so that detection of slow flow is maximized. Because portal vein flow increases after eating, postprandial scans can also help in detecting slow portal venous flow. If flow remains undetectable despite these maneuvers, portal vein thrombosis is probably present. However, slow flow remains a possibility, and other tests should be obtained to help make this distinction. Contrast enhanced Doppler should also help with this distinction. Another pitfall of color Doppler is that it can obscure focal nonobstructive thrombus that may be easy to see on grey-scale imaging alone.

Lymphoma

1. Both images show multiple hypoechoic solid masses around the mesenteric vessels and the aorta and cava. This is typical of lymphadenopathy.

2. Lymphoma and metastatic disease are the primary considerations for this degree of lymphadenopathy.

3. Whenever lymphoma is a consideration, biopsy specimens should be placed in saline (rather than formalin) so that flow cytometry can be performed. This is necessary to subcategorize the type of lymphoma.

4. Although it occurs, it is unusual to see liquefied areas in lymphoma.

References

Fisher AJ, Paulson EK, Sheafor DH, et al: Small lymph nodes of the abdomen, pelvis and retroperitoneum: Usefulness of sonographically guided biopsy. *Radiology* 1997;205:185–190.

Jing BS: Diagnostic imaging of abdominal and pelvic lymph nodes in lymphoma. *Radiol Clin North Am* 1990;28:801–831.

Cross-Reference

Genitourinary Radiology: THE REQUISITES, p 181.

Comment

The differential diagnosis of abdominal adenopathy is similar to that of adenopathy elsewhere in the body. Inflammatory and infectious conditions should be considered because they are the most common cause. Sarcoidosis is a frequently forgotten cause of abdominal adenopathy. Lymphoma and metastatic disease also must be considered, especially when nodes are as large as the ones shown in this case. Retroperitoneal and periportal adenopathy is very nonspecific, but bulky adenopathy in the mesentery is usually due to non-Hodgkin's lymphoma.

Abdominal adenopathy is often overlooked on sonography. This is probably because enlarged nodes are usually close to isoechoic when compared to the organs in the abdomen. They must be recognized as rounded or ovoid masses separate from the solid organs and the bowel. In the retroperitoneum and mesentery, nodes are best seen when the overlying structures are compressed with transducer pressure. Compression is also critical in performing ultrasound guided biopsies, which allows for biopsy of even small nodes.

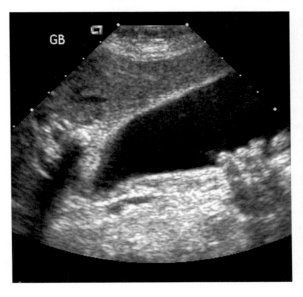
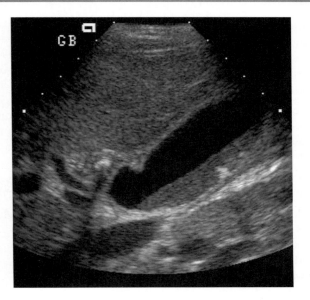

Longitudinal views of the gallbladder in two patients.

1. What is unusual about both patients?
2. What are the causes of a false-negative ultrasound in detection of gallstones?
3. What is the predictive value of a positive ultrasound in diagnosing gallstones?
4. Would cholescintigraphy be valuable in these patients?

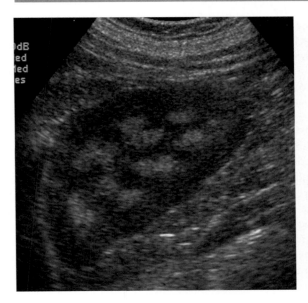
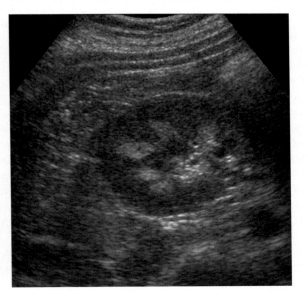

Longitudinal and transverse views of the right kidney. The left kidney had a similar appearance.

1. Describe the abnormality.
2. Is this a mild or severe form of the disease?
3. What are the three most common etiologies of this condition?
4. What would you expect to see on an abdominal radiograph?

Stones Impacted in the Gallbladder Neck

1. Both patients have stones and/or sludge layering into the dependent aspect of the gallbladder (GB). In addition, they both have impacted stones at the junction of the GB neck and cystic duct.

2. Contracted GB, extensive right upper quadrant bowel gas, very small stones, obesity, patient immobility and stones in the gallbladder neck can cause false-negative results on an ultrasound scan.

3. Almost nothing can simulate a gallstone. Therefore, the positive predictive value is close to 100%.

4. Cholescintigraphy is useful when the sonographic findings are confusing or indeterminant. It is unlikely that cholescintigraphy would be useful in these patients because an impacted stone is clearly present in both.

Reference
Middleton WD: Right upper quadrant pain. In Bluth EI, Benson C, Arger P, et al (eds): *The Practice of Ultrasonography.* New York, Thieme, 1999, pp 3-16.

Cross-Reference
Ultrasound: THE REQUISITES, pp 38-40.

Comment
A gallstone is usually quite easy to identify as an echogenic focus contrasted in the anechoic background of the intraluminal bile. However, when a stone is located in the GB neck or the cystic duct, it is not surrounded by bile and is not as obvious. In most individuals, the neck is the most posterior portion of the GB, so it is not uncommon for stones to rest in the neck in supine patients. In most cases, stones can be moved out of the neck by positioning the patient so that the neck is not the most dependent aspect of the GB. This can be accomplished in most patients by rolling the patient into a left lateral decubitus or a prone position. The left lateral decubitus position is especially beneficial because the GB is generally easiest seen with patients in this position, while it can be difficult to see well with patients in the prone position. Even when the GB is not well seen in the prone position, it is still useful to have patients roll into that position and then roll back to a left lateral decubitus position because stones may be seen rolling from the fundus back into the GB body with this maneuver. Another maneuver that may help is to have the patient stand upright and, if necessary, bend forward at the waist.

Despite these maneuvers, some stones in the GB neck will not move. As might be expected, nonmobile stones in the GB neck are one of the causes of a false-negative ultrasound. This situation occurs with obstructing stones that are impacted in the neck or with stones

that are transiently trapped behind prominent junctional folds between the GB neck and the cystic duct. To avoid overlooking this variety of stone, it is important to carefully look at the region of the gallbladder neck. A variety of approaches can be used to image the GB neck. Scanning from a subcostal approach through the fundus of the GB is often very useful. Another approach is to scan from a lateral intercostal space using the liver as a window.

Medullary Nephrocalcinosis

1. Both views show increased echogenicity of the medullary pyramids.

2. This is a mild case because the pyramids produce no shadowing. The absence of shadowing indicates that the extent of calcification is minimal.

3. Medullary sponge kidney, hyperparathyroidism, and distal renal tubular acidosis are the common causes of medullary nephrocalcinosis.

4. Radiographs are normal with mild nephrocalcinosis. In more advanced cases, radiographs show small calcifications in the expected regions of the renal pyramids.

Reference
Glazer GM, Callen PW, Filly RA: Medullary nephrocalcinosis: Sonographic evaluation. *AJR Am J Roentgenol* 1982;138:55-57.

Cross-Reference
Ultrasound: THE REQUISITES, pp 104-105.

Comment
Nephrocalcinosis refers to renal calcification outside of the collecting system. Most commonly it occurs in the medullary pyramids and is caused by hyperparathyroidism, renal tubular acidosis, or medullary sponge disease. Other, less common causes include milk alkali syndrome, sarcoidosis, and hypervitaminosis D.

On sonography, the pyramids appear hyperechoic. As the calcification progresses, shadowing is detected in some of the pyramids. Continued progression results in more pronounced shadowing from all of the pyramids. Sonography appears to be unusually sensitive in detection of medullary nephrocalcinosis. Sonographic findings clearly precede radiographic changes and are often more dramatic than the findings on CT. The best way to detect medullary nephrocalcinosis is to get a longitudinal view of the kidney just lateral to the renal sinus. In this view, the echogenic pyramids can be seen and are easier to distinguish from the echogenic renal sinus fat.

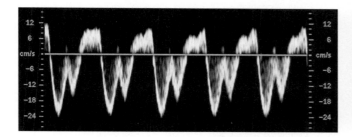
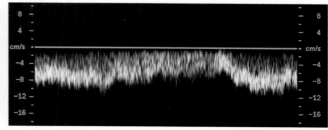

Pulsed Doppler waveforms from two veins.

1. Which waveform is from a normal hepatic vein, and which is from a peripheral systemic vein?
2. Why do the waveforms have a different appearance?
3. Identify ventricular systole, ventricular diastole, and atrial contraction on the first waveform.
4. What effect does a deep inspiration have on the hepatic vein waveform?

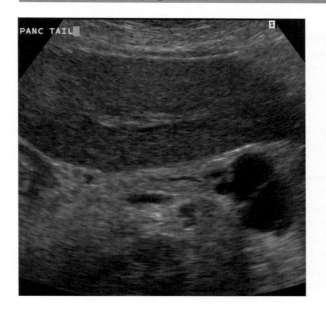
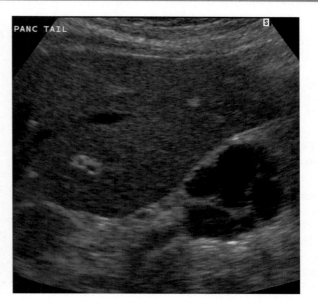

Transverse and longitudinal views of the pancreas.

1. Is this a typical location for this lesion?
2. Is this lesion benign or malignant?
3. Would you consider another diagnosis if this patient were a man?
4. At what age is this lesion most frequently seen?

Normal Hepatic Venous Waveform

1. The triphasic pattern in the first waveform is typical of a normal hepatic vein waveform. The slow respiratory phasicity of the second waveform is typical of a peripheral vein.

2. The hepatic veins are very close to the right atrium, and the pulsatility of the right atrium is readily transmitted into the hepatic veins. The peripheral extremity veins are more remote from the right atrium, and the pressure fluctuations are much more blunted or are absent.

3. Ventricular systole is the larger, first pulse below the base line. Ventricular diastole is the smaller, second pulse below the base line. Atrial contraction is the short pulse above the base line.

4. Deep inspiration causes some blunting of the normal triphasic pattern. In some cases, it eliminates all of the pulsatility.

Reference

Abu-Yousef MM: Normal and respiratory variation of the hepatic and portal venous duplex Doppler waveforms with simultaneous electrocardiographic correlation. *J Ultrasound Med* 1992;11:263-268.

Cross-Reference

Ultrasound: THE REQUISITES, pp 19-21.

Comment

Because the hepatic veins are so close to the right atrium, the pressure fluctuations in the atrium are transmitted back into the hepatic veins. This effect can be seen in the hepatic venous waveform. During right atrial contraction there is a short period where the blood flow in the hepatic vein actually reverses and heads back into the liver. This is seen as the short phase of flow above the base line. As the right atrium relaxes (corresponding to ventricular systole), blood flow rapidly exits the liver and enters the atrium, producing flow below the base line. As the atrium starts to fill up, the flow out of the liver slows, and the waveform starts to approach the base line. Then the tricuspid valve opens (at the beginning of ventricular diastole), and the right atrium starts to decompress into the right ventricle. This leads to another period of rapid outflow from the liver into the right atrium, resulting in a second pulse of flow below the base line. Finally, the right atrium starts to contract again, and the process repeats itself. The end result is a triphasic pattern with one retrograde pulse above the base line (during atrial contraction) and two antegrade pulses below the base line. The first antegrade pulse is usually the largest and occurs during ventricular systole. The second antegrade pulse is usually smaller and occurs during ventricular diastole.

The second waveform in this case came from a superficial femoral vein. Because it is so far away from the right atrium, the pulsatility related to the heart is lost. In its place is mild phasicity related to respiratory changes.

Mucinous Macrocystic Pancreatic Neoplasm

1. Mucinous macrocystic neoplasms are usually located in the body and tail of the pancreas. It is unusual to see them in the head of the pancreas.

2. This lesion is malignant or potentially malignant.

3. Yes. Mucinous macrocystic neoplasms are seen almost exclusively in women.

4. This lesion is most frequently seen in middle age.

Reference

Buetow PC, Rao P, Thompson LDR: From the archives of the AFIP: Mucinous cystic neoplasms of the pancreas: Radiologic-pathologic correlation. *Radiographics* 1998; 18:433-449.

Cross-Reference

Ultrasound: THE REQUISITES, pp 137-139.

Comment

The macrocystic mucinous pancreatic neoplasm is seen much more commonly in women than in men. They are usually located in the body or more often in the tail of the pancreas. The majority manifest in middle age. Although some of these tumors have benign histologic features, they should all be considered potentially malignant. Some experts believe that this tumor is a variety of mucin-producing pancreatic neoplasm where the abnormal ductal epithelium originated in a peripheral side branch and lost its communication with the main pancreatic duct. Even when these tumors are malignant, the prognosis is much better than it is for ductal adenocarcinoma of the pancreas. In fact, complete surgical resection results in up to 90% long-term survival.

Mucinous macrocystic tumors tend to be very large and may be either unilocular or multilocular. Solid mural nodules can occur and make the chance of frankly malignant histology more likely. When the lesion is multiloculated, the individual locules are usually larger than 2 cm. Focal areas of calcification are seen in the wall of the mass in less than 10% of patients. Unlike the microcystic pancreatic neoplasm, central calcification is rare.

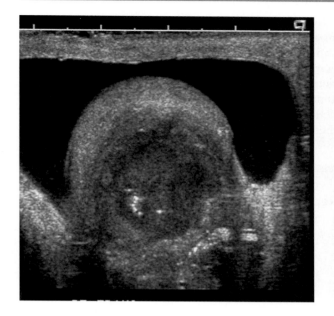
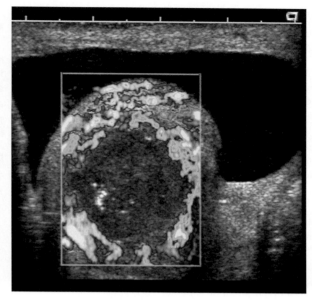

Transverse grey-scale and power Doppler views of the testis.

1. What are the major findings in this case?
2. Are these abnormalities most likely due to a neoplastic or nonneoplastic etiology?
3. Does the age of the patient help in establishing the differential diagnosis?
4. What question would you like to ask the urologist who referred the patient?

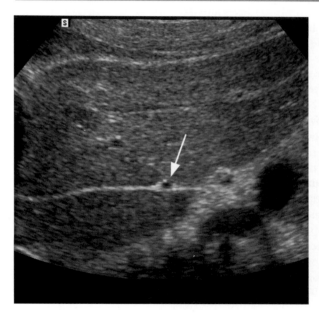
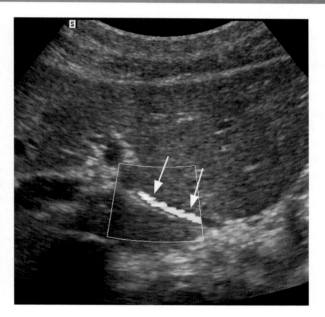

Longitudinal grey-scale view and transverse color Doppler view of the left lobe of the liver.

1. Is the structure indicated by the arrows normal?
2. Would a Doppler waveform demonstrate arterial or venous flow?
3. Is this seen commonly on ultrasound?
4. From where does this structure originate?

Testicular Abscess

1. The images show an avascular intratesticular mass, a hydrocele, and increased testicular vascularity.

2. These abnormalities are most likely nonneoplastic. Tumors would be expected to have some detectable internal flow and would not produce increased flow to the rest of the testis.

3. Tumors are less common in older men.

4. The most important clinical information is whether the lesion is palpable. Intratesticular lesions that can be palpated are much more likely to be tumors.

Reference

Horstman WG: Scrotal imaging. *Urol Clin North Am* 1997;24:653–671.

Cross-Reference

Ultrasound: THE REQUISITES, pp 445–446.

Comment

A testicular tumor (especially malignant tumors but also benign tumors) should always be considered when an intratesticular lesion is seen on sonography. However, there are many nonneoplastic conditions that can also appear as an intratesticular mass and simulate a tumor. Included in this list are hematomas, abscesses, infarctions, contusions, necrosis, inflammatory lesions, and granulomatous diseases. There is so much overlap in the grey-scale appearance of these conditions and tumors that it is not possible to rely much on the grey-scale features.

On the other hand, Doppler findings can be useful to a certain extent. Provided that appropriate transducers are used and appropriate technical adjustments are made to optimize detection of low blood flow, most tumors have at least some detectable flow, and many are hypervascular. Inflammatory lesions may also be vascular, but most other nonneoplastic lesions are avascular. This is true of fluid collections, such as hematomas and abscesses, and also of infarctions, contusions, and necrosis.

Findings on physical examination and other clinical features can be very valuable in further defining the etiology of intratesticular lesions. The most important clinical information is whether the lesion is palpable or not. Most nonneoplastic lesions are nonpalpable, and most tumors are palpable. Clinical evidence of infection or inflammation is clearly helpful in patients with orchitis or an abscess. A history of trauma certainly would lead one toward a diagnosis of hematoma or contusion, whereas a history of tuberculosis or sarcoid would suggest that an intratesticular abnormality was a granulomatous lesion.

In the final management of intratesticular lesions, surgery is usually performed if either the clinical or the sonographic findings suggest a tumor. If the sonographic, Doppler and clinical findings all suggest a nonneoplastic condition, surgery can usually be avoided and replaced with a series of follow-up sonograms to determine whether the lesion responds to conservative therapy in the expected manner.

Replaced Left Hepatic Artery

1. The arrows indicate a replaced or accessory left hepatic artery. This is a normal variant.

2. A Doppler waveform would show an arterial signal with the flow directed into the liver.

3. Because the left lobe of the liver provides such a convenient window, it is usually very easy to see the fissure for the ligamentum venosum. Because of this, replaced left hepatic arteries are also very easy to see. Careful evaluation of this region will reveal this variant in approximately 15% of patients.

4. Replaced/accessory left hepatic arteries arise from the left gastric artery.

Reference

Lafortune M, Patriquin H: The hepatic artery: Studies using Doppler sonography. *Ultrasound Q* 1999; 15(1):9–26.

Cross-Reference

Ultrasound: THE REQUISITES, pp 3–5.

Comment

A number of common vascular variants may be found in the upper abdomen. Variations in the arterial supply to the liver are among the most common. Normally, the common hepatic artery arises as a branch of the celiac axis. After the takeoff of the gastroduodenal artery, the common hepatic artery is referred to as the proper hepatic artery. The proper hepatic artery supplies the arterial flow to the liver via its right and left branches. However, both the right and left hepatic artery may arise from sites other than the proper hepatic artery.

The left hepatic artery occasionally arises from the left gastric artery. In such cases, it enters the liver through the fissure for the ligamentum venosum. It then travels to the origin of the umbilical segment of the left portal vein and enters the left lobe adjacent to this vein. It is rare to see any other vascular structures in the fissure for the ligamentum venosum, but it is common to see this arterial variant.

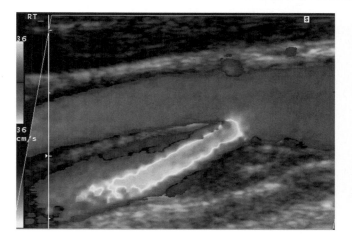
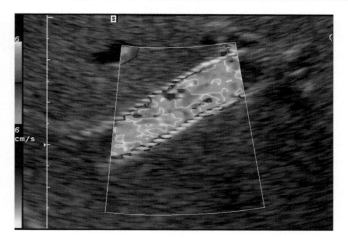

Longitudinal color Doppler view of the carotid bifurcation and a transjugular intrahepatic porto-systemic shunt. (See color plates.)

1. Where is the artifact located in the first image?
2. Where is the artifact located in the second image?
3. How can this artifact be distinguished from true flow reversal?
4. How can this artifact be eliminated?

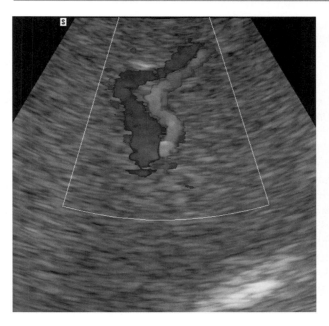
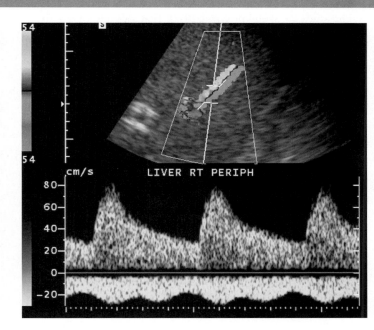

Magnified color Doppler view and pulsed Doppler waveform of the right lobe of the liver in two patients. (See color plates.)

1. What is the abnormality common to both of these patients?
2. Is it normal to see any pulsations in the portal vein?
3. Does the abnormality shown in this case occur most often in the right or in the left portal vein?
4. Is this abnormality seen early or late in the underlying disease process?

Aliasing

1. The first image shows aliasing in the center of the internal carotid artery.

2. The second image shows severe aliasing throughout the lumen of the stent.

3. With aliasing, the color conversion occurs from the high frequency shifts on one side of the scale to the high frequency shifts on the other side of the scale. This is shown on the first image as conversion from light red to light blue. True flow reversal occurs from the low frequency shifts. This is shown on the first image at the periphery of the internal carotid origin.

4. Aliasing can be eliminated or decreased by increasing the Doppler angle, increasing the Doppler scale, or decreasing the transmitted frequency.

Reference

Middleton WD: Color Doppler image optimization and interpretation. *Ultrasound Q* 1998;14:194–208.

Cross-Reference

Ultrasound: THE REQUISITES, p 474.

Comment

Aliasing is a well-known artifact that occurs when the Doppler sampling rate (i.e., the pulse repetition frequency or PRF) is less than twice the Doppler frequency shift. When aliasing occurs on color Doppler images, there is a wrap-around effect so that the color representing the highest positive frequency shift changes to the color representing the highest negative frequency shift, or vice versa. This change in color assignment can be distinguished from true flow reversal because the change is between light color shades rather than between dark color shades. When aliasing is severe, there can be multiple wrap-arounds of the color assignment, and this can produce an appearance of random color assignment that simulates noise or severe flow turbulence (as seen in the TIPS shunt). Although aliasing is artifactual, when properly recognized, it can be useful because it dramatically identifies areas of high frequency shifts, and these areas of high frequency shifts often correspond to areas of high flow velocity.

Aliasing can be diminished or eliminated by increasing the PRF. In most instances, the maximum PRF is limited by the depth of the vessel, because it takes a finite amount of time to deliver the Doppler pulse to the vessel and wait for the echo to return to the transducer before the next pulse is transmitted. Another means of decreasing or eliminating aliasing is to decrease the observed frequency shift. This can be done by manipulating the transducer so that the vessel is scanned at a Doppler angle closer to 90 degrees or by switching to a lower frequency transducer.

Portal Vein Flow Reversal

1. The color Doppler view shows parallel vessels. The only vessels that travel in a parallel fashion are the hepatic arteries and portal veins. The different color assignments indicate that flow in the artery and vein are in opposite directions. The waveform shows simultaneous arterial flow and venous flow on different sides of the base line. This also indicates that flow is in different directions. In the liver, flow in both vessels should be in the same direction, that is, into the liver. In this case the portal venous flow is reversed.

2. There are mild pulsations in the portal venous signal. This is within normal limits. Severe portal vein pulsations indicate right heart dysfunction.

3. A common portal systemic collateral in patients with portal hypertension is the recanalized umbilical vein, which is supplied by the left portal vein. A common finding in these patients is reversed right portal flow that crosses the portal bifurcation and contributes to antegrade left portal flow and ultimately to flow into the umbilical vein.

4. Reversal of portal venous flow is a late sign of portal hypertension.

Reference

Ralls PW: Color Doppler sonography of the hepatic artery and portal venous system. *AJR Am J Roentgenol* 1990;155:517–525.

Cross-Reference

Ultrasound: THE REQUISITES, pp 19–23.

Comment

Under normal circumstances, portal venous blood flow travels into the liver. With diffuse liver disease such as cirrhosis, the resistance to portal vein flow increases. Increased portal pressures then develop in an attempt to maintain constant portal perfusion of the liver. As the portal pressure rises, portal-systemic collaterals start to develop. As the liver disease progresses, resistance to flow increases to the point that hepatic arterial flow cannot effectively cross the sinusoidal bed of the liver. At this point, hepatic artery flow is shunted into the portal vein system, and the portal vein flow reverses. In essence, the portal vein becomes an outflow tract for the liver. With advanced portal hypertension, portal vein flow reversal initially starts in the peripheral portal veins. If the process progresses, flow reversal may start to effect the central portal veins and even the main portal vein.

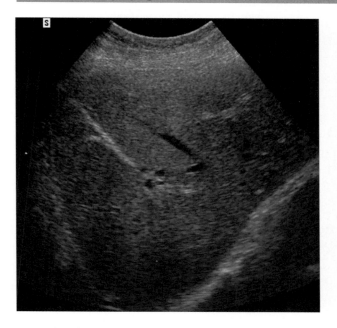
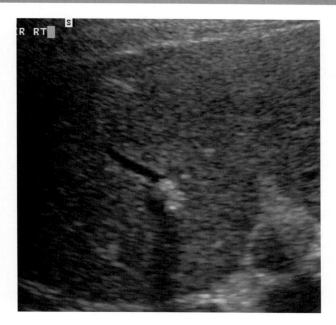

Standard and magnified transverse views of the right lobe of the liver.

1. What is the abnormality?
2. What is the differential diagnosis?
3. What underlying abnormality would you suspect if this patient were Asian?
4. Which test would be most useful in further management of this patient, CT, ultrasound guided biopsy, or endoscopic retrograde cholangiopancreatography (ERCP)?

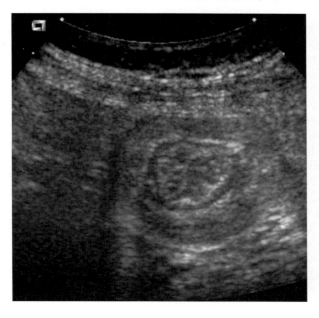
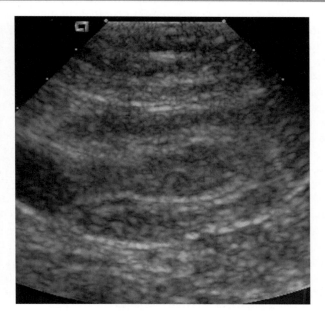

Views of the left mid abdomen.

1. Describe the abnormality shown on these images.
2. What is the differential diagnosis?
3. Is this abnormality more common in children or in adults?
4. Does color Doppler have a role in evaluating patients with this abnormality?

Intrahepatic Bile Duct Stones

1. The first image shows a branching, hyperechoic linear structure in the periphery of the right lobe. The magnified image shows a dilated intrahepatic duct and three adjacent stones with slight shadowing.

2. The differential diagnosis includes intrahepatic duct stone, biliary air, and calcified intrahepatic arteries.

3. Oriental cholangiohepatitis (also known as recurrent pyogenic cholangitis) would be suspected.

4. ERCP would be the most helpful next test.

Reference

Kirby, CL, Horrow MM, Rosenberg HK, Oleaga JA: US case of the day: Oriental cholangiohepatitis. *Radiographics* 1995;15:1503–1506.

Cross-Reference

Ultrasound: THE REQUISITES, pp 61–63.

Comment

Intrahepatic duct stones usually occur in the setting of abnormal bile ducts. The classic condition associated with intrahepatic duct stones is recurrent pyogenic cholangitis, also known as Oriental cholangiohepatitis. In this disease, bile stasis is believed to cause infection, which results in deconjugation of bile and precipitation of calcium bilirubinate crystals that ultimately form multiple intrahepatic pigmented stones. These stones are soft (muddy) and may form a cast of the bile duct lumen. When they shadow, the diagnosis is usually evident. However, they may not produce enough acoustic attenuation to cause shadowing, and thus they may be confused with blood clots or tumors of the duct. Other conditions that cause biliary stasis can result in stones that form primarily in the ducts. Sclerosing cholangitis and Caroli's disease are two examples.

One of the conditions easiest to mistake for intrahepatic stones is biliary air. Both can appear as shadowing echogenic material in the bile ducts. However, air is usually more echogenic, more mobile, casts a dirtier shadow, or produces a ring-down artifact. Intrahepatic stones rarely are mobile and never cause a ring-down artifact. It is important to realize that patients can have both air and stones in the bile ducts. If there is a significant amount of pneumobilia, it may be impossible to determine whether the intrahepatic ducts are dilated and also if there are stones present. Calcified arteries can also cause confusion. Visualization of more central arterial calcification in the larger vessels can point to the correct diagnosis.

Intussusception

1. A target-like lesion with multiple concentric rings. This is a typical appearance for an intussusception.

2. The differential diagnosis includes bowel wall thickening from any cause, feces in the colon, intramural hematoma, or, potentially, a volvulus.

3. Intussusception is much more common in early childhood than in adults.

4. Color Doppler can help because lack of detectable blood flow predicts the need for surgery and increases the likelihood of bowel wall necrosis.

Reference

Del-Pozo G, Albillos JC, Tejodor D: Intussusception: US findings with pathologic correlation: The crescent in doughnut sign. *Radiology* 1996;199:688–692.

Cross-Reference

Gastrointestinal Radiology: THE REQUISITES, pp 132–133.

Comment

Intussusception represents the invagination of one loop of bowel into another loop of bowel. The proximal segment that enters the intussusception is called the intussusceptum, and the distal segment that receives the intussusceptum is called the intussuscipiens. A variety of causes give rise to intussusception. In children, they are most often idiopathic and located at the ileocolic junction. In adults, they are often associated with a lead mass (polyps, lipomas, metastases, lymphomas, cancer), Meckel's diverticulum, or celiac disease. However, the increased use of ultrasound and CT has led to increased detection of transient idiopathic intussusceptions in adults. In this case, a small bowel series was performed two hours after the ultrasound, and the intussusception was resolved and no mass was seen.

The sonographic appearance of an intussusception is predictable. Three concentric layers of bowel wall result in multiple concentric, hypoechoic, and echogenic rings. In many cases, the intussuscepted mesentery can be seen in the proximal aspect of the intussusception as a slightly eccentric echogenic structure. The appearance of an intussusception has been variously compared to a target, a bull's eye, a doughnut, a pseudokidney, and a sandwich.

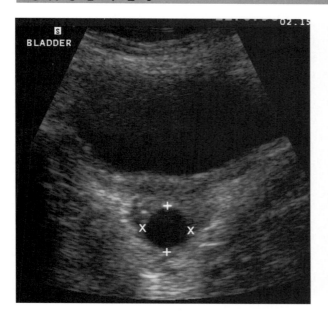 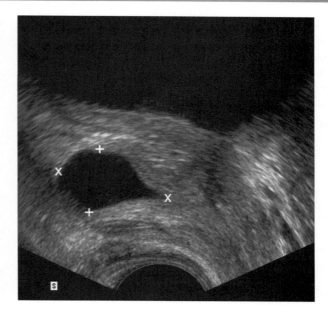

Transverse transabdominal view of the bladder and sagittal endorectal view of the prostate.

1. Describe the abnormality.
2. What is the differential diagnosis?
3. What type of cyst in this area is associated with congenital anomalies of the genitourinary system?
4. How often does prostate cancer have cystic components?

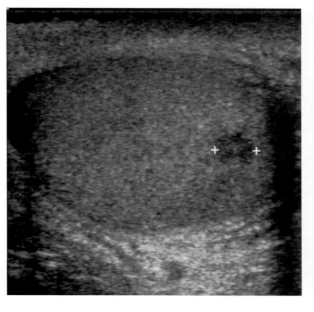 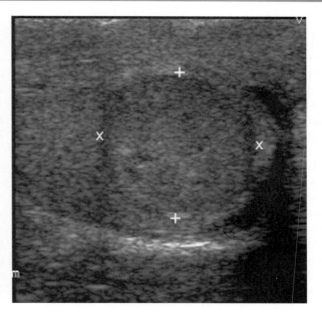

Views of the scrotum in two patients with the same abnormality.

1. What is the differential diagnosis?
2. What is the most likely diagnosis if these were boys with precocious puberty?
3. If these lesions are tumors, are they likely to be palpable?
4. If these lesions are inflammatory, are they likely to be palpable?

CASE 120

Prostatic Cyst

1. The transabdominal image shows a simple-appearing cyst posterior to the bladder. The endorectal view shows that the cyst is located in the midline, has a teardrop shape, and arises from the prostate.

2. The most likely diagnosis is a prostatic utricle cyst or a müllerian duct cyst. An ejaculatory cyst is also a consideration, although that type of cyst tends to deviate more from the midline.

3. Seminal vesicle cysts are believed to arise from an embryologic abnormality of the mesonephric duct that can also lead to ipsilateral agenesis of the kidney and vas deferens and ectopic ureteral insertion. Utricle cysts can also be associated with hypospadias, cryptorchidism, and renal agenesis.

4. Prostate cancer only rarely has significant cystic components.

Reference
Ngheim HT, Kellman GM, Sandberg SA, Craig BM: Cystic lesions of the prostate. *Radiographics* 1990;10:635–650.

Cross-Reference
Ultrasound: THE REQUISITES, pp 461–462.

Comment
A variety of cysts can occur within or adjacent to the prostate. Utricle cysts and müllerian duct cysts appear in the midline and originate within the prostate. Utricle cysts are typically fairly small. Müllerian duct cysts may become larger and extend above the prostate. It is difficult to distinguish these cysts sonographically. Utricle cysts communicate with the urethra and can cause postvoid dribbling.

Ejaculatory cysts occur near the midline along the course of the ejaculatory duct. They may be congenital or due to obstruction of the ejaculatory duct. They are typically asymptomatic, although when they enlarge, they can cause perineal pain, pain with ejaculation, dysuria, and hematospermia. They contain spermatozoa, so aspiration can help to distinguish them from other prostatic cysts.

Cysts of the seminal vesicles are distinguishable from prostatic cysts because they are located superior to the prostate and are lateral to the midline. As mentioned previously, they are associated with other genitourinary anomalies. They are also associated with autosomal dominant polycystic kidney disease. Dilatation of the seminal vesicle can be confused with a seminal vesicle cyst. Seminal vesicle dilatation can occur as a result of obstruction of the seminal vesicle or ejaculatory duct and can be due to benign prostatic hypertrophy or may follow prostatic surgery.

CASE 121

Leydig Cell Tumor

1. Intratesticular lesions that are hypoechoic, round, and well defined are usually tumors. Germ cell tumors are most common. In the proper clinical setting, lymphoma and metastases are considerations. Primary benign stromal tumors are much less common but should also be considered. Nonneoplastic lesions such as abscess, hematoma, focal orchitis, and granulomatous disease are also possibilities that should be considered if the history is appropriate.

2. Leydig cell tumors can manifest with precocious puberty.

3. Most testicular tumors are palpable. In this case, the smaller lesion was too small to feel.

4. Inflammatory conditions that cause focal testicular lesions are usually not palpable.

Reference
Horstman WG, Haluszka MM, Burkhard TB: Management of testicular masses incidentally discovered by ultrasound. *J Urol* 1994;151:1263–1265.

Cross-Reference
Ultrasound: THE REQUISITES, pp 439–440.

Comment
Stromal cell tumors of the testis account for approximately 5% of testicular neoplasms. They may contain Leydig, granulosa, thecal, or lutein cells. Ninety percent of stromal cell tumors are histologically benign. The majority of stromal cell neoplasms are Leydig cell tumors. These occur most often between the ages of 20 and 50 years. Androgens, estrogens, or combinations of both may be secreted by these tumors. Therefore, patients may present with gynecomastia, precocious puberty, impotence, and loss of libido.

Sonographically, stromal cell tumors are indistinguishable from germ cell tumors. They tend to be homogeneous, solid, and hypoechoic. Cystic areas and calcifications are uncommon unless the tumor is large and has undergone hemorrhage and/or necrosis. Like other testicular tumors, they usually have detectable internal blood flow and they are usually palpable unless they are quite small. Interestingly, small stromal cell tumors are the most common incidental, nonpalpable lesion discovered in patients being scanned for other reasons.

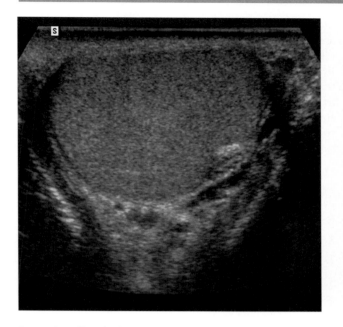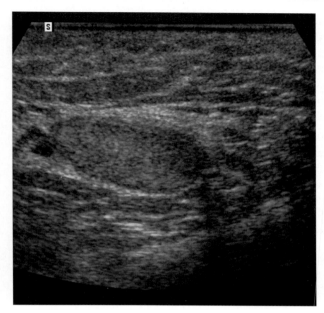

Longitudinal views of the right and left testes.

1. What is the most likely explanation for the difference in appearance of the two testes in this patient?
2. What are two important complications of this condition?
3. How often is the condition bilateral?
4. Under what circumstances is this a surgical condition?

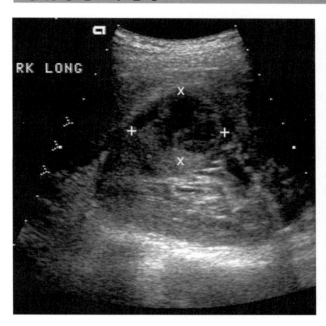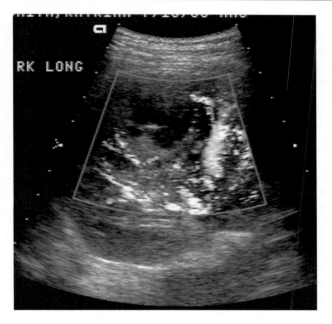

Longitudinal grey-scale and color Doppler view of the right kidney.

1. What is the sonographic abnormality seen in these images?
2. If this patient had pyuria, what would be the most likely diagnosis?
3. If this patient had hematuria, what would be the most likely diagnosis?
4. If this patient had a history of trauma, what would be the most likely diagnosis?

Undescended Testis

1. The smaller testis with more overlying soft tissue is undescended and located in the inguinal canal. Obviously, making this diagnosis is much easier when scanning the patient yourself, when you can observe that the abnormal testis is not located in the scrotum.

2. Infertility and development of malignant germ cell tumors are two important complications.

3. Approximately 10% are bilateral.

4. Surgery is usually performed if the condition persists after 1 year of age or if a testicular tumor is identified.

Reference

Horstman WG: Scrotal imaging. *Urol Clin North Am* 1997;24:653–671.

Cross-Reference

Genitourinary Radiology: THE REQUISITES, pp 319–320.

Comment

Undescended testes, also referred to as cryptorchid testes, occur in approximately 4% of term infants and 30% of premature infants. In premature babies, the testis will usually descend into the scrotum by 3 months of age. At 1 year of age, the incidence is about 1%. Approximately 80% of undescended testes are located in the inguinal region. Most of these are just distal to the external inguinal ring, and the rest are in the inguinal canal. Intra-abdominal testes are located in the retroperitoneum anywhere along the path of testicular descent, from the lower pole of the kidney to the more common location near the internal inguinal ring.

Many undescended testes are histologically abnormal and demonstrate altered spermatogenesis. This leads to a high rate of infertility. They are also predisposed to germ cell tumors of the testis, especially seminoma. The risk of germ cell tumors in the cryptorchid testis is as much as 40 times higher than in the normal testis, and intra-abdominal testes have an even higher risk of cancer than intrainguinal testes. Additional complications of undescended testes include torsion and inguinal hernias. Given the likelihood of eventual descent into the scrotum, undescended testes are usually not treated until 1 year of age. Between ages 1 and 5, the risk of cancer can be eliminated by performing orchiopexy. Between the ages of 5 and 10, the impact of orchiopexy on the risk of cancer diminishes, so complete orchiectomy is usually considered.

The tissue covering an undescended testis is almost always thicker than normal scrotal tissue. This finding can be a clue to the diagnosis even when the anatomic location of the scans is uknown. Intra-abdominal testes are often located immediately adjacent to the external iliac vessels, and this is another clue to the diagnosis. In some cases, the echogenicity of an undescended testis is heterogeneous, but a discrete mass is not seen. In other cases, the depth of the testes and the small size of the testis precludes adequate evaluation with sonography. In both these situations, MRI may be helpful for further evaluation.

Renal Abscess

1. A complex cystic lesion in the kidney.

2. Renal abscess.

3. Renal tumor, especially renal cell cancer.

4. Renal hematoma.

Reference

Baumgarten DA, Baumgarten BR: Imaging and radiologic management of upper urinary tract infections. *Urol Clin North Am* 1997;24:545–569.

Cross-Reference

Ultrasound: THE REQUISITES, pp 99–100.

Comment

This case illustrates the differential diagnosis of complex fluid collections in the kidney. Given the nonspecific appearance on ultrasound, lesions such as this require careful correlation with the clinical history.

Renal abscesses occur most often as the result of inadequate treatment of pyelonephritis. The typical situation in which imaging is requested is a patient with pyelonephritis who has not responded after 72 hours of antibiotic treatment. Patients at increased risk for abscess formation include those with obstructed collecting systems, stones, diabetes, and a history of intravenous drug abuse.

Sonographically, renal abscesses are usually solitary, round, complex collections. They may have a visible, thick wall. Depending on the amount of fluid and the composition of the fluid, there may be detectable posterior acoustic enhancement. When an abscess is well walled off, low-level echoes may be seen diffusely throughout the lesion or may settle to the dependent portion of the lesion and form a fluid level. Occasionally gas bubbles form and produce typical bright reflectors, sometimes with ring-down artifacts. Although ultrasound can detect most significant renal abscesses, contrast enhanced CT is clearly superior and should be considered when the ultrasound is negative and clinical suspicion remains high.

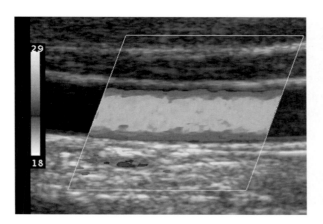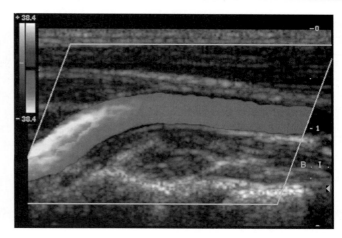

Color Doppler views of the common carotid artery and the vertebral artery. (See color plates.)

1. On what is color coding based?
2. Why is the color in the periphery of the common carotid artery different than in the center of the vessel?
3. Why is the color in the normal vertebral artery different in the proximal and distal segments?
4. On what is the Doppler frequency shift dependent?

CASE 125

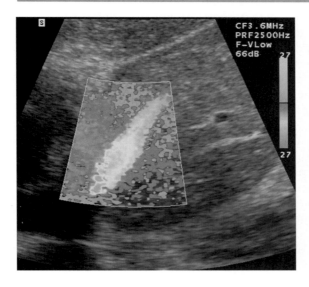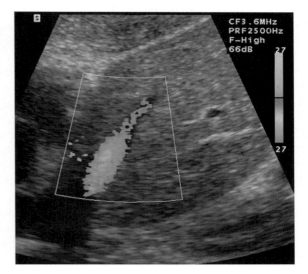

Longitudinal color Doppler views of the left hepatic lobe and left hepatic vein. (See color plates.)

1. What causes the extravascular color assignment on the first image?
2. How has the extravascular color assignment been eliminated on the second image?
3. What is another way to eliminate artifactual color assignment that obscures background tissues?
4. Is it possible to suppress Doppler signals from flowing blood?

Changes in Color Shading

1. Color coding is based on the mean Doppler frequency shift.

2. The color variations in the common carotid artery are due to differences in the flow velocity along the wall of the vessel and in the center of the vessel.

3. The color changes in the vertebral artery are due to changes in the direction of the vessel and resulting changes in the Doppler angle.

4. The Doppler frequency is dependent on the velocity, Doppler angle, transmitted frequency, and speed of sound.

Reference
Middleton WD: Color Doppler image optimization and interpretation. *Ultrasound Q* 1998;14:194–208.

Cross-Reference
Ultrasound: THE REQUISITES, pp 464–470.

Comment
The Doppler equation, which follows, indicates that the Doppler frequency shift is proportional to the blood flow velocity:

$$Fd = Ft \times V \times \cos\theta \times 1/C \times 2$$

where, Fd = Doppler frequency shift, Ft = transmitted Doppler frequency, V = velocity of blood flow, θ = angle between the transmitted Doppler pulse and the direction of blood flow, and C = speed of sound.

Therefore, higher flow velocities produce higher frequency shifts and are assigned lighter color shades. In situations where the blood vessel is straight and the orientation of the Doppler pulse is constant, the primary color assignment is usually constant throughout the vessel, and any variation in color shading indicates a change in velocity.

The Doppler equation also indicates that the frequency shift is proportional to the cosine of θ. Because of this, the Doppler frequency shift is maximal for a given velocity when the direction of the Doppler pulse is parallel to the direction of the flow velocity ($\theta = 0°$) because the cosine of 0 degrees is 1. When the Doppler pulse and the flow velocity are oriented perpendicular to each other ($\theta = 90°$), the cosine of 90° is 0, and there is little, if any, detectable Doppler shift. Because of this angle effect, vessels that have a uniform flow velocity may vary in their color shading owing to changes in the Doppler angle. This situation arises frequently with curving vessels. Likewise, the color assignment and color shade may change when the direction of the Doppler pulse changes, as with sector or curvilinear probes.

Use of the Wall Filter to Suppress Tissue Motion

1. The extravascular color assignment is caused by tissue motion related to cardiac pulsations.

2. The wall filter has been increased. This is shown on the display of technical parameters as F–VLow (filter very low) and F–High (filter high).

3. Adjust the color priority.

4. Improper adjustment of both the wall filter and the color priority can suppress Doppler signals from intravascular blood flow as well as from moving soft tissues.

Reference
Middleton WD: Color Doppler image optimization and interpretation. *Ultrasound Q* 1998;14:194–208.

Cross-Reference
Ultrasound: THE REQUISITES, pp 464–470.

Comment
Doppler techniques are intended to detect moving blood cells in the vascular system. Since moving reflectors produce a Doppler shift, blood that is flowing in a sufficient quantity and at a sufficient velocity can be detected with Doppler techniques. Unfortunately, tissues in the body other than blood also move to some degree. In this case, cardiac contractions have resulted in movement of the left hepatic lobe. This movement has produced enough of a Doppler shift to be detected by the ultrasound equipment, and thus, color has been assigned to nonvascular portions of the left lobe. Respiratory motion, bowel peristalsis, fetal movement, and muscular contraction are other examples of nonvascular motion that can produce unwanted Doppler signals. In the vascular system, movement of the vessel wall can also produce a Doppler signal.

In situations such as those just described, eliminating unwanted signals or artifactual signals is more important than detecting low-volume or low-velocity flow. One control that is intended to filter out frequency shifts arising from pulsating vessel walls or moving soft tissues is called the wall filter, a high pass filter that allows frequency shifts above a certain level to be displayed while frequency shifts below that level are not displayed. Use of this filter can produce the desired effect of reducing or eliminating tissue motion. It is important to recognize however, that if the wall filter is adjusted improperly, it can also filter out true low-level blood flow. Therefore, in situations where there is little tissue motion and not much background noise, the wall filter can be lowered to ensure that low-velocity or low-volume flow is detected.

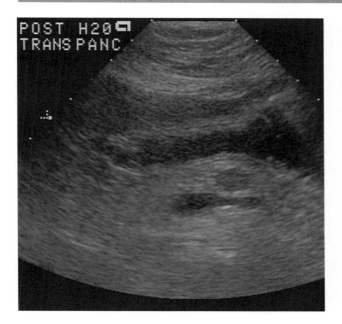
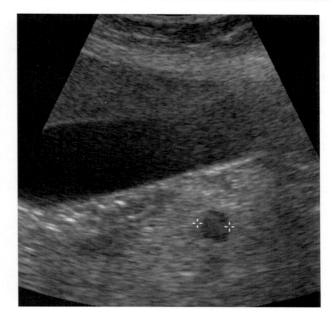

**Transverse view of the pancreatic body and longitudinal view
of the pancreatic head in two patients.**

1. What are the two tumors that should be considered first in your differential diagnosis?

2. Which of these tumors is more likely to contain calcifications?

3. Which of these tumors is hypovascular?

4. Which of these tumors most often obstructs the pancreatic duct?

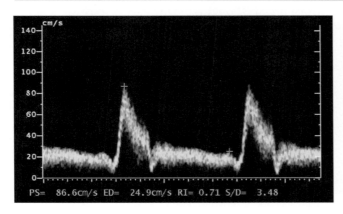
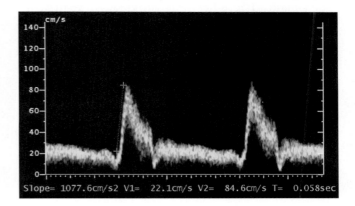

Pulsed Doppler waveform with two spectral measurements.

1. What is being measured in the first image?

2. Is this measurement dependent on the Doppler angle?

3. What is being measured in the second image?

4. Is this measurement dependent on the Doppler angle?

Islet Cell Tumor of the Pancreas

1. Adenocarcinoma and islet cell tumors are the most likely possibilities.

2. Islet cell tumor is more likely to contain calcifications.

3. Adenocarcinoma is hypovascular.

4. Adenocarcinoma more commonly obstructs the duct.

Reference

Beutow PC, Miller DL, Parrino TV, Buck JL: Islet cell tumors of the pancreas: Clinical radiologic and pathologic correlation in diagnosis and localization. *Radiographics* 1997;17:453-471.

Cross-Reference

Ultrasound: THE REQUISITES, pp 136-138.

Comment

Islet cell tumors are much less common than ductal adenocarcinoma of the pancreas. The most common type of islet cell tumor is the insulinoma. In approximately 90% of cases this occurs as a solitary lesion. Approximately 10% of cases are multiple, and 10% are malignant. Owing to hypersecretion of insulin, patients usually present at an early stage, when the tumor is small (typically 1.5 cm or less), with symptoms of hypoglycemia such as headaches, fainting, fatigue, drowsiness, seizures, and personality changes.

Gastrinomas are the next most common type of islet cell tumor. They differ from insulinomas in that they are most often malignant, they are frequently multiple, and they occur most often in the head of the pancreas and the wall of the duodenum. They are the most common islet cell tumor in patients with multiple endorine neoplasia (MEN) type I syndrome. Other rare islet cell tumors include glucagonomas, vipomas, somatostatinomas, and nonfunctioning tumors. Nonfunctioning tumors manifest later and are therefore more likely to be large and often contain cystic areas of necrosis as well as calcification.

On sonography, functioning islet cell tumors usually appear as small, well-marginated, homogeneous, hypoechoic lesions. Central calcification or cystic changes can occur and increase the likelihood of malignancy. The lesions are usually hypervascular on contrast enhanced CT or angiography, but this vascularity is usually not detectable on transabdominal Doppler. Although the imaging features overlap with those of ductal adenocarcinoma, islet cell tumors are usually smaller and better defined and lack the tendency to encase adjacent arteries and obstruct the pancreatic and bile ducts. Liver metastases from islet cell cancers are sometimes hyperechoic, and this is unusual for metastases from adenocarcinoma of the pancreas.

Spectral Doppler Measurements

1. The first measurement is the resistive index (RI).

2. The RI is independent of the Doppler angle.

3. The second measurement is the systolic acceleration.

4. The acceleration is dependent on the Doppler angle.

Reference

Nelson TR, Pretorius DH: The Doppler signal: Where does it come from and what does it mean? *AJR Am J Roentgenol* 1988;151:439-447.

Cross-Reference

Ultrasound: THE REQUISITES, pp 464-470.

Comment

A number of measurements are used to analyze arterial waveforms. The most common is the resistive index (RI), defined as:

$$RI = 1 - (D/S) = (S - D)/S$$

where S is the peak systolic velocity (or frequency shift) and D is the end diastolic velocity (or frequency shift). The RI goes up when resistance to flow goes up. When there is no diastolic flow, the RI is 1. Because the calculation depends only on the ratio of systolic to diastolic flow, it is independent of Doppler angle. Parenchymal organs should normally have a resistive index of less than 0.7.

Another common measurement is the pulsatility index, defined as:

$$PI = (S - D)/M$$

where M is the mean flow velocity throughout the cardiac cycle. The pulsatility index is probably a truer indication of vascular resistance than the resistive index, but because it is harder to measure, it has not gained widespread use. Like the RI, pulsatility index is independent of Doppler angle.

In addition to these measurements of vascular resistance, measurements of systolic upstroke are also becoming more widely used as a means of detecting proximal arterial stenosis. The early systolic acceleration is one such parameter. It is obtained by measuring the slope (change in velocity divided by change in time) of the early systolic upstroke. Unlike the RI and the pulsatility index, systolic acceleration requires determination of an absolute difference in velocities and thus must be calculated from an *angle-corrected* velocity waveform.

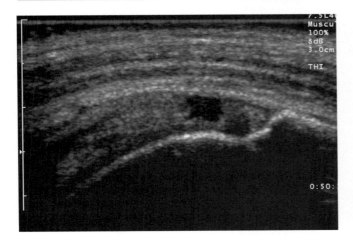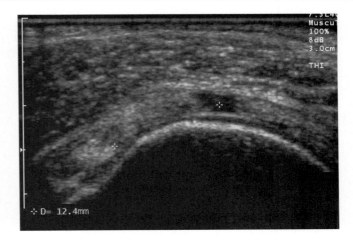

Longitudinal and transverse views of the shoulder.

1. Is the abnormality shown in these images a common or uncommon cause of shoulder pain?
2. Is this patient likely to be younger than 40 years old?
3. What tendon(s) is/are involved?
4. What is the sensitivity of ultrasound in establishing this diagnosis?

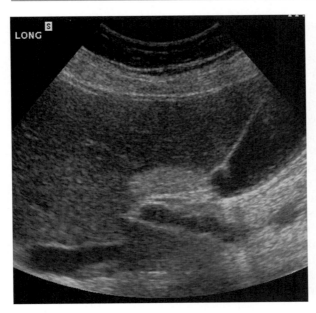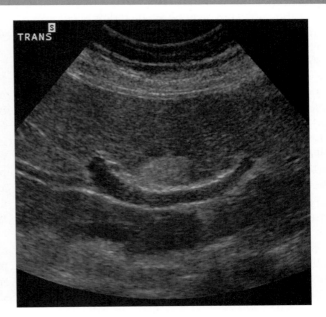

Longitudinal and transverse views of the liver in the region of the portal vein bifurcation.

1. What comes to mind when you see an echogenic lesion anywhere in the body?
2. What is the differential diagnosis for hyperechoic liver masses?
3. What is most characteristic about this lesion?
4. If necessary, how would you confirm the diagnosis?

C A S E 1 2 8

Full Thickness Rotator Cuff Tear

1. Rotator cuff disorders are the most common cause of shoulder pain and dysfunction.

2. Full thickness rotator cuff tears are uncommon in patients younger than 40 years old, unless there is a history of unusual athletic activity.

3. The transverse view shows that the tear is located 12 mm from the biceps tendon. This is in the territory of the supraspinatus.

4. Ultrasound is capable of detecting close to 100% of full thickness rotator cuff tears.

Reference

Teefey SA, Middleton WD, Yamaguchi K: Shoulder sonography: State of the art. *Radiol Clin North Am* 1999;37:767-786.

Cross-Reference

Ultrasound: THE REQUISITES, pp 455-457.

Comment

Full thickness rotator cuff tears refer to tears that extend from the deep surface of the cuff to the superficial surface of the cuff. They may be small and only involve a tiny region of a single tendon, or they may be large and involve multiple tendons. The majority of tears originate at the site of insertion of the supraspinatus tendon to the greater tuberosity. From there, they may extend posteriorly to involve the infraspinatus, extend medially to involve the more proximal supraspinatus, or extend in both directions. The subscapularis tendon may also be involved with massive full thickness rotator cuff tears. However, it is rare to have an isolated tear of the subscapularis tendon in the absence of a prior anterior shoulder dislocation or a dislocated biceps tendon.

The sonographic appearance of full thickness rotator cuff tears depends on whether there is a significant amount of fluid in the joint. When fluid is present, the tear appears as a fluid-filled defect. This type of tear is referred to as a wet tear, and these are generally very easy to identify, and the appearance is easy to understand. Such is the case in the images shown here.

Once a full thickness tear has been identified, it is important to determine which tendons are involved. If the tear just involves the first 1.5 cm of cuff behind the biceps tendon, then it is isolated to the supraspinatus. If it extends to involve the cuff more than 1.5 cm behind the biceps, then the infraspinatus is also involved. These measurements are made on the short axis (transverse) views. The degree of retraction of the cuff from the greater tuberosity is measured on the long axis (longitudinal) view.

C A S E 1 2 9

Focal Fatty Infiltration of the Liver

1. Things that cause increased echogenicity in a lesion include air, calcification, fat (usually mixed with soft tissue or liquid), and multiple interfaces.

2. The basic differential diagnosis for hyperechoic liver masses includes hemangioma, focal fat, metastatic disease, and hepatocellular cancer. Adenoma and focal nodular hyperplasia (FNH) are less likely possibilities. Gas-containing abscesses are a consideration in the proper clinical setting.

3. The characteristic features in this case of focal fat infiltration are the typical location in the preportal region of the liver and the nonspherical shape.

4. Fatty infiltration of the liver can be confirmed with a high degree of certainty with MRI.

Reference

Yoshikawa J, Matsui O, Takashima T, et al: Focal fatty change of the liver adjacent to the falciform ligament: CT and sonographic findings in five surgically confirmed cases. *AJR Am J Roentgenol* 1987;149:491-494.

Cross-Reference

Ultrasound: THE REQUISITES, pp 16-20.

Comment

Focal fatty infiltration of the liver is a relatively common condition that produces areas of increased echogenicity in the hepatic parenchyma. It may be multifocal or isolated. When it is multifocal, it is typically geographic in shape and produces no mass effect on adjacent structures. When it is solitary, it usually localizes to the preportal portion of the liver (as in this case), or to the anterior aspect of the left hepatic lobe adjacent to the ligamentum teres. Nonspherical echogenic lesions in these locations require no further workup.

In addition to these typical appearances, fatty infiltration occasionally looks very nodular and localizes to nonspecific areas of the liver. In such cases, the diagnosis cannot be made by sonography. MRI with chemical shift imaging, using in- and out-of-phase (opposed phase) sequences, can establish a confident diagnosis of fatty infiltration in most of these cases.

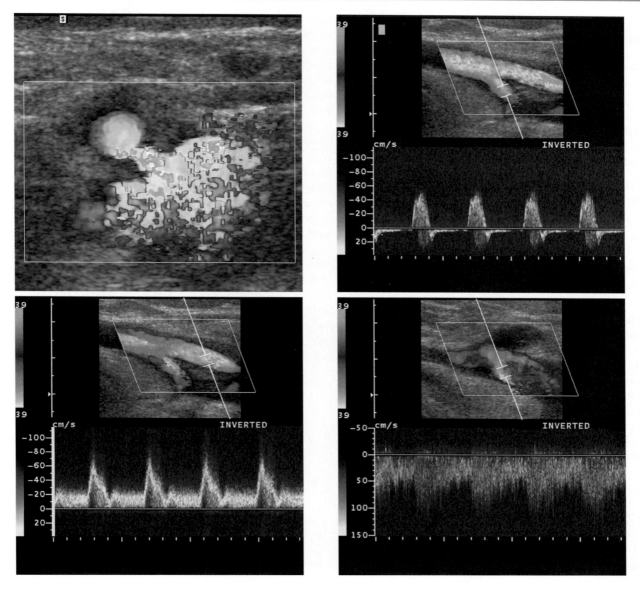

Transverse color Doppler view of the groin and pulsed Doppler waveforms from the profunda femoral artery, superficial femoral artery, and the femoral vein. (See color plates.)

1. Describe the important findings.

2. Is this abnormality seen most often above or below the femoral bifurcation?

3. What are the typical grey-scale findings in this condition?

4. How do these patients usually present clinically?

Femoral Arteriovenous Fistula

1. The color Doppler views show perivascular tissue vibration centered over the femoral vein. The profunda femoral artery waveform shows a normal waveform for an extremity artery. The superficial femoral artery waveform shows an abnormally high level of diastolic flow. The femoral vein shows an arterialized waveform with a turbulent appearance. These findings are all typical of a fistula between the superficial femoral artery and the femoral vein.

2. Arteriovenus fistula (AVF) is almost always located below the femoral bifurcation.

3. It is very unusual to see any grey-scale changes associated with AVFs. When AVFs are chronic and large, there may be enlarged tortuous vessels leading to and exiting from the fistula.

4. Patients with AVFs usually come to attention when a bruit is detected following a femoral puncture. AVFs may also be detected during the evaluation of postcatheterization pain and swelling.

Reference

Middleton WD: Duplex and color Doppler sonography of postcatheterization arteriovenous fistulas. *Semin Interv Radiol* 1990;7:192–197.

Cross-Reference

Ultrasound: THE REQUISITES, pp 481–483.

Comment

Like pseudoaneurysms, AVFs have become more common since the use of larger catheters and anticoagulation for vascular interventional procedures. They rarely cause symptoms, although large fistulas can potentially cause high output stress on the heart or can cause ischemic symptoms in the lower extremity. They are rarely located below the femoral bifurcation because at that level the femoral artery and vein are side by side, and it is difficult to puncture the artery and the vein simultaneously. On the other hand, below the bifurcation the femoral vein starts to travel behind the artery, so that it becomes easier to puncture both vessels simultaneously. In addition, a branch of the femoral vein frequently travels right between the superficial femoral artery and the profunda artery, and this can be the vein that is involved in the fistula.

Unlike pseudoaneurysms, AVFs essentially exhibit no grey-scale changes. Therefore, the hemodynamic changes that are detectable with Doppler are the only way to make the diagnosis. The most dramatic change seen on color Doppler is the perivascular tissue vibration caused by the turbulent blood flow. This is essentially the color Doppler equivalent of a thrill, and the typical mixture of random red and blue color assignment is well shown in this case. Although this can be seen with arterial stenoses, it is usually much more pronounced with AVFs. Another hemodynamic change in the artery is related to the bypass of the high resistance arterial bed afforded by the direct communication with the vein. Therefore, the arterial waveform changes from the typical, high-resistance, triphasic pattern to a low-resistance pattern with more diastolic flow. On color Doppler, continuous flow is seen in the artery immediately adjacent to the fistula, while no flow is seen during diastole in the segments of the artery that are not close to the fistula. On the venous side, the jet of arterial flow entering the compliant vein causes a marked flow disturbance in the vein. This is seen as a haphazard arrangement of intraluminal color and as a very distorted venous waveform. In some cases, like the one shown here, an arterial pattern can be seen in the venous waveform. Finally, it is sometimes possible to actually visualize the tract that connects the artery and the vein on color Doppler. Even when the communication is not seen, the localized hemodynamic changes just described provide convincing evidence that an AVF is present.

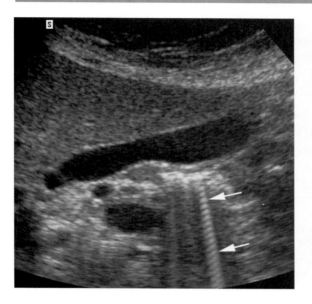
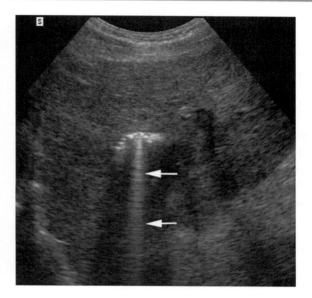

Views of the right upper quadrant and the liver in two patients.

1. Do the bright lines indicated by the arrows correspond to an anatomic structure?

2. What is the etiology?

3. What is the most common cause of this finding?

4. Should you be concerned if you saw this adjacent to the bile duct in a patient 3 months after a cholecystectomy?

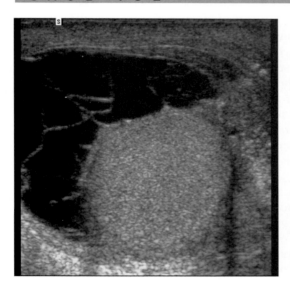
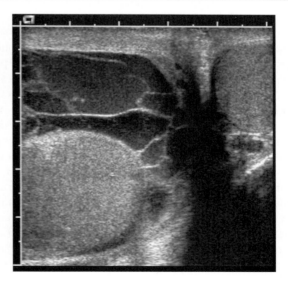

Views of the scrotum in two patients.

1. What are the two most reasonable potential diagnoses in these patients?

2. Is it possible to tell the difference with ultrasound?

3. What are the most common causes for these conditions?

4. Do these conditions typically cross the midline?

C A S E 1 3 1

Ring-down Artifact

1. The lines are nonanatomic. They represent artifacts caused by ring-down.

2. The sound pulse causes something in the body to resonate. Like a tuning fork, the resonating object transmits sound back to the transducer. The returning sound is interpreted as coming from deeper tissues, and a bright line is formed deep to the resonating structure.

3. Gas bubbles are the most common cause of ring-down artifact.

4. Ring-down artifact can also be produced by metallic objects such as surgical clips, so it is commonly seen following cholecystectomy and should not arouse concern.

Reference

Middleton WD: Ultrasound artifacts. In Siegel MJ (ed): *Pediatric Sonography,* 2nd ed. New York, Raven Press, 1994.

Cross-Reference

Ultrasound: THE REQUISITES, p 63.

Comment

Ring-down is one of the most conspicuous ultrasound artifacts, and when it is recognized and properly interpreted, it can greatly assist in certain diagnoses. This is because ring-down artifact occurs most frequently as a result of gas. When a sound pulse interacts with gas bubbles, it excites the fluid that is trapped between the bubbles. This causes the fluid to resonate, or ring, in a manner analogous to hitting a tuning fork with a hammer. Although gas is the most common cause of ring-down, metallic objects, such as surgical clips, hardware, or foreign bodies can also produce this artifact.

Because the ringing starts after the sound pulse arrives at the gas, the sound produced by the ringing follows the returning echo back to the transducer. This constant stream of sound returning to the transducer is interpreted as arising from reflectors deep to the gas. Therefore, a continuous set of echoes is written on the image deep to the gas. This produces the bright line that is called a ring-down artifact. As is demonstrated in this case, the linear artifact is oriented parallel to the scan lines on the image.

In certain clinical situations, it is very useful to know that gas is present. For instance, a complex fluid collection could be many things, but if gas is present, the likelihood of an abscess becomes very high. Another example is a highly echogenic gallbladder wall with shadowing. This could be a porcelain gallbladder, but if air is identified due to a ring-down artifact, then a diagnosis of emphysematous cholecystitis should be made. Therefore, it is important to look for and recognize ring-down artifact when it is present.

C A S E 1 3 2

Complex Hydroceles

1. Pyocele and hematocele are the most reasonable diagnoses.

2. In most cases, it is very difficult to distinguish a pyocele from a hematocele.

3. Epididymitis is the most common cause of pyocele. Trauma is the most common cause of hematocele.

4. Hydroceles, pyoceles, and hematoceles are confined to one side of the scrotum by the median raphe. Although they can occur bilaterally, they do not cross the midline.

Reference

Feld R, Middleton WD: Recent advances in sonography of the testis and scrotum. *Radiol Clin North Am* 1992;30:1033–1051.

Cross-Reference

Ultrasound: THE REQUISITES, pp 446–448.

Comment

The first thing to consider when analyzing fluid collections in the scrotum is to decide if they are in the testis or outside of the testis. If they are outside of the testis, one should then decide if they are in the sac formed by the tunica vaginalis or within the scrotal wall. In the two images shown in this case, the fluid is in contact with the testis and is crescent-shaped. This is typical of any fluid within the tunica vaginalis. The internal septations and the low-level echoes indicate that these are not simple hydroceles. As elsewhere in the body, the presence of complex fluid in the scrotum initially raises the possibility of a hemorrhagic collection or an infected collection. Few ways exist to distinguish the two on ultrasound. If the collection contains very bright reflectors with ring-down artifacts, then gas should be diagnosed, and the presence of gas indicates either infection with a gas-forming organism, communication with a gas-containing viscus, or some type of prior instrumentation. Infected fluid may also incite an inflammatory reaction in the surrounding tissues that can be recognized on color Doppler as hyperemia. However, once a complex fluid collection is seen in the scrotal sac, clinical features are required to help distinguish blood from pus.

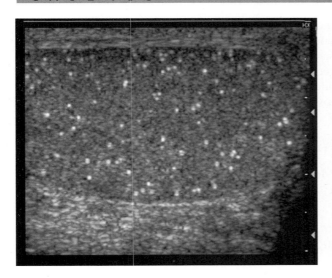 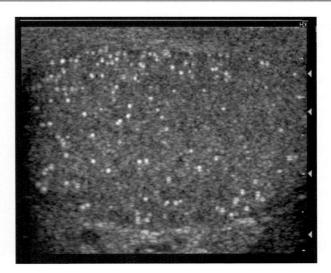

Views of the right and left testis.

1. Where exactly are these bright reflectors located?
2. How is this condition graded?
3. Does this patient require further workup or surgery?
4. Is this condition usually unilateral or bilateral?

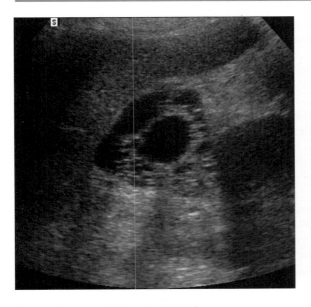 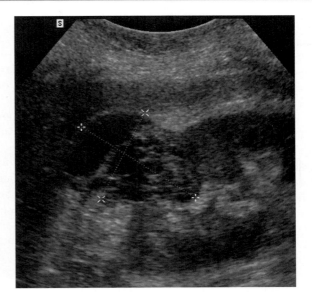

Two views of the right kidney.

1. What is the primary differential diagnosis for this renal lesion?
2. What is the management of this type of lesion?
3. Is percutaneous biopsy valuable?
4. Would knowing the patient's gender help in favoring one diagnosis over the other?

Classic Testicular Microlithiasis

1. The calcifications are located in the lumen of the seminiferous tubules.

2. Microlithiasis is classified as classic if it is possible to see five or more microliths on at least one view of the testis. It is classified as limited if all views of the testis show fewer than five microliths.

3. Data from the second reference below indicates that regular follow-up ultrasounds are low yield for detecting tumors. It probably makes more sense to do regular self-examinations and annual physical examinations, and reserve sonography for cases that develop a palpable abnormality.

4. Microlithiasis is usually bilateral.

References

Backus ML, Mack LA, Middleton WD, et al: Testicular microlithiasis: Imaging appearances and pathologic correlation. *Radiology* 1994;192:781–785.

Bennett HF, Middleton WD, Bullock AF, Teefey SA: Testicular microlithiasis. US follow-up. *Radiology* 2001; 218:359–363.

Cross-Reference

Ultrasound: THE REQUISITES, pp 443–444.

Comment

Testicular microlithiasis refers to laminated concretions that are located within the lumen of the seminiferous tubules. Microlithiasis has been reported to be associated with a number of abnormalities, the most important of which is germ cell tumor of the testis. Although the original report found that 40% of patients with microlithiasis had a tumor, it is now clear that significantly fewer patients with microlithiasis have a coexistent tumor.

In addition to the coexistence of tumors and microlithiasis at the time of the initial ultrasound, several case reports have documented the subsequent development of a germ cell tumor in patients who had sonographically documented microlithiasis but no tumor on the initial sonogram. These reports have raised concern that microlithiasis may be a premalignant condition in some individuals. For this reason, it is now common practice to recommend annual sonographic follow-up in patients with microlithiasis. As indicated in the second reference cited in this case, we have found that the yield of follow-up sonograms is extremely low. Therefore, our current approach is to recommend careful regular self-examinations, annual examinations by a physician, and periodic sonograms only when a palpable abnormality develops.

One unusual situation that occasionally arises is the patient who has a tumor in one testis and bilateral microlithiasis. In these patients, there is a significant increased risk of intratubular germ cell neoplasia in the contralateral testis. Since intratubular germ cell neoplasia frequently progresses to a macroscopic tumor, we recommend that the contralateral testis be explored and biopsied at the time of the orchiectomy for the ipsilateral tumor.

Multilocular Cystic Nephroma

1. Cystic renal cell carcinoma and multilocular cystic nephroma are the primary considerations in a multiloculated cystic renal mass.

2. Lesions with this appearance require surgical excision because of the possibility of cystic renal cell cancer.

3. Percutaneous biopsy is not recommended because a negative biopsy result does not exclude a renal cell carcinoma.

4. In adults, multilocular cystic nephroma is much less common in men.

Reference

Agrons GA, Wagner BJ, Davidson AJ, Suarez ES: From the archives of the AFIP: Multilocular cystic renal tumor in children: Radiologic-pathologic correlation. *Radiographics* 1995;15:653–669.

Cross-Reference

Ultrasound: THE REQUISITES, pp 96–97.

Comment

Multilocular cystic nephroma is considered by most to be a benign renal neoplasm. As the name implies, it consists of multiple cystic spaces that do not communicate with each other or with the renal collecting system. The cysts are epithelium-lined and separated by fibrous septations. The lesion is usually well encapsulated. The condition tends to affect young boys (typically 3 months to 4 years of age) and adult women (over age 30).

Multilocular cystic nephroma has no malignant potential, and if a confident diagnosis could be made with ultrasound or a combination of imaging tests, then surgery would not be necessary. Unfortunately, there is overlap in the appearance of some varieties of cystic renal cell carcinoma and multilocular cystic nephroma. Percutaneous biopsies are not indicated because a negative biopsy result does not exclude the possibility of renal cell cancer. Because it is not possible to confidently distinguish these lesions, surgery is usually necessary.

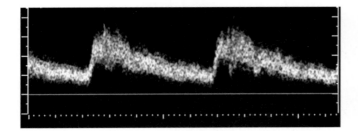
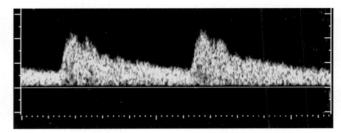

Pulsed Doppler waveforms from two arteries.

1. Would you characterize these waveforms as high or low resistance?

2. What is the difference in these two waveforms?

3. Which of these waveforms is likely to have come from a normal internal carotid artery, and which is likely to have come from a normal arcuate artery in the kidney?

4. What parameter is displayed on the vertical axis?

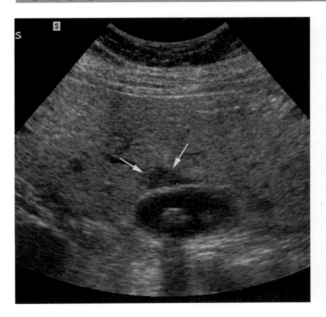
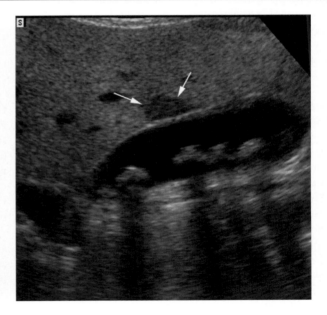

Two views of the liver.

1. Describe the abnormality indicated by the arrows.

2. Is this condition seen more often on ultrasound or on CT?

3. Where else is this abnormality typically seen?

4. What can be done to help increase diagnostic confidence?

Low Resistance Arterial Waveforms with and without Spectral Broadening

1. Both waveforms have low resistance characteristics.

2. The second waveform has signal that extends from the base line all the way to the maximum. The first waveform has a clean window under the signal.

3. The clean signal is typical of a larger superficial artery, such as the internal carotid artery, and the broadened signal is typical of a smaller, deeper artery, such as the renal arcuate artery.

4. The vertical axis represents the Doppler frequency shift. If the direction of blood flow is known, a Doppler angle can be determined, and the frequency shift information can be converted to velocity information.

Reference

Nelson TR, Pretorius DH: The Doppler signal: Where does it come from and what does it mean? *AJR Am J Roentgenol* 1988;151:439-447.

Cross-Reference

Ultrasound: THE REQUISITES, pp 464-470.

Comment

Both of the waveforms shown demonstrate relatively broad systolic peaks, slow systolic deceleration into diastole, and well-maintained diastolic flow throughout the cardiac cycle. This is typical of an artery that supplies a vascular territory with a low resistance to blood flow. The solid parenchymal organs of the body are the structures that have low resistance flow. Therefore, this type of waveform could be seen from the brain, kidney, liver, spleen, testes, and so forth.

The difference in the two waveforms is the continuous signal extending from the base line to the maximum for the renal arcuate artery. This occurs because a broad range of velocities is being sampled, which produces a broad range of frequency shifts. This phenomenon is known as spectral broadening and was originally used as a sign of disordered or turbulent blood flow. However, spectral broadening is also typical of small parenchymal vessels. In the internal carotid artery, the range of frequency shifts is much narrower and concentrated near the maximum, so that there is a clear window between the signal and the base line. This difference is at least partially related to the relative size of the vessel and the size of the sample volume. In a small vessel, the slow flow at the edge of the vessel wall and the faster flow in the center of the lumen are being sampled simultaneously. In a larger vessel only the faster flow in the center is being sampled. In addition to large sample volumes, high Doppler gain and high power outputs can also produce spectral broadening in normal vessels.

Fatty Infiltration with Focal Sparing

1. Both images show an area of apparently decreased echogenicity in the liver parenchyma immediately adjacent to the gallbladder. This is typical of focal sparing in an otherwise diffusely fatty liver.

2. Ultrasound is more sensitive than CT for fatty infiltration. Therefore, focal fatty sparing is seen more often on ultrasound.

3. Fatty sparing typically occurs around the gallbladder and anterior to the portal bifurcation.

4. To further confirm fatty sparing, it is useful to compare the liver to the right kidney and pancreas in order to confirm that the rest of the liver is fatty-infiltrated.

Reference

White EM, Simeone JF, Mueller PR, et al: Focal periportal sparing in hepatic fatty infiltration: A cause of hepatic pseudomass on ultrasound. *Radiology* 1987;162:57-59.

Cross-Reference

Ultrasound: THE REQUISITES, pp 16-18.

Comment

Fatty infiltration of the liver is usually a diffuse process. However, it is relatively common to have small regions of liver parenchyma that are spared. This is probably most common in the liver parenchyma immediately adjacent to the gallbladder. It is also very common in segment 4 of the liver, immediately anterior to the portal bifurcation.

The problem with fatty sparing is that it is easy to assume that the echogenic fatty-infiltrated liver is normal and the less echogenic spared area is abnormal. When this happens, the spared areas can be confused with a number of abnormalities that are hypoechoic, such as neoplasms, infarcts, infections, and so forth. Recognition that the liver is fatty-infiltrated is extremely helpful. In addition, several clues can help to avoid this pitfall. Fatty sparing produces no mass effect, is not spherical, is usually in typical locations, and often changes dramatically on short-term follow-up.

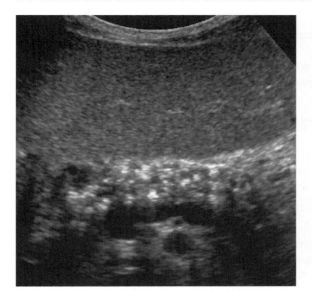
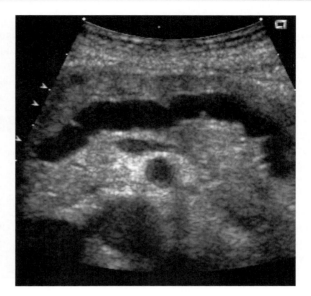

Transverse views of the pancreas in two patients with different manifestations of the same disease.

1. Describe the abnormal findings?
2. What might be seen on endoscopic retrograde cholangiopancreatography (ERCP)?
3. Are these patients likely to have gallstones?
4. What would your diagnosis be if you saw a pancreatic cyst in these patients?

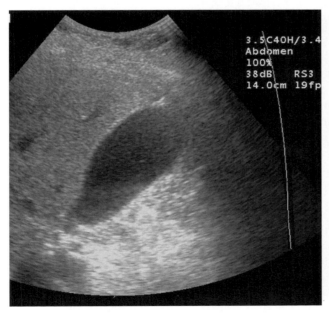
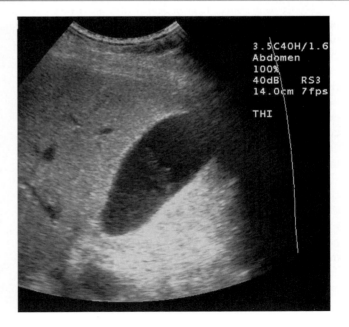

Two views of the gallbladder.

1. What technique was used to allow the gallbladder sludge to be better seen on the second image?
2. Is this technique theoretically more important in thin patients or in obese patients?
3. Is this technique theoretically more important for high or low frequency transducers?
4. Is this technique possible on all transducers?

Chronic Pancreatitis

1. The first image shows diffuse punctate calcifications in the pancreas. The second image shows irregular dilatation of the pancreatic duct and parenchymal atrophy. These abnormalities are all consistent with chronic pancreatitis.

2. ERCP would show irregular dilatation and short strictures of the pancreatic duct, with ectatic side branches and possibly filling defects due to intraductal concretions.

3. Chronic calcific pancreatitis is caused by alcohol abuse, not by gallstones.

4. A pseudocyst. Approximately 25% to 40% of patients with chronic pancreatitis develop pseudocysts.

Reference

Taylor AJ, Bohorfoush AG (eds): Pancreatic duct in inflammation of the pancreas. In *Interpretation of ERCP with Associated Digital Imaging Correlation.* Philadelphia, Lippincott-Raven, 1997, pp 231–260.

Cross-Reference

Ultrasound: THE REQUISITES, pp 126–133.

Comment

Chronic calcific pancreatitis is a complication of prolonged alcohol abuse. It is believed that alcohol predisposes to the precipitation of proteins in the side branches of the pancreatic duct. These proteins attract calcium carbonate and form stones that obstruct the peripheral side branches, resulting in an inflammatory response that causes parenchymal damage and, ultimately, periductal fibrosis. Side branch strictures and ectasia result from the scarring and from the intraductal concretions. With more advanced disease, the main pancreatic duct becomes involved, with alternating strictures and dilatation.

On sonography, chronic pancreatitis is seen as some combination of parenchymal changes and alteration in the main pancreatic duct. The ductal dilatation is usually irregular, sometimes producing a "chain of lakes" appearance. The parenchyma appears heterogeneous and may become extremely atrophic. Punctate foci of increased echogenicity reflect underlying calcification, which may be focal or diffuse. They may produce no detectable shadowing or may shadow so much that the deeper aspects of the gland cannot be visualized.

Up to one third of patients with chronic pancreatitis have a focal inflammatory mass in the pancreas. These masses are usually located in the pancreatic head and may cause dilatation of the common bile duct and the pancreatic duct. Therefore, they can be difficult to distinguish from pancreatic carcinoma. The presence of calcifications strongly supports the diagnosis of chronic pancreatitis. When calcifications are absent and especially when the mass is hypoechoic, ERCP and biopsy should be considered to further evaluate for possible malignancy.

Tissue Harmonic Imaging

1. The second image used tissue harmonic imaging (THI) to improve visualization of the sludge.

2. THI has a greater impact in obese patients, but it can help in thin patients as well.

3. THI is theoretically more important for low frequency transducers.

4. THI can be installed on all transducers.

Reference

Choudhry S, Gorman B, Charboneau JW, et al: Comparison of tissue harmonic imaging with conventional US in abdominal disease. *Radiographics* 2000;20:1127–1135.

Comment

Conventional ultrasound transmits pulses of a certain fundamental frequency spectrum and receives echoes at the same frequency. As the sound pulse interacts with the tissues that it travels through, harmonic signals that are multiples of the fundamental frequency are generated. This is analogous to the overtones of a musical note. These harmonic components build up at increased depth and then decrease owing to attenuation. Although multiple harmonic frequencies are present, the higher harmonics are very low in amplitude. With current harmonic imaging technology, only the second harmonic, which is twice the fundamental frequency, is used. In this case, the image was created by transmitting at 1.6 MHz and analyzing the 3.2 MHz harmonic signal after the 1.6 MHz echoes were filtered out.

Because the harmonic signal is a higher frequency, axial resolution improves with harmonic imaging. Additionally, the harmonics allow for better focusing, which also improves lateral resolution. Side lobes and scattering are both less prominent with harmonic frequencies, and this leads to less artifacts. Finally, harmonic signals are generated beyond the body wall, and this helps to avoid the defocusing effects of the body wall.

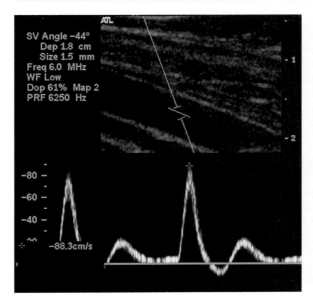
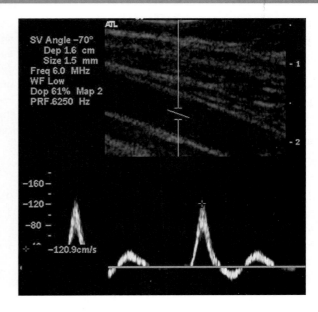

Pulsed Doppler waveforms from the femoral artery.

1. Which velocity is more reliable?
2. What happens to the Doppler frequency shift when the Doppler angle approaches 0 degrees?
3. What happens to the Doppler frequency shift when the Doppler angle approaches 90 degrees?
4. How can the Doppler angle be changed?

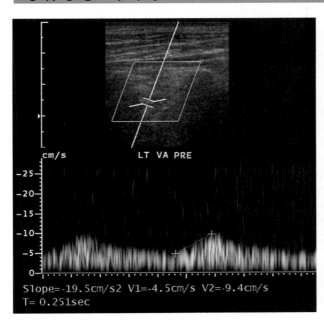
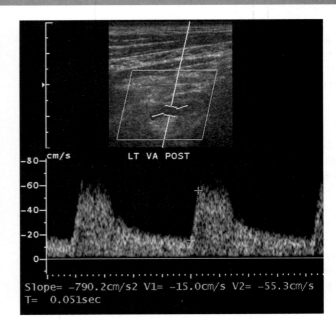

Waveforms of the vertebral artery taken 1 day apart.

1. Which of the waveforms is abnormal?
2. What is the significance of this waveform abnormality?
3. What would you consider if this waveform abnormality were seen in multiple abdominal and peripheral arteries?
4. What would you consider if this waveform abnormality were seen in the lower pole of a kidney while a normal waveform was seen in the upper pole?

Relationship of Velocity Calculation Accuracy to Doppler Angle

1. The first velocity is more accurate because the Doppler angle is less than 60 degrees. The second velocity should not be trusted because the Doppler angle is greater than 60 degrees.

2. The frequency shift is maximized as the Doppler angle approaches 0 degrees.

3. The frequency shift is minimized as the Doppler angle approaches 90 degrees.

4. With linear array transducers, it is possible to steer the Doppler beam to one side or the other (as was done in the first image) so that the Doppler angle will change. With other transducers, the only way to change the Doppler angle is to change the position of the transducer so that the orientation of the Doppler beam with respect to the vessel also changes.

Reference

Taylor KJW, Holland S: Doppler US: Part I. Basic principles, instrumentation, and pitfalls. *Radiology* 1990; 174:297–307.

Cross-Reference

Ultrasound: THE REQUISITES, pp 467–468.

Comment

In many situations, it is important to calculate blood flow velocities. This can be done by rearranging the Doppler equation to solve for velocity, as shown:

$$V = Fd \times 1/Ft \times C \times 1/\cos\theta \times 1/2$$

In this equation, V = velocity, Fd = Doppler frequency shift, Ft = transmitted frequency, C = the speed of sound, and θ = Doppler angle. If it were possible to determine the exact Doppler angle, then an accurate velocity could be calculated almost regardless of the Doppler angle. Unfortunately, it is not possible to determine the exact Doppler angle. Part of the problem is that there is always some degree of error in the angle estimation when the angle indicator line is rotated parallel to the axis of the vessel. In addition, blood flow is rarely oriented directly along the long axis of the vessel. Some flow is oriented toward the vessel walls, and some is oriented out of the imaging plane. Therefore, there is always an unavoidable error in the determination of the precise Doppler angle.

This inherent error has important implications in calculating flow velocities. As can be seen from the preceding equation, velocity is proportional to $1/\cos\theta$. If one were to draw a graph that plots $1/\cos\theta$ with respect to θ, it would show that at Doppler angles less than 60 degrees, there is little change in $1/\cos\theta$ despite large differences in the angle θ. However, above 60 degrees, small differences in the angle θ produce large differences in the value of $1/\cos\theta$. Therefore, it is important to maintain a Doppler angle of 60 degrees or less when attempting to calculate flow velocities. When this is not possible, it should be recognized that significant errors can be made.

Parvus-Tardus Waveform

1. The first is abnormal.

2. In the proper clinical setting, it indicates a proximal arterial stenosis. In this case, a second image demonstrates a normal waveform obtained after a vertebral artery stent was placed across a proximal stenosis.

3. Aortic valvular stenosis or coarctation should be considered.

4. Stenosis of an accessory artery to the lower pole should be considered.

Reference

Bude RO, Rubin JM, Platt et al: Pulsus tardus: Its cause and potential limitations in detection of arterial stenosis. *Radiology* 1994;190:779–784.

Cross-Reference

Ultrasound: THE REQUISITES, pp 111–112.

Comment

Normal arterial waveforms demonstrate an extremely rapid early systolic upstroke because there is fast acceleration of blood at the initiation of systole. The first waveform shown in this case demonstrates a very slowed systolic upstroke and a systolic peak that is reduced when compared to the amount of diastolic flow. These changes are referred to as parvus (reduced amplitude) and tardus (delayed). This type of waveform is also frequently described as being blunted.

Parvus-tardus waveforms are most frequently the result of a significant proximal stenosis. The maximum effect of the stenosis occurs during systole when the pressure is the greatest. The overall velocity in peak systole is reduced beyond the stenosis, and the time it takes to reach maximum velocity (acceleration) is also reduced. Since pressure is lower during diastole, the effect on diastolic flow is less. Therefore, the difference between systolic flow and diastolic flow is less than normal, and the waveform appears blunted. In severe cases, the difference between systole and diastole may be so minimal that the arterial waveform appears more like a venous waveform.

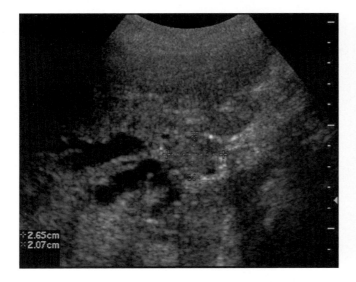
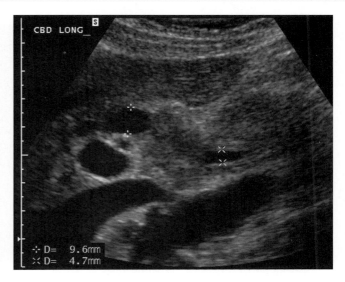

Views of the intrahepatic and extrahepatic portion of the liver hilum in two patients.

1. What is the abnormality in the first image?
2. What is the abnormality in the second image?
3. What is the most common location for this lesion?
4. How is the diagnosis confirmed?

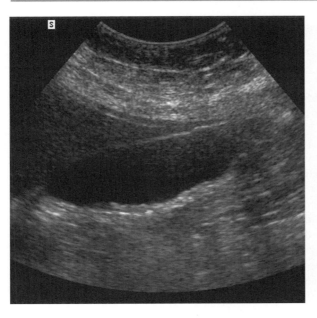
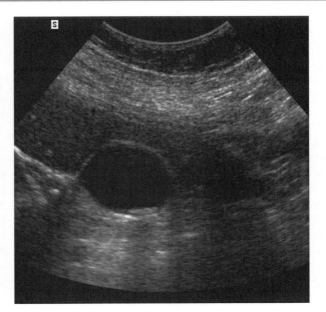

Longitudinal and transverse views of the gallbladder.

1. If this patient had intermittent bouts of severe right upper quadrant pain lasting a few hours, would a cholecystectomy be indicated?
2. What is the major sonographic difference between stones and sludge?
3. What is the sonographic sensitivity for gallstones?
4. What is the sonographic negative predictive value for gallstones?

Cholangiocarcinoma

1. Dilated intrahepatic ducts abruptly terminate at the level of a soft tissue mass.

2. A dilated common hepatic duct terminates abruptly at the level of a suprapancreatic mass. The distal duct is normal in diameter.

3. Cholangiocarcinomas most commonly occur at the confluence of the left and right bile ducts. The lesion in the first image is located here. The lesion in the second image is in the mid duct.

4. The diagnosis is confirmed either by intraluminal brush biopsies or by percutaneous biopsy with ultrasound guidance. Pathology is notoriously difficult; therefore, a negative biopsy result should not be considered definitive, especially in the presence of convincing imaging tests.

Reference

Bloom CM, Langer B, Wilson SR: Role of US in the detection, characterization, and staging of cholangio-carcinoma. *Radiographics* 1999;19:1199–1218.

Cross-Reference

Ultrasound: THE REQUISITES, pp 63–66.

Comment

Cholangiocarcinoma (CCa) is relatively rare, accounting for less than 1% of malignant neoplasms. It generally occurs in the sixth or seventh decade of life. In the majority of cases, there is no known etiology. However, predisposing factors include cystic disease of the bile ducts (choledochal cysts and Caroli's disease), sclerosing cholangitis, ulcerative colitis, Thorotrast exposure, and hepatic parasitic infection. The prognosis is dismal, with a 5-year survival rate of approximately 1%. Even with curative resection, the 5-year survival rate is only 20%.

Cholangiocarcinoma most often affects the extra-hepatic ducts. As many as 70% of cases occur at the bifurcation of the common hepatic duct. Tumors in this location are often referred to as Klatskin tumors. Typically, Klatskin tumors are small at the time of pre-sentation. They tend to infiltrate the wall of the duct, the adjacent vessels, and the adjacent liver parenchyma. Involvement of adjacent vessels and extension into the more peripheral aspects of the bile ducts beyond the bifurcation determine whether the tumor is resectable and what type of resection can be performed.

Sonographically, most Klatskin tumors appear as a relatively isoechoic mass in the liver hilum. In many cases the margins of the mass are best identified by noting the location of transition of the dilated bile ducts. An important aspect of the sonographic examination is determining the extent of invasion of the adjacent ves-sels. Soft tissue encasement of the vessels is a reliable sign of invasion.

Ten percent to 20% of cholangiocarcinomas occur in the intrahepatic bile ducts. In this location they usually grow to be quite large, since they do not produce early symptoms. Sonographically they appear as nonspecific solid masses that vary in their echogenicity.

The remainder of cholangiocarcinomas occur in the common bile duct and common hepatic duct below the bifurcation. These tumors may be infiltrative or polypoid in nature. Tumors in the most distal aspect of the duct can be easily confused both clinically and pathologically with ampullary, duodenal, and pancreatic cancers. There-fore, this group of tumors is often referred to as periampul-lary. In this location, surgical resection is much more likely to be possible and to be successful.

Gallstones

1. This patient has multiple small stones. Intermittent bouts of right upper quadrant pain represent biliary colic as these stones pass through the cystic duct. This patient would almost certainly benefit from cholecystectomy.

2. Sludge does not shadow, and all but the smallest gallstones do shadow.

3. Sonographic sensitivity for gallstones is greater than 95%.

4. Negative predictive value for gallstones is greater than 95%.

Reference

Middleton WD: Right upper quadrant pain. In Bluth EI, Benson C, Arger P, et al (eds): *The Practice of Ultrasonography.* New York, Thieme, 1999, pp 3–16.

Cross-Reference

Ultrasound: THE REQUISITES, pp 38–41.

Comment

In this case, a thin layer of small stones rests along the dependent wall of the gallbladder. Notice that the stones are much easier to appreciate on the transverse view than on the longitudinal view. On the longitudinal view, it is easy to confuse the echogenic layer of stones for the back wall of the gallbladder. This is less of a problem on the transverse view. In addition, the shadow caused by the stones is narrower on the transverse view and is easier to pick out from the adjacent tissues. In a case such as this, it is important to image the patient in different positions because the stones may rearrange into a configuration that is easier to appreciate.

III Challenge

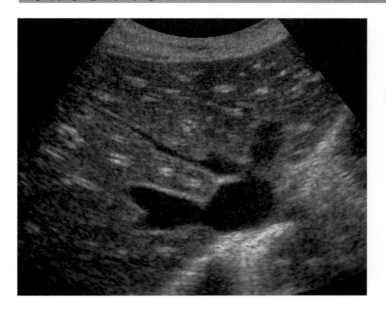
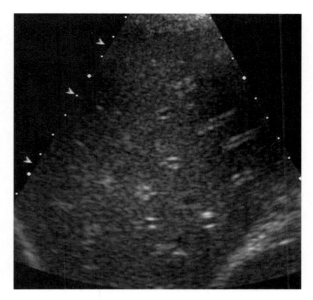

Views of the liver in two patients.

1. Describe the abnormality.

2. What is the descriptive term for this finding?

3. With what is this finding classically associated?

4. How useful is this finding?

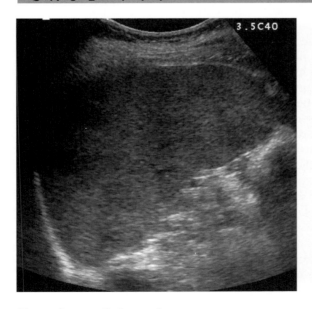
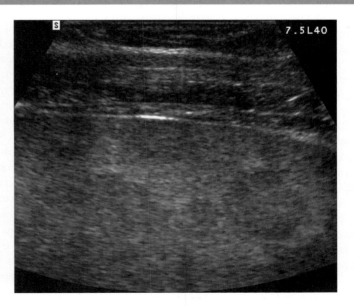

Two views of the spleen.

1. Describe the abnormality.

2. What is your differential diagnosis?

3. If this patient were African American and had mediastinal and bilateral hilar adenopathy, what would be your leading diagnosis?

4. What other abdominal findings might you expect?

Hepatitis

1. Both views show increased echogenicity of the portal triads in the periphery of the liver.

2. This is referred to as the "starry sky" sign.

3. The starry sky sign is classically associated with hepatitis.

4. Usefulness of this sign is limited because (unlike this case) it is usually very subtle, and it can be seen in patients who have no other clinical or laboratory evidence of hepatitis.

Reference

Kurtz AB, Rubin CS, Cooper HS, et al: Ultrasound findings in hepatitis. *Radiology* 1980;136:717-723.

Cross-Reference

Ultrasound: THE REQUISITES, pp 112-115.

Comment

Patients with right upper quadrant pain and abnormal liver function tests often are referred for sonographic evaluation. The main goal in this group of patients is to determine whether there are gallstones and whether there is any evidence of biliary obstruction. In the absence of either of these abnormalities, the next consideration is usually diffuse liver parenchymal disease.

Except for fatty infiltration, ultrasound is not a good way of evaluating or quantitating diffuse liver disease. Hepatitis is no exception. Nevertheless, there are some sonographic findings that are seen in patients with hepatitis. Perhaps the most common abnormality is thickening of the gallbladder wall (see case 13). In fact, hepatitis can produce dramatic gallbladder wall thickening. It is also characteristic of patients with hepatitis for the gallbladder lumen to be contracted. Another finding seen commonly is mildly enlarged lymph nodes in the porta hepatis, around the celiac axis, and in the peripancreatic area. Unfortunately, mildly enlarged nodes are very common in these areas and can be associated with many other inflammatory or infectious conditions in the right upper quadrant. They are also common in liver diseases other than hepatitis, such as primary biliary cirrhosis and sclerosing cholangitis.

This case demonstrates the starry sky sign in the liver. Decreased echogenicity of the liver parenchyma around the portal veins is felt to be the cause, although increase in the echogenicity of the periportal tissues may also be at least partially responsible. Regardless of the cause, when the portal tracts are imaged in cross section in the periphery of the liver, the net result is small focal areas of increased echogenicity on a darker background, simulating stars in the night sky. Although this finding was described in association with hepatitis, it is not terribly helpful owing to poor sensitivity and a limited positive predictive value. In addition, when it is present, it is usually subtle enough that diagnostic confidence is limited. The changes seen in this case are considerably more striking than are usually seen.

Splenic Sarcoid

1. Patchy hypoechoic areas in the spleen.

2. The differential diagnosis includes lymphoma, metastatic disease, sarcoidosis, infarction, and infection.

3. Sarcoidosis would be most likely, although lymphoma would also be a consideration.

4. Abdominal sarcoid also affects the liver and causes lymphadenopathy.

Reference

Warshaur DM, Molina PL, Hamman SM, et al: Nodular sarcoidosis of the liver and spleen: Analysis of 32 cases. *Radiology* 1995;195:757-762.

Cross-Reference

Ultrasound: THE REQUISITES, p 145.

Comment

Sarcoidosis is a disease of unknown etiology that affects primarily the chest but can involve virtually any organ in the body. It is characterized by noncaseating granulomas in lymph nodes as well as in organs with a rich lymphatic supply. Approximately 50% of patients are asymptomatic at the time of diagnosis, so the disease can be detected as an incidental finding during abdominal sonography.

Sarcoidosis involves the abdominal lymph nodes in approximately 30% of cases. Lymph nodes are commonly seen in the region of the porta hepatis, celiac axis, pancreas, and retroperitoneum. Involvement of the liver and spleen is also seen in approximately 30% of cases. This is usually manifest as diffuse enlargement of the liver or spleen, but focal lesions can also be seen. It is extremely difficult to distinguish abdominal sarcoidosis from abdominal lymphoma purely on the basis of imaging findings.

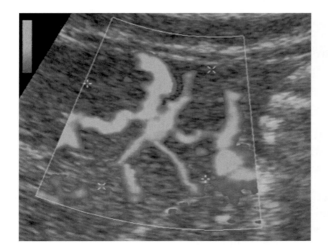
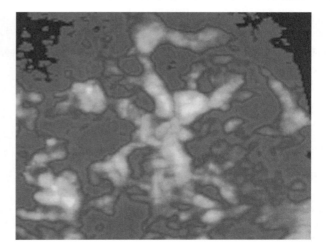

Two-dimensional and three-dimensional power Doppler views of the liver in two patients. (See color plates.)

1. Describe the findings.
2. What is the natural history of this lesion?
3. What is the best way of confirming the diagnosis?
4. Would the presence of central calcification change your approach to this lesion?

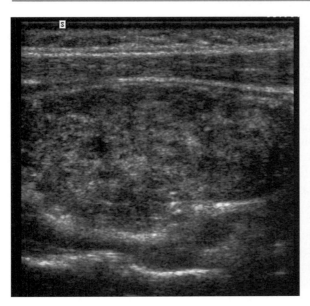
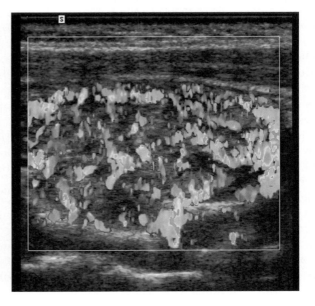

Longitudinal grey-scale and color Doppler views of the thyroid. (See color plates.)

1. Describe the abnormality shown on the grey-scale view.
2. Describe the abnormality shown on the color Doppler view.
3. Is this condition more common in men or in women?
4. Would you be surprised if this patient were hypothyroid?

Hepatic Focal Nodular Hyperplasia

1. The first image shows a collection of vessels arranged in a spokewheel configuration. The underlying grey-scale appearance of the liver is barely distorted. The second image also shows a spokewheel configuration in three dimensions.

2. Focal nodular hyperplasia rarely causes clinical symptoms and has no malignant potential.

3. Currently the most definitive imaging means for confirming the diagnosis is sulfur colloid scanning.

4. Central calcification suggests the diagnosis of fibrolamellar hepatocellular carcinoma and would prompt a more aggressive approach

Reference

Buetow PC, Pantograg-Brown L, Buck JL, et al: From the archives of the AFIP: Focal nodular hyperplasia of the liver: Radiologic-pathologic correlation. *Radiographics* 1996;16:369–388.

Cross-Reference

Ultrasound: THE REQUISITES, p 14.

Comment

Focal nodular hyperplasia (FNH) is a benign tumor of the liver that is composed of Kupffer cells, hepatocytes, and biliary structures. It is hypothesized that it develops from a congenital vascular malformation that promotes hepatocellular hyperplasia. Pathologically, it often has a central, stellate scar. It is supplied by an internal arterial network that is arranged in a spokewheel pattern.

FNH is usually detected as an incidental mass on CT or on ultrasound. Like hepatic adenoma, FNH is more common in women. Unlike hepatic adenoma, it is not related to the use of birth control pills. The nodules seldom bleed or cause any clinical symptoms, although pain may be encountered when the lesions are large.

Although the appearance of FNH varies on sonography, most FNHs are isoechoic or nearly isoechoic to liver parenchyma. The central stellate scar, which is frequently seen on CT and MRI, is uncommonly seen on ultrasound. However, the spokewheel pattern of internal vascularity is better displayed on color or power Doppler than on CT or MRI.

When FNH is suspected based on ultrasound, hepatic scintigraphy with sulfur colloid can be very useful. Due to the concentration of Kupffer cells, approximately 60% of FNHs are either hot (more intense than adjacent liver) or warm (isointense to adjacent liver). The typical features on ultrasound and these findings on sulfur colloid scans are sufficient to make the diagnosis with a high degree of certainty. If the lesion is cold on sulfur colloid scans, then FNH remains a possibility, but other lesions also need to be considered.

Hashimoto's Thyroiditis

1. The thyroid is mildly enlarged, hypoechoic, and diffusely heterogeneous, without discrete focal nodules.

2. The thyroid is very hypervascular.

3. Hashimoto's thyroiditis is much more common in women.

4. Hashimoto's thyroiditis is the most common cause of hypothyroidism in the United States.

Reference

Yeh HC, Futterweit W, Gilbert P: Micronodulation: Ultrasonographic sign of Hashimoto's thyroiditis. *J Ultrasound Med* 1996;15:813–819.

Cross-Reference

Ultrasound: THE REQUISITES, p 452.

Comment

Hashimoto's thyroiditis (also called chronic autoimmune lymphocytic thyroiditis) is believed to be due to autoantibodies to thyroid proteins, especially thyroglobulin. Therefore, the diagnosis is often made serologically. The gland is infiltrated with lymphocytes and plasma cells, with an associated fibrotic reaction. Patients may be euthyroid initially but generally become hypothyroid owing to replacement of functioning thyroid parenchyma. It has a peak incidence between the ages of 40 and 60 years and is six times more common in women than in men. Other autoimmune disorders such as Sjögren's syndrome, systemic lupus erythematosus, rheumatoid arthritis, fibrosing mediastinitis, sclerosing cholangitis, and pernicious anemia may coexist with Hashimoto's thyroiditis. There appears to be a slight increased risk of thyroid lymphoma in patients with Hashimoto's thyroiditis.

On sonography, the gland is hypoechoic and usually enlarged. Generally the normal homogeneous echotexture is replaced by a more heterogeneous texture. Thin, echogenic fibrous strands may cause a multilobulated or micronodular appearance. Often the gland is extremely hypervascular. Hashimoto's thyroiditis can cause nodules, and other types of benign and malignant nodules can coexist with Hashimoto's thyroiditis. In the end stage, the gland becomes atrophic.

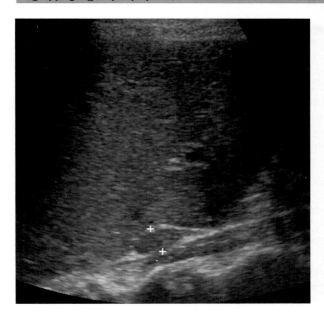
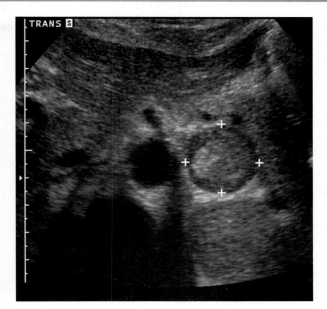

Longitudinal view of the right upper quadrant and transverse view of the aorta and left upper quadrant in two patients.

1. What do these two patients have in common?
2. What is included in the differential diagnosis?
3. If there were a history of hypertension, what would be the most likely diagnosis?
4. If there were a history of medullary cancer of the thyroid, what would be the most likely diagnosis?

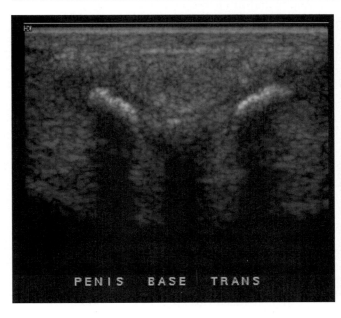
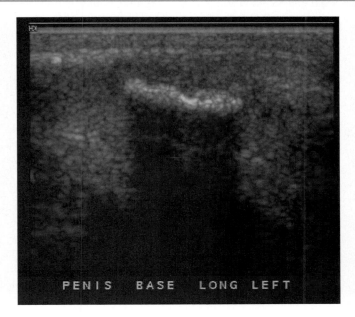

Transverse and longitudinal views of the penis.

1. Describe the abnormality.
2. What is the physical examination of the penis likely to reveal?
3. What symptoms is this patient likely to have?
4. Is this more common along the dorsal or ventral surface of the penis?

Adrenal Masses

1. The first image shows a mass posterior to the liver. A portion of the normal adrenal gland is seen extending inferior to this mass. The second image shows a mass lateral to the aorta.

2. The differential diagnosis for adrenal masses includes adenomas, pheochromocytomas (second image), myelolipomas, adrenal cancer, metastases (first image), lymphoma, and hematomas.

3. Hypertension can be caused by pheochromocytomas and by functioning adenomas that secrete aldosterone (Conn's disease).

4. Medullary thyroid cancer and an adrenal mass should suggest multiple endocrine neoplasia (MEN), type II. The adrenal mass would then be a pheochromocytoma.

Reference

Krebs TL, Wagner BJ: MR imaging of the adrenal gland: Radiologic-pathologic correlation. *Radiographics* 1998;18:1425-1440.

Cross-Reference

Genitourinary Radiology: THE REQUISITES, pp 346-355.

Comment

Ultrasonography generally does not image normal adrenal glands. Nevertheless, ultrasound frequently identifies masses in the right adrenal gland and infrequently identifies left adrenal gland masses. Right adrenal masses can be imaged from an intercostal or a subcostal approach. Masses appear immediately adjacent to the posterior surface of the liver and lateral to the inferior vena cava. Right adrenal masses are usually superior to the upper pole of the kidney. Left adrenal masses are located in a left para-aortic location at the level of the upper pole of the kidney. They are best identified from a left coronal intercostal approach, using the spleen or kidney as a window, or from an anterior subxiphoid approach.

The most common adrenal mass is the adenoma. Autopsy series identify adenomas in 3% of the population. Adenomas are usually asymptomatic but can produce Cushing's syndrome (excessive glucocortisol) and Conn's syndrome (hyperaldosteronism). They contain significant amounts of lipid and are typically low attenuation lesions on CT. They are usually less than 3 cm in size and homogeneous. Despite their small size, the adrenals are the fourth most common site of metastases. Metastases are usually larger than adenomas and are heterogeneous. Pheochromocytomas produce symptoms of hypertension, headache, tachycardia, anxiety, and palpitations. They are referred to as "the 10% tumor" because 10% are malignant, 10% are extra-adrenal, 10% are bilateral, and 10% occur with MEN syndromes.

Pheochromocytomas are typically large, vascular, heterogeneous tumors. Primary adrenal carcinomas are very rare tumors. They are typically very large masses that present with pain or symptoms due to the mass effect. Necrosis, hemorrhage, and calcification are common. Myelolipomas are benign tumors that contain hematopoietic and fatty elements. They rarely cause symptoms and can be small or large.

There is significant overlap in the sonographic appearance of various solid adrenal masses. In most cases, sonographic detection of an adrenal mass is followed by CT or MRI for further characterization. In some instances, laboratory studies are sufficient to determine the etiology of an adrenal mass. In this case, the lesion shown in the first image was a right adrenal metastasis in a patient with lung cancer. The lesion shown in the second image was a left adrenal pheochromocytoma in a patient referred for a renal artery Doppler scan. Urinary catecholamine levels documented the diagnosis.

Peyronie's Disease

1. Calcification of the tunica albuginea of the corpora cavernosa.

2. Localized firmness and thickening at the site of the plaque.

3. Painful and/or curved erections.

4. This is most common on the dorsal side of the penis.

Reference

Balconi G, Angeli E, Nessi R, et al: Ultrasonographic evaluation of Peyronie's disease. *Urol Radiol* 1988; 10:85-88

Cross-Reference

Ultrasound: THE REQUISITES, pp 112-115.

Comment

Peyronie's disease is fibrosis of the tunica albuginea of the corpora cavernosa. It is idiopathic and typically affects men older than 45 years. Since the tunica albuginea cannot stretch in the area of fibrosis, the penis bends toward the plaque during erection. Pain and penile curvature can make intercourse impossible.

On sonography, the plaques appear as localized areas of thickening of the tunica albuginea. They are often hyperechoic and may be calcified. The typical location is along the dorsum of the penis near the base, but Peyronie's disease can also involve the lateral margins and the septum.

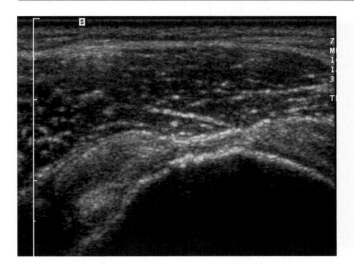
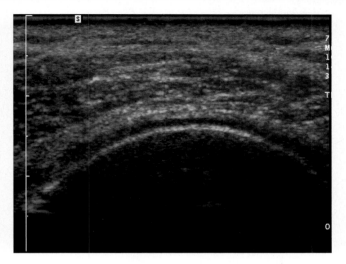

Transverse views of the shoulder in two patients.

1. What do these patients have in common?

2. Which patient requires further imaging for confirmation of the diagnosis?

3. How does ultrasound compare to MRI in making this diagnosis?

4. In which patient is the diagnosis most likely to be apparent on radiographs of the shoulder?

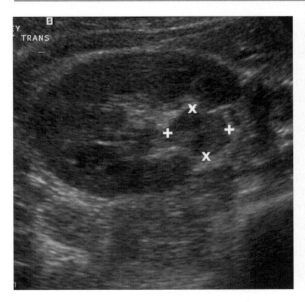
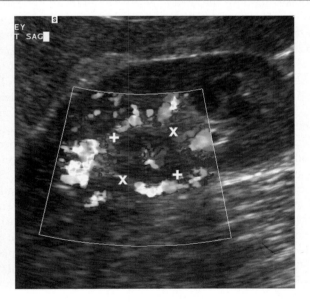

Transverse grey-scale view and longitudinal color Doppler view of the right kidney. (See color plates.)

1. Describe the abnormality.

2. What is the most likely diagnosis?

3. Is this the most common location for this lesion?

4. How is this lesion treated?

C A S E 1 4 9

Full Thickness Rotator Cuff Tear

1. Both patients have full thickness rotator cuff tears. The first image shows a contour concavity, and the second shows nonvisualization of the cuff.

2. The findings on sonography are diagnostic in both cases. No further imaging is required.

3. In the hands of experienced sonologists and experienced MRI readers, ultrasound and MRI are equivalent for detection of full thickness rotator cuff tears.

4. The patient with nonvisualization (second image) is likely to have superior migration of the humeral head detectable on shoulder radiographs.

Reference

Teefey SA, Hasan SA, Middleton WD, et al: Ultrasonography of the rotator cuff: A comparison of ultrasonography and arthroscopic surgery in one hundred consecutive cases. *J Bone Joint Surg* 2000;82(A):498–504.

Cross-Reference

Ultrasound: THE REQUISITES, pp 455–457.

Comment

Full thickness rotator cuff tears are classified as wet or dry, depending on whether there is a significant amount of joint fluid surrounding the torn edges of the cuff. In the patients shown in this question, the tears are dry. The appearance of dry tears is somewhat more difficult to understand than wet tears. When the defect created by the tear is not filled with fluid, it must be filled with something else. In most cases, the overlying subdeltoid bursa and peribursal fat drops into the defect. This produces a concavity in the reflections from the bursa and fat. In most cases, this concavity is readily visible at rest. If the torn ends of the tendon have not retracted from each other, a concavity may not be visible at rest. In such a case, compression of the shoulder with the transducer can push the bursa and peribursal fat into the defect at the same time that it produces some separation of the tendon ends. Compression can also exaggerate some tears that are otherwise subtle because they are filled with hypertrophied synovial tissue. This is presumably due to the greater compressibility of the thickened synovium compared to the rotator cuff. In the absence of a tear, the normal rotator cuff does not compress at all.

When there is a massive tear with extensive retraction of the torn tendon, the humeral head becomes completely uncovered by cuff tissue. In such a situation, there is no sonographically visible cuff on standard images. This is referred to as nonvisualization of the cuff. In these cases, the subdeltoid bursa, peribursal fat, and deltoid muscle come into direct contact with the articular cartilage and humeral head.

C A S E 1 5 0

Transitional Cell Carcinoma

1. The first image shows a solid mass in the renal hilum. The second image shows the mass with minimal internal vascularity and multiple hilar vessels draped around its margins.

2. Both of the findings should suggest transitional cell carcinoma.

3. No. Most transitional cell cancers occur in the bladder.

4. Upper tract transitional cell cancer is treated with nephrectomy and ureterectomy.

Reference

Wong-You-Cheong JJ, Wagner BJ, Davis CJ, Jr: From the archives of the AFIP: Transitional cell carcinoma of the urinary tract: Radiologic-pathologic correlation. *Radiographics* 1998;18:123–142.

Cross-Reference

Ultrasound: THE REQUISITES, pp 94–95.

Comment

Transitional cell cancer (TCC) is typically divided into tumors that involve the bladder and tumors that involve the upper urinary tract (ureter, renal pelvis, and intrarenal collecting system). Bladder tumors are much more common than upper tract tumors, and tumors of the renal pelvis are more common than tumors of the ureter. Approximately 90% of renal pelvis tumors and 99% of ureteral tumors are TCC.

Patients most often present with gross hematuria. Flank pain is uncommon and usually indicates obstruction and hydronephrosis. Colicky pain may develop during periods of clot passage. Patients with advanced disease may present with constitutional symptoms such as weight loss and anorexia.

Sonography is not a primary means of evaluating patients with TCC of the upper urinary tract. However, it may be the first test obtained in a patient with hematuria, and thus the initial identification of the tumor may be with ultrasound. TCC has a variety of sonographic appearances. It may appear as a solid mass within a dilated renal pelvis, as a solid mass distorting the renal sinus fat, or as an area of uroepithelial thickening. In general, the sonographic findings are non-specific, and the differential diagnosis includes blood clots, sloughed papillae, and pyelonephritis. Detection of internal vascularity confirms that the lesion is viable soft tissue and almost always indicates a tumor of some sort. Further evaluation with intravenous urography, retrograde pyelography, or ureteroscopy is generally required.

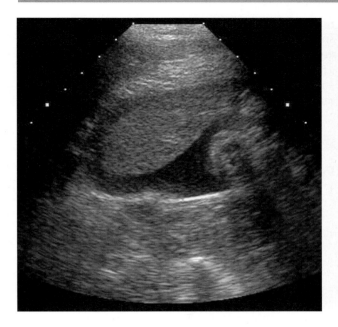 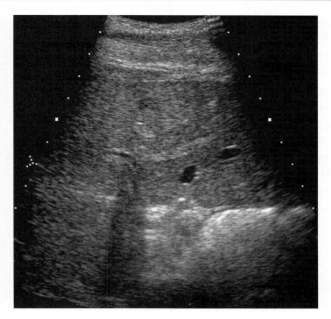

Transverse views of the liver.

1. Describe the abnormalities in these images.
2. If there is a history of trauma, what is the most likely diagnosis?
3. How effective is ultrasound in establishing this diagnosis?
4. What role, if any, does ultrasound have in evaluating trauma patients?

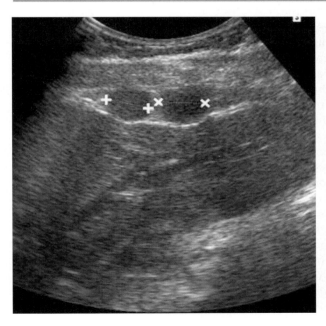 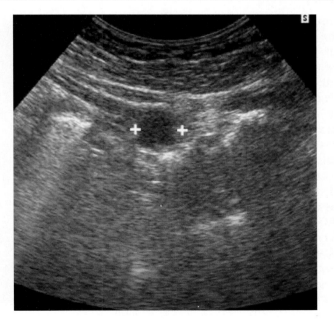

Longitudinal view of the right upper quadrant and transverse view of the mid abdomen.

1. Describe the abnormality.
2. What is the differential diagnosis?
3. What is the best way to confirm the diagnosis?

Liver Laceration and Hemoperitoneum

1. The first image shows peritoneal fluid around the liver. The second image shows mild distortion of the liver echotexture.

2. In the setting of trauma, any peritoneal fluid should be assumed to be a hemoperitoneum. The subtle changes in the liver indicate that the liver is the likely source as a result of a hepatic laceration.

3. Ultrasound is good at identifying hemoperitoneum. It is not very good at identifying an acute laceration of a parenchymal organ such as the liver, spleen, or kidney.

4. The role of ultrasound in the setting of blunt abdominal trauma is controversial and in evolution. It is clear that ultrasound can substitute for the diagnostic peritoneal lavage. Given this, some believe that ultrasound should be used to identify patients with hemoperitoneum.

Reference
Richards JR, McGahan JP: Ultrasound for blunt abdominal trauma in the emergency department. *Ultrasound Q* 1999;15(2):60–72.

Cross-Reference
Gastrointestinal Radiology: THE REQUISITES, pp 174–175.

Comment
The use of ultrasound in the evaluation of blunt abdominal trauma is increasing world-wide. Ultrasound is a rapid and effective means of detecting hemoperitoneum and has become one of the initial checkpoints in the triage of blunt abdominal trauma patients. If the patient has fluid detectable on ultrasound, has a positive physical examination, and is hemodynamically unstable, then an emergency abdominal exploration is performed to identify and correct the site of bleeding. If the patient is stable, further evaluation may be obtained with either CT, follow-up ultrasound, or laparotomy. If the patient has no fluid, or has fluid but is stable and has a negative physical examination, then he or she is observed clinically. If the clinical status deteriorates, then CT, follow-up ultrasound, or laparotomy is performed. If the patient remains stable and improves, no further evaluation is carried out.

Problems in the use of ultrasound include its limited ability to identify and grade liver, splenic, renal, pancreatic, mesenteric, and bowel lacerations. As shown in this case, acute hemorrhage in solid organs may be very subtle on sonography. In addition, hemoperitoneum may be absent with isolated retroperitoneal injuries and may initially be minimal or absent with injuries to the bowel, mesentery, or contained injuries to the liver and spleen. On the other hand, simple ascites may be present and simulate hemoperitoneum. Finally, quality-degrading factors such as obesity, excessive bowel gas, subcutaneous emphysema, and pneumoperitoneum may limit the examination.

Peritoneal Metastases

1. The first image shows two solid, hypoechoic masses between the surface of the liver and the abdominal wall. The second image shows a similar mass in the mid abdomen, also adjacent to the anterior abdominal wall. This appearance is typical of peritoneal metastases. This patient had a primary bronchogenic cancer.

2. Other possibilities include splenosis, endometriosis, mesothelioma, and tuberculosis.

3. If confirmation of the diagnosis were necessary, ultrasound guided biopsy would be the most straightforward approach.

Reference
Yeh HC: Ultrasonography of peritoneal tumors. *Radiology* 1979;133:419–424.

Comment
Peritoneal metastases most often arise from gynecologic tumors or tumors of the gastrointestinal tract (especially colon, stomach, and pancreas). Breast cancer, lung cancer, and melanoma are also capable of metastasizing to the peritoneum. Peritoneal metastases are often small and not visualized by any imaging technique. When they reach 1 cm or greater in size, they can be detected sonographically. As shown in this case, peritoneal tumor implants typically appear as discrete masses that are separate from bowel. The best way to identify them is to use a transducer with high near-field resolution, such as a linear or curved array transducer. Tumor implants are most often seen immediately deep to the abdominal wall, so it is important to focus attention to this superficial area. As the transducer is swept up and down the abdomen, peritoneal nodules will appear and disappear from view. This distinguishes them from bowel loops, which are continuous and connected to other bowel loops.

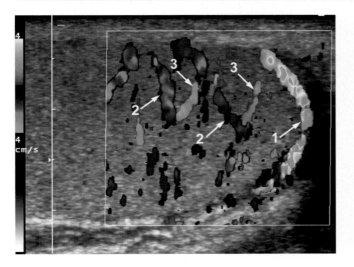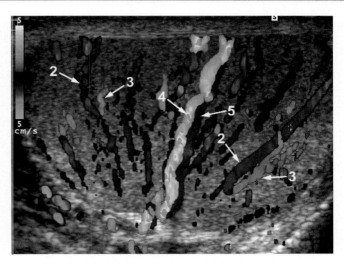

Longitudinal and transverse color Doppler views of the testis. (See color plates.)

1. Identify the vessels that are labeled on the images in this case.

2. How is testicular blood flow different from blood flow in other organs?

3. Is the testis as vascular as the epididymis?

4. What arteries are located in the spermatic cord?

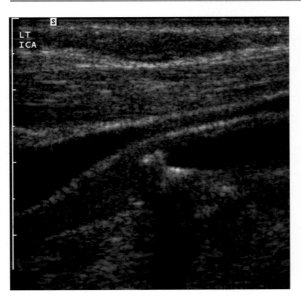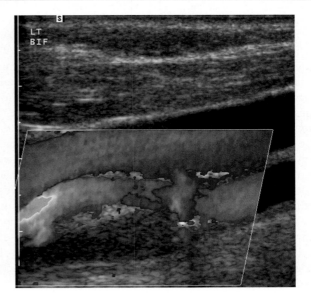

Longitudinal grey-scale view of the internal carotid artery and longitudinal color Doppler view of the carotid bifurcation. (See color plates.)

1. Describe the abnormal findings.

2. Does treatment differ for an internal carotid artery (ICA) with a total occlusion compared to an artery with a high-grade subtotal occlusion?

3. What happens to the common carotid artery waveform when the ICA is totally occluded?

4. What might cause a patent ICA to appear totally occluded?

Normal Testicular Vasculature

1. 1 = Capsular artery, 2 = Centripetal artery, 3 = Recurrent ramus, 4 = Transmediastinal artery, 5 = Transmediastinal vein.

2. The largest testicular arteries are located on the surface of the organ.

3. The testis demonstrates more vascularity than the epididymis on color Doppler.

4. In addition to the testicular artery, the cremasteric artery and the deferential artery are located in the spermatic cord.

Reference

Middleton WD, Bell MW: Analysis of intratesticular arterial anatomy with emphasis on transmediastinal arteries. *Radiology* 1993;189:157–160.

Cross-Reference

Ultrasound: THE REQUISITES, p 435.

Comment

Arterial supply of the scrotum is via the testicular artery (which is the primary supply to the testis), the deferential artery (which is the primary supply to the vas deferens and epididymis), and the cremasteric artery (which supplies the scrotal wall). The testicular artery typically divides into two to four branches that travel along the periphery of the testis. These are called capsular arteries and are the largest arteries of the testis. Capsular arteries supply branches called centripetal arteries that head into the testis and travel toward the mediastinum. Centripetal arteries branch into vessels called recurrent rami that curve back away from the mediastinum. In approximately 50% of testes, one or more of the capsular arteries actually travels through the mediastinum and crosses inside the testicular parenchyma before it reaches the surface of the testis on the opposite side. These arteries are called transmediastinal arteries, and a typical example is seen on the transverse image shown in this case. Doppler waveform analysis from the various testicular arteries shows a low resistance pattern typical of a solid parenchymal organ.

Detectable testicular veins are less numerous than testicular arteries. However, they can be seen on many normal testicular Doppler examinations. Some testicular veins drain out of the mediastinum and some drain peripherally into capsular veins. It is not uncommon to see a large transmediastinal vein running parallel to a transmediastinal artery, as shown in this case.

Complete Occlusion of the Internal Carotid Artery

1. The grey-scale view shows partially calcified plaque in the internal carotid origin and low level echoes in the proximal ICA. The color Doppler view shows flow in the jugular vein (blue) and in the common and external carotid arteries (red), but no detectable flow in the ICA.

2. Patients with total occlusions are not candidates for endarterectomies, but patients with subtotal occlusions are candidates for this procedure.

3. The common carotid artery waveform starts to look like that of the external carotid artery.

4. A subtotal occlusion with slow flow can be mistaken for a complete occlusion. Other causes include extensive calcification with shadowing and a very deeply situated ICA.

Reference

Gortter M, Niethammer R, Widder B: Differentiating subtotal carotid artery stenoses from occlusion by colour-coded duplex sonography. *J Neurol* 1994; 241:301–305.

Cross-Reference

Ultrasound: THE REQUISITES, p 473.

Comment

Patients with a high-grade stenosis must be distinguished from patients with a totally occluded ICA because the former are candidates for endarterectomy and the latter are not. This is a potential problem for Doppler analysis because the flow distal to a very high-grade stenosis may be very slow and difficult to detect. Fortunately, Doppler sensitivity improved dramatically throughout the 1990s, and it is now very uncommon to mistake a high-grade stenosis for a complete occlusion. Nevertheless, this mistake does occur, and for this reason it is common practice to perform a carotid angiogram to confirm any questionable Doppler diagnosis of complete occlusion.

Techniques that can be used to improve the detection of flow in a high-grade stenosis are similar to those used elsewhere in the body. One common problem in the carotids arises when the internal carotid is deep and high in the neck. In such cases, it usually helps to switch to a lower frequency probe and perhaps to a curved array rather than a linear array. Another technique that can help is to eliminate lateral beam steering so that the beam is directed straight down. Power Doppler can theoretically improve detection of slow flow. Intravenous microbubble contrast agents are being developed and refined and will undoubtedly improve the situation in the future.

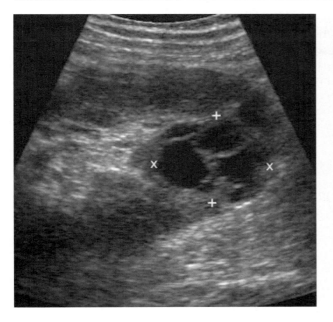 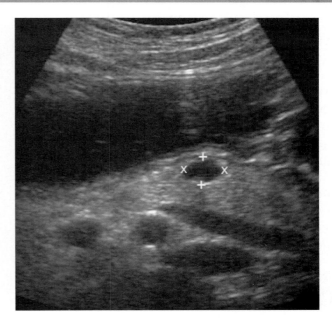

Longitudinal view of the lower pole of the left kidney and transverse view of the pancreas in the same patient.

1. What abnormalities are shown in this case?

2. What is the most likely diagnosis?

3. What other abnormalities are associated with this disorder?

4. Are family members at risk?

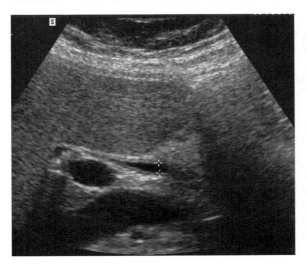 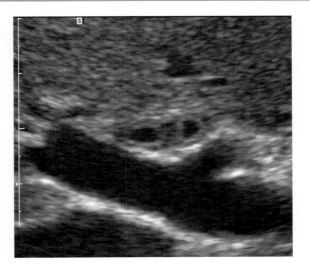

Longitudinal view of the common hepatic duct and magnified transverse view of the bile duct bifurcation in two patients.

1. What abnormal finding is shown in this case?

2. What is the differential diagnosis?

3. Which of the possibilities would be most likely if the patient had a history of ulcerative colitis?

4. Which of the possibilities would be most likely if the lumen of the duct was completely obliterated?

Von Hippel-Lindau Disease

1. The first image shows a complex renal cyst with thick irregular septations. The second image shows a cyst in the body of the pancreas.

2. This combination of findings should suggest the diagnosis of von Hippel-Lindau disease with a cystic renal cell cancer.

3. Associated abnormalities include pheochromocytomas, retinal angiomas, cerebellar hemangioblastomas, and pancreatic islet cell tumors.

4. Von Hippel-Lindau disease is inherited as an autosomal dominant trait, so family members are at risk.

Reference

Choyke PL, Glenn GM, Walther MM, et al: Von Hippel-Lindau disease: Genetic, clinical, and imaging features. *Radiology* 1995;194:626-642

Cross-Reference

Ultrasound: THE REQUISITES, pp 88-89.

Comment

Von Hippel-Lindau (VHL) disease is an inherited disorder caused by a defect on the short arm of the third chromosome that confers on patients a susceptibility to various neoplasms and visceral cysts. More than 25 different lesions have been reported associated with this condition. However, the significant lesions that are most common are renal cell carcinoma (25% to 50% of patients), retinal angioma (60% of patients), central nervous system hemangioblastoma (more than 50% of patients), and pheochromocytoma (20% of patients). Renal cysts are also extremely common, and pancreatic cysts are common in certain kindreds. The diagnosis is made by finding a hemangioblastoma and at least one other lesion of the VHL complex, or at least one lesion in a patient with a family member who has a hemangioblastoma.

Patients most often present with symptoms due to hemangioblastomas of the cerebellum or spinal cord, or with symptoms due to visual defects related to retinal angiomas. Hemangioblastomas account for approximately 50% of deaths, and renal cell carcinoma for approximately 35% of deaths in these patients.

Renal cell cancers are diagnosed at a younger age in patients with VHL. In 75% of patients, renal cell carcinoma is bilateral, and in 90% of patients it is multiple. In patients with VHL, renal cell cancer may be entirely solid, or it may develop in the walls of otherwise simple cysts. Identification of renal cell carcinoma is complicated by the typical presence of multiple cysts. In most patients with VHL, CT is superior to ultrasound in the detection of renal cell carcinoma. However, because of the difference in cost, ultrasound is frequently used instead of, or in addition to, CT in the screening of patients with VHL. In addition, ultrasound is very useful in characterizing complex lesions that are indeterminate on CT. Intraoperative ultrasound is also quite helpful because it can identify cancers that are not detected with preoperative CT or ultrasound.

Bile Duct Wall Thickening

1. Both images show a hyperechoic inner layer and a hypoechoic outer layer of the bile ducts. This indicates wall thickening.

2. The causes of bile duct thickening include sclerosing cholangitis, bile duct stones, irritation from indwelling stents, AIDS cholangitis, oriental cholangiohepatitis, pyogenic cholangitis, cholangiocarcinoma, and pancreatitis.

3. Sclerosing cholangitis is associated with ulcerative colitis.

4. Associated luminal obliteration suggests cholangiocarcinoma.

Reference

Middleton WD: The bile ducts. In Goldberg BB (ed): *Diagnostic Ultrasound.* Baltimore, Williams & Wilkins, 1993, pp 146-172.

Cross-Reference

Ultrasound: THE REQUISITES, pp 66-68.

Comment

The wall of the common bile duct is normally so thin that it is seen only as a reflection from the interface between the wall and the bile in the lumen of the duct. Whenever it is possible to resolve the thickness of the bile duct wall, the wall should be considered to be abnormally thick. In most cases, the thickened wall itself will appear hypoechoic, in contrast to the bright reflections from the internal surfaces of the anterior and posterior walls. Although ultrasound can detect bile duct wall thickening, careful correlation with clinical information is necessary to narrow the differential diagnosis. In many patients, further imaging with CT, magnetic resonance cholangiopancreatography, or endoscopic retrograde cholangiopancreatography is helpful in establishing the diagnosis and determining the extent of the disease process. In both of these patients the diagnosis was sclerosing cholangitis.

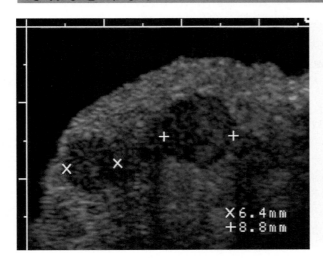
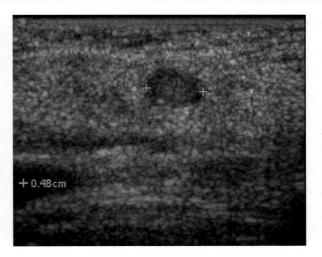

Two views of the pancreas in different patients.

1. What is the most likely reason for doing these scans?
2. How good is ultrasound in this situation?
3. What are the two most common subtypes of this lesion?
4. Are these lesions benign or malignant?

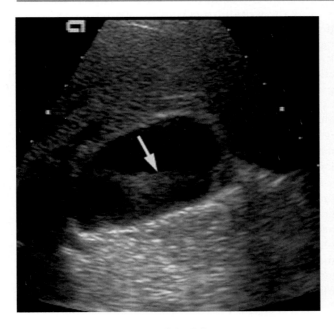
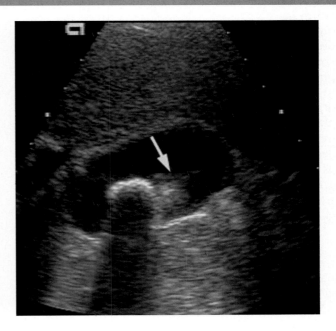

Two views of the gallbladder.

1. What is the cause of the echoes (*arrows*) shown in the lumen of the gallbladder?
2. Explain how these echoes are generated.
3. How can these echoes be eliminated?
4. Are echoes such as these seen more often in solid or in cystic structures?

Intraoperative Scans of Pancreatic Islet Cell Tumors

1. These scans are performed to localize an islet cell tumor for surgical resection.

2. Very good. The combination of intraoperative ultrasound and palpation detects close to 100% of intrapancreatic islet cell tumors. Approximately 30% of gastrinomas are peripancreatic, and these are more difficult to detect with intraoperative ultrasound.

3. The most common islet cell tumors are insulinomas and gastrinomas.

4. Insulinomas are usually benign, and gastrinomas are usually malignant.

Reference

Beutow PC, Miller DL, Parrino TV, Buck JL: Islet cell tumors of the pancreas: Clinical radiologic and pathologic correlation in diagnosis and localization. *Radiographics* 1997;17:453–471.

Cross-Reference

Ultrasound: THE REQUISITES, pp 136–138.

Comment

Preoperative localization of islet cell tumors is generally more reliable with CT than with ultrasound because often the entire pancreas is not well visualized on sonography. Spiral CT with early arterial phase imaging and MRI are almost certain to further improve the noninvasive preoperative detection of islet cell tumors. Angiography and venous sampling are invasive techniques that have also been reported to have sensitivity in the same range as CT. Although ultrasound is not used routinely, it is capable of detecting most islet cell tumors that are 2 cm or larger and many tumors that are smaller. Ultrasound is also a very valuable problem solving technique for the portions of the pancreas that are usually well visualized sonographically, especially the body of the pancreas and most of the pancreatic head. In fact, for the areas that can be easily seen, ultrasound is probably as good as, or superior to, CT and MRI in visualizing islet cell tumors.

Unfortunately, all of the preoperative techniques are limited, and it is not uncommon for a surgeon to operate without being sure where the tumor is. Intraoperative ultrasound is clearly the best way of localizing islet cell tumors. When ultrasound is combined with intraoperative palpation, virtually all intrapancreatic lesions can be detected. Islet cell tumors in the wall of the duodenum or in adjacent lymph nodes, a frequent occurrence with gastrinomas, are more difficult to detect with intraoperative ultrasound.

Side Lobe Artifact

1. The echoes are due to side lobe artifact.

2. When the center of the sound beam is traveling through the lumen of the gallbladder, weak side lobes from the center sound beam are reflecting off strong reflectors from the surface of the gallstone. The weak returning echo is interpreted as coming from the center beam and is therefore placed in the lumen of the gallbladder next to the gallstone.

3. Side lobe artifacts can be very difficult to eliminate. Reducing power and gain may help but often do not completely eliminate the artifact.

4. Side lobe artifacts, like most other artifacts, are seen more often in the black background of cystic structures than in the grey background of solid structures.

Reference

Middleton WD: Ultrasound artifacts. In Siegel MJ (ed): *Pediatric Sonography,* 2nd ed. New York, Raven Press, 1994.

Comment

Most of the energy in the sound pulses that are generated by the transducer is concentrated in the center of the pulse. However, there are weak side lobes that radiate out at an angle from the center beam and surround the center beam throughout its 360-degree circumference. Side lobes are always present to some degree, but in most situations, the reflections generated by side lobes are so weak that they do not produce any identifiable echoes on the image. If the weak side lobe reflects off a very strong reflector, the resulting echo may be of sufficient intensity to cause an effect on the image. Side lobes are generally only a problem when they occur near fluid-filled structures, simply because they are more easily appreciated in the anechoic background of fluid-filled structures than in the echogenic background of solid structures. In the images shown in this case, a gallstone produces enough of an echo that the side lobe reflection can be seen in the anechoic lumen of the gallbladder. Gas in the lumen of the bowel frequently causes side lobe artifacts in the gallbladder and the urinary bladder.

It is important to realize that the bright reflector that causes the side lobe artifact may be located immediately adjacent to, but not within, the imaging plane. This can occur because the side lobes extend completely around the center beam (both in the plane of imaging and out of the plane of imaging). This explains why the artifact is present on the first image even though the gallstone is not seen.

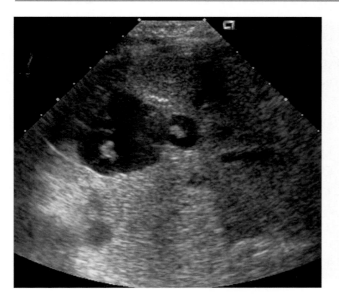
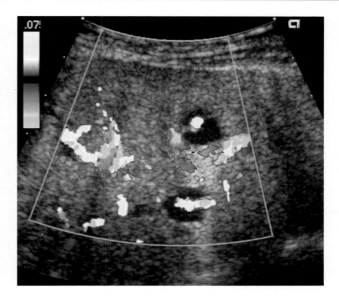

Grey-scale and color Doppler views of the liver. (See color plates.)

1. What sonographic sign is demonstrated on these scans?
2. What disease causes this sign?
3. To what is this patient predisposed?
4. What other organ is usually affected with this disease?

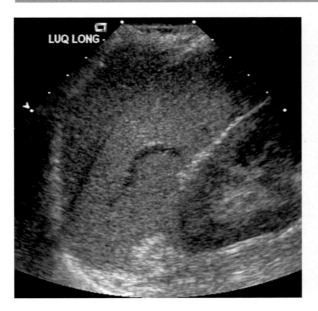
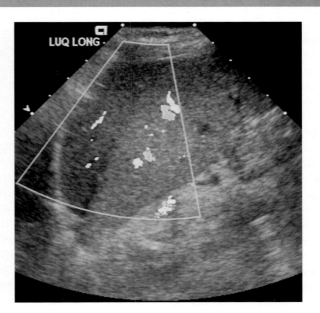

Longitudinal grey-scale and color Doppler images of the left upper quadrant. (See color plates.)

1. What is unusual about these images?
2. With what is this often confused?
3. How can this best be confirmed?
4. Should this finding prompt further investigation?

Caroli's Disease

1. The images show cystic lesions with central solid components containing blood flow. This is called the "central dot" sign.

2. This sign is characteristic of Caroli's disease.

3. Caroli's disease is associated with biliary stones, bile duct obstruction, cholangitis, liver abscess, and cholangiocarcinoma.

4. The kidneys are also affected with a variety of cystic diseases.

Reference

Miller WJ, Sechtin AG, Campbell WL, Pieters PC: Imaging findings in Caroli's disease. *AJR Am J Roentgenol* 1995;165:333–337.

Cross-Reference

Ultrasound: THE REQUISITES, pp 69–70.

Comment

Caroli's disease is a congenital disorder that typically manifests first in children and adolescents. Some believe that it is a continuum with hepatic fibrosis and autosomal recessive (infantile) polycystic kidney disease. In the classification scheme of choledochal cysts, it is classified as type V. In its pure form, Caroli's disease consists of multiple areas of focal, saccular dilatation of the intrahepatic bile ducts. The stasis of bile in the saccular areas predisposes the patient to stone formation, intrahepatic duct obstruction, cholangitis, and liver abscesses. In the more common form of Caroli's disease, there is associated hepatic fibrosis that leads to portal hypertension and ultimately to liver failure. Cystic disease of the kidneys is often associated with Caroli's disease, and the clinical presentation is sometimes dominated by renal failure rather than by hepatic problems. As with the other categories of choledochal cysts, patients with Caroli's disease are predisposed to cholangiocarcinoma.

The key to the diagnosis on ultrasound is to recognize that the cystic appearing areas of saccular dilatation communicate with either normal or ectatic bile ducts. A unique feature of the focally dilated ducts is that instead of displacing the hepatic artery and portal vein, they sometimes surround these structures. In such cases, the vessels produce the appearance of a central dot in the lumen of the dilated duct. When seen, the central dot sign is highly suggestive of Caroli's disease. The sonographic appearance of Caroli's disease is usually typical, and the diagnosis can be made without additional tests. However, in some instances the focal saccular nature of the dilated ducts may be difficult to appreciate on ultrasound, and an erroneous diagnosis of biliary obstruction may be considered. In other cases, it may not be apparent that the cystic spaces communicate with the bile ducts, and an erroneous diagnosis of liver cysts may be made. In such cases, hepatobiliary scintigraphy and cholangiography can be useful in establishing the correct diagnosis.

Normal Variant: Left Hepatic Lobe Over Spleen

1. A crescent-shaped hypoechoic structure is present superior to the spleen.

2. This finding is often confused with complex perisplenic or subcapsular fluid.

3. The etiology can best be confirmed by using Doppler to document the vessels in this structure.

4. This is a normal variant and requires no further evaluation.

Reference

Li DK, Cooperberg PL, Graham MF, Callen P: Pseudo perisplenic "fluid collection": A clue to normal liver and spleen echogenic texture. *J Ultrasound Med* 1986;5:397–400.

Cross-Reference

Ultrasound: THE REQUISITES, pp 147–148.

Comment

In some individuals, the left lobe of the liver extends into the left upper quadrant. When this happens, it insinuates itself between the spleen and the diaphragm. Longitudinal views of the left upper quadrant then show the liver immediately above the spleen. Because the normal liver is significantly less echogenic than the normal spleen, the liver can be mistaken for a subcapsular or perisplenic hematoma. It is usually not possible to trace the left lobe in continuity with the remainder of the liver because of interference from the left ribs and costal cartilages and from left upper quadrant bowel gas. However, knowledge of this normal variant usually allows for a confident diagnosis. Correct interpretation can be aided by identifying vessels in the left lobe of the liver and by watching the two organs slide with respect to each other during respiration.

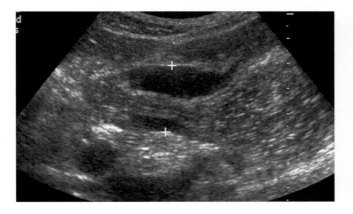 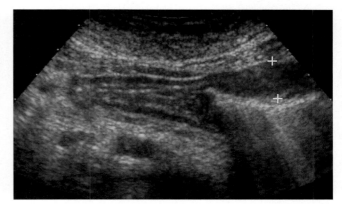

Views of the stomach in two patients.

1. What is the normal gut signature on sonography?
2. What abnormality is present in both images?
3. What is the differential diagnosis?
4. What would be an appropriate next test?

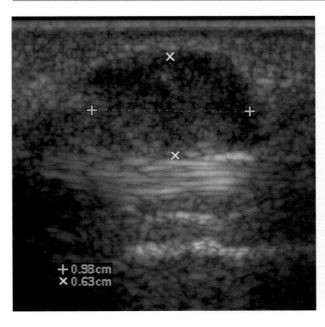 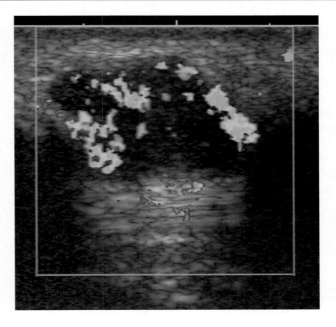

Longitudinal grey-scale and color Doppler views of the thumb in a patient with a palpable mass along the volar surface. (See color plates.)

1. Is this mass solid or cystic?
2. What is its relationship to the tendon?
3. What is the most likely diagnosis?
4. The histologic appearance of this lesion is identical to what other lesion?

Gastric Wall Thickening

1. Intestinal structures appear echogenic centrally and hypoechoic peripherally.

2. Both images show thickening of the gastric wall.

3. The differential diagnosis includes peptic ulcer disease, inflammation, or neoplastic infiltration.

4. Because ultrasound cannot determine the cause of gastric thickening, an upper gastrointestinal tract examination or endoscopy should be performed.

Reference

Wilson SR: Gastrointestinal tract sonography. *Abdom Imaging* 1996;21:1-8.

Cross-Reference

Pediatric Radiology: THE REQUISITES, pp 79-80.

Comment

Because of the presence of gas in the intestinal lumen, ultrasound is generally not used as a primary way of evaluating the bowel. Nevertheless, ultrasound is often capable of detecting bowel-centered pathology. With gentle pressure, normal bowel loops can be compressed, and air can be pressed out of the lumen. When the bowel is well visualized on sonography, five layers are visible. The central layer is the hyperechoic reflection between the luminal contents and the mucosa. The next layer is hypoechoic, and it represents the mucosa itself and the muscularis mucosa. The third layer is hyperechoic and represents the submucosa. The fourth layer is hypoechoic and represents the muscularis propria. The last and most peripheral layer is hyperechoic and represents the serosa or adventitia. In many patients transabdominal scanning shows only two layers.

Normal bowel wall has a thickness of 3 to 5 mm. Localized thickening of the bowel can produce a "pseudokidney" sign, where the luminal gas or the coapted mucosa causes a central hyperechoic region, and the thickened wall produces a surrounding hypoechoic layer. The etiology of bowel wall thickening is often not evident on sonography, and the patient's clinical history must be considered along with the sonographic findings. In general, the differential diagnosis includes infectious and inflammatory conditions, neoplastic infiltration, edema, and ischemia.

Although ultrasound is not sensitive to gastric ulcers, many patients with pain from ulcer disease will undergo sonography early in their workup for evaluation of the other abdominal organs. Therefore, ultrasound may be the initial study that detects the ulcer. In addition to gastric wall thickening, ulcer craters that contain gas may appear as bright intramural echoes with associated dirty shadowing or ring-down artifacts. In almost all cases, an upper gastrointestinal barium examination or endoscopy must be performed to confirm and further evaluate suspected gastric ulcers detected on sonography.

Giant Cell Tumor of the Tendon Sheath

1. It is solid with internal vascularity.

2. It is intimately associated with the tendon.

3. This is most likely a giant cell tumor of the tendon sheath.

4. The appearance of this lesion is similar to pigmented villonodular synovitis.

Reference

Middleton WD, Teefey SA, Boyer MI: Hand and wrist sonography. *Ultrasound Q* 2001;17:21-36.

Cross-Reference

Musculoskeletal Radiology: THE REQUISITES, pp 236-238.

Comment

After ganglion cyst, giant cell tumor (GCT) represents the most common cause of a mass in the hand. Giant cell tumors are a benign disorder of proliferative synovium arising from the tendon sheaths. It is not clear if they are reactive or neoplastic. Histologically, giant cell tumors of the tendon sheaths are identical to pigmented villonodular synovitis. Giant cell tumors are most common in 30- to 50-year-olds and are seen more often in women than in men. They occur typically along the volar surface of the first three fingers and are usually isolated lesions. They are slow-growing and relatively painless. Approximately 10% produce a pressure erosion on the adjacent bone. The treatment of choice is surgical resection. Approximately 20% recur following surgery.

Sonographically, giant cell tumors are solid, homogeneous, hypoechoic masses located adjacent to tendons. Frequently they partially surround the tendon. However, because they arise from the sheath and not the tendon, they do not move with the tendon when the finger is flexed and extended. High frequency color Doppler generally shows readily detectable internal blood flow.

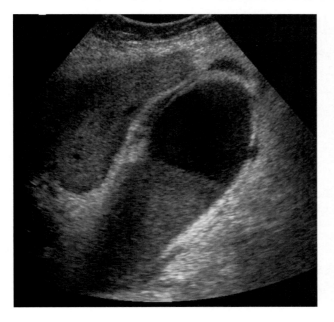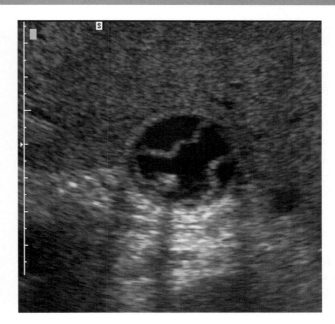

Longitudinal views of the gallbladder in two patients.

1. Describe the gallbladder abnormalities.
2. What is the significance of these abnormalities?
3. Are these findings common?
4. Would your diagnosis change if the sonographic Murphy's sign were negative?

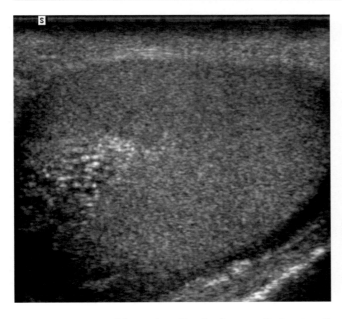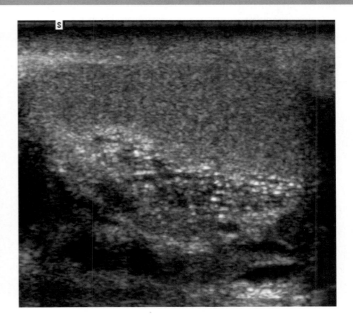

Transverse and longitudinal views of the testis.

1. Does this patient need further workup or surgery?
2. Is this lesion likely to be palpable?
3. What is a commonly associated lesion?
4. Is this condition usually unilateral or bilateral?

Gangrenous Cholecystitis

1. The first image shows thickening of the gallbladder wall, a focal area of mucosal ulceration along the inferior margin, and a small region of pericholecystic fluid. The second image shows sloughed mucosal membranes.

2. Both patients have acute cholecystitis. The mucosal ulceration and the sloughed membranes indicate gallbladder wall necrosis.

3. Localized mucosal ulceration and sloughed membranes are both rare.

4. Patients with gangrenous cholecystitis often have a negative Murphy's sign.

Reference

Middleton WD: The gallbladder. In Goldberg BB (ed): *Diagnostic Ultrasound.* Baltimore, Williams & Wilkins, 1993, pp 116–142.

Cross-Reference

Ultrasound: THE REQUISITES, pp 41–45.

Comment

Complications of acute cholecystitis include gallbladder wall necrosis (manifested as mucosal ulceration, hemorrhage, or desquamation) and perforation. Typical cases of acute cholecystitis produce relatively uniform wall thickening and gallbladder enlargement. As the disease progresses, wall thickening may become more eccentric and assume a layered appearance. As the mucosa starts to break down, discontinuities may appear on sonography. This is demonstrated in the first image. Bile or blood may dissect under the mucosa and cause mucosal desquamation into the gallbladder lumen. These sloughed membranes are demonstrated on the second image. Both of these findings are very uncommon, but it is important that they be recognized because they indicate gallbladder wall necrosis and gangrenous cholecystitis. The perforation rate and mortality are both higher in gangrenous cholecystitis, so these patients require more urgent and aggressive care. Another sign of gangrenous cholecystitis is a focal bulge in the gallbladder wall. This is likely due to the combined effects of progressive increase in intraluminal pressure and focal weakening of the gallbladder wall. Actual perforation of the gallbladder causes focal collections of fluid adjacent to the gallbladder, often tracking up over the edge of the liver or down into the right lower quadrant. Small pericholecystic collections are usually due to focal peritonitis and indicate more advanced disease but do not imply perforation.

Tubular Ectasia of the Rete Testes

1. The sonographic appearance is sufficiently specific for tubular ectasia that it is not necessary to obtain further workup or to perform surgery.

2. Tubular ectasia is not palpable.

3. Spermatoceles are commonly associated with tubular ectasia.

4. Tubular ectasia is usually bilateral, but it may be very asymmetric.

Reference

Weingarten BJ, Kellman GM, Middleton WD, Gross ML: Tubular ectasia within the mediastinum testis. *J Ultrasound Med* 1992;11:349–353.

Cross-Reference

Ultrasound: THE REQUISITES, pp 438–439.

Comment

The rete testes are a complex collection of small tubules that are located in the mediastinum of the testis. Fluid from the seminiferous tubules drains into the rete testis and then exits the rete testis via the efferent ductules. The efferent ductules then converge into the head of the epididymis.

Tubular ectasia of the rete testes is believed to be caused by some degree of outflow obstruction of the seminiferous fluid. Perhaps this is the reason that it is frequently associated with testicular cysts and spermatoceles of the epididymal head. It is also more commonly seen in patients with a history of inguinal surgery, such as hernia repairs and vasectomies. Like testicular cysts, tubular ectasia of the rete testes is more common in elderly patients.

Normally, the tubules of the rete testes are so small that they are not resolved as specific structures in the mediastinum. However, when there is ectasia, the tubules can become resolved as small, fluid-filled, cystic spaces. In most cases, the cystic spaces appear round and do not take on a tubular appearance. When the ectasia is mild, the bright refections from the back wall of the fluid-filled tubules may be more prominent than the cystic changes. When the ectasia becomes more advanced, as in this case, the cystic changes are the predominant feature.

The key to making the diagnosis and distinguishing tubular ectasia of the rete testes from cystic testicular tumors is to note the bilateral involvement when present and to recognize the elongated shape on long-axis views of the testis.

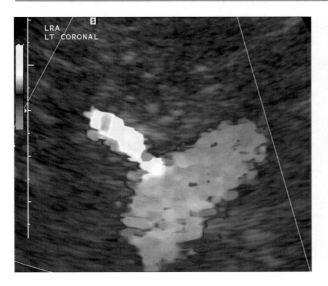
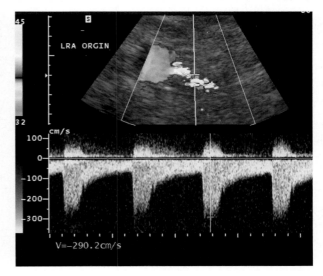

The first image is a coronal magnified color Doppler view of the aorta and the left renal artery. The second image is a transverse color Doppler view of the left renal artery and a pulsed Doppler waveform. (See color plates.)

1. What is the upper limit of normal for renal artery peak systolic velocity?
2. What is the normal ratio of renal artery to aortic peak systolic velocity?
3. How often are the renal arteries seen with ultrasound?
4. How common are accessory renal arteries?

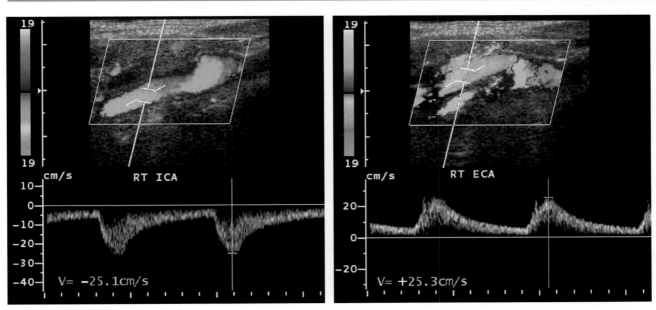

Longitudinal color Doppler views and corresponding pulsed Doppler waveforms of the internal and external carotid arteries. (See color plates.)

1. In what direction is the flow in the external carotid artery?
2. In what direction is the flow in the internal carotid artery?
3. What are the implications of these findings?
4. What are the potential sources of flow in the external carotid artery?

Increased Renal Artery Velocity Due to Arterial Stenosis

1. The upper limit of normal for renal artery velocity is 180 to 200 cm/sec.

2. The upper limit of normal for renal to aortic ratio is 3.0 to 3.5.

3. Visualization of renal arteries varies from report to report, but the average is around 80% to 90%.

4. Approximately 20% of patients have an accessory renal artery.

Reference

House MK, Dowling RJ, King P, Gibson RN: Using Doppler sonography to reveal renal artery stenosis: An evaluation of optimal imaging parameters. *AJR Am J Roentgenol* 1999;173:761-765.

Cross-Reference

Ultrasound: THE REQUISITES, pp 111-112.

Comment

Hypertension affects up to 60 million people in the United States and is one of the most common diseases in the world. Three-fourths of cases are mild and controlled by diet and diuretics. Almost all of these patients have primary hypertension. Severe hypertension that is poorly controlled or controlled only with multiple medications is more likely to be caused by a secondary factor such as renal artery stenosis (RAS). Although RAS accounts for only 5% of the total number of patients with hypertension, it is potentially curable. Therefore, attempts at developing a noninvasive screening test that can identify patients with RAS are important.

Doppler evaluation of the kidneys is one approach. There are two basic ways that Doppler can detect RAS. One is analogous to evaluation of the carotid arteries, where an attempt is made at detecting elevated velocities in the stenotic portion of the artery. Another is detection of changes in the arterial waveform distal to the stenosis.

In this case, the first image shows color Doppler aliasing at the origin of the left renal artery. This identifies the site of maximum velocity. The waveform obtained from this area yields a velocity of 290 cm/sec. This clearly exceeds the upper limit of normal of 180 to 200 cm/sec and allows for a diagnosis of RAS.

The use of Doppler sonography in the evaluation of suspected RAS is controversial. Based on my experience through the late 1990s, I have come to the conclusion that it is a valuable technique that can work in the majority of patients. However, it takes a great deal of experience and may not be appropriate for all practices.

Common Carotid Occlusion

1. Flow in the external carotid artery (ECA) is reversed.

2. Flow in the internal carotid artery (ICA) is antegrade.

3. This combination of findings occurs in patients with occlusion of the common carotid artery (CCA) when retrograde flow in the ECA provides collateral flow to the ipsilateral ICA.

4. The ECA receives collateral flow from the ipsilateral thyrocervical trunk (inferior thyroidal to superior thyroidal), the ipsilateral vertebral artery (muscular branches), and the contralateral ECA (ascending pharyngeal, occipital, facial, and temporal).

Reference

Stasst J, Cavanaugh BC, Siegal TL, et al: US case of the day: Occlusion of the CCA with segmental reversal of ECA flow and a patent ICA. *Radiographics* 1995;15:1235-1238.

Cross-Reference

Ultrasound: THE REQUISITES, pp 470-477.

Comments

Occlusion of the CCA is an uncommon finding in populations of symptomatic patients with extracranial carotid artery disease. CCA occlusion is usually associated with concomitant occlusion of the ipsilateral ICA and ECA. As is shown in this case, in a minority of patients, the vessels above the bifurcation can remain patent. When this occurs, retrograde flow in the ECA crosses the bifurcation to supply antegrade flow to the ICA. Since the flow is supplied entirely by collaterals, the velocities are low, and the arterial signals are blunted with a parvus-tardus appearance. In addition, since the ECA is now supplying the ICA and the brain, the waveform from the ECA will appear similar to that of the ICA.

In the setting of a totally occluded CCA, detection of a patent ICA has important clinical implications because bypass procedures can be performed. Although Doppler techniques are a reliable way of assessing patency of the ICA, angiography is also necessary in the preoperative evaluation of these patients in order to determine the status of the aortic arch, the contralateral vessels, and the intracranial vessels.

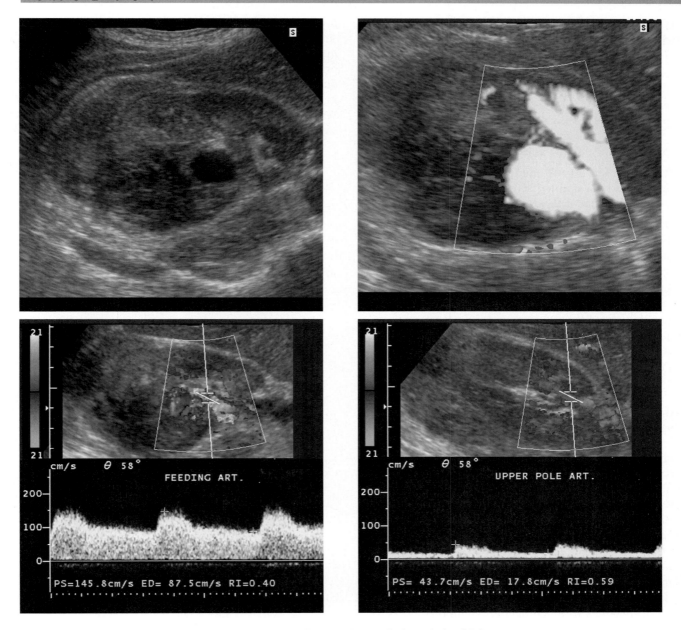

cm/s   θ 58°   FEEDING ART.

200—

100—

0—

PS=145.8cm/s ED= 87.5cm/s RI=0.40

cm/s   θ 58°   UPPER POLE ART.

200—

100—

0—

PS= 43.7cm/s ED= 17.8cm/s RI=0.59

Transverse grey-scale view of the interpolar region of the right kidney followed by a power Doppler view at the same level. The two pulsed Doppler waveforms are from segmental arteries supplying the interpolar kidney and the upper pole, respectively. (See color plates.)

1. Describe the findings in the first two images.

2. Why is there such discrepant flow seen in the two waveforms?

3. How might this patient have presented?

4. What would you recommend be done next in this patient?

Posttraumatic Renal Pseudoaneurysm and Arteriovenous Fistula

1. The grey-scale view shows a complex fluid collection arising from the right kidney. In addition, there is a simple-appearing, round, cystic structure within the otherwise complex collection. The power Doppler view shows flow in the apparent cyst. All of these findings are consistent with a pseudoaneurysm and adjacent hematoma.

2. The increased flow to the interpolar region is not explained by a simple pseudoaneurysm. There must be an associated arteriovenous fistula.

3. This patient may have had trauma or a recent renal biopsy and presented with flank pain and hematuria.

4. The next test should be an arteriogram with embolization.

Reference

Middleton WD, Kellman GM, Melson GL, Madrazo B: Postbiopsy renal transplant arteriovenous fistulas: Color Doppler US characteristics. *Radiology* 1989;171:253–257.

Cross-Reference

Ultrasound: THE REQUISITES, pp 115–116.

Comment

Renal pseudoaneurysm (PA) occurs as a result of laceration of an artery, usually from biopsy or penetrating trauma, but also from blunt trauma. Arteriovenous fistulas (AVF) may develop if there is coexistent injury to an adjacent vein. PA and AVF of the groin have both been illustrated previously (case 63 and 130), and the same principles apply in the kidney. Unfortunately, the classic to-and-fro pattern of flow in a PA neck is much harder to document in the kidney than in the groin because the abnormality is so much deeper. Therefore, the diagnosis of a PA is made based on detection of a cystic lesion with blood flow throughout the cyst lumen. Although a PA communicates with the arterial system, the typically narrow neck usually limits inflow and outflow. In addition, the arterial flow jet that enters during systole dissipates rapidly in the large lumen cavity. Therefore, waveforms from the PA lumen usually display low velocity signals that are pulsatile but do not appear classically arterial in nature unless the sample volume is positioned close to the entering jet.

In this case, the waveform in the PA (not shown) was a strong and large arterial signal. This suggests that outflow, and correspondingly inflow, is brisk and should raise the possibility of an associated AVF. Other clues should then be sought. If an AVF is present, the arterial flow to the segment of the kidney containing the AVF should be increased compared to other normal segments. This can be seen as a prominent supplying artery on color Doppler and discrepant waveforms from the different segments. In some cases, the draining vein may also be apparent as an unusually prominent vessel. Waveforms from the vein will show an inverted arterial signal if the sample volume is placed close to the AVF.

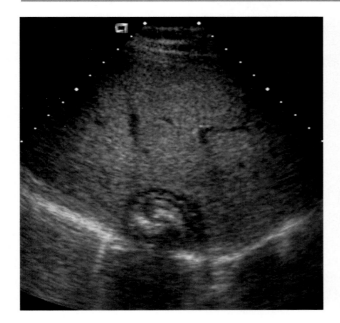
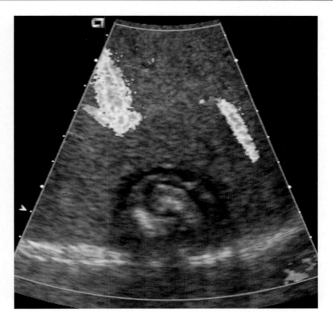

Transverse grey-scale and magnified color Doppler scan from a patient with prostate carcinoma. CT scan showed a single lesion in the liver but no other abnormalities. Bone scan was negative. (See color plates.)

1. How likely is this liver lesion to be a prostate metastasis?

2. What other abnormalities should be considered?

3. What specific information would you like to know about this patient?

4. What else could be done to help establish the diagnosis?

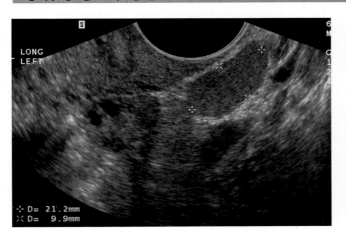
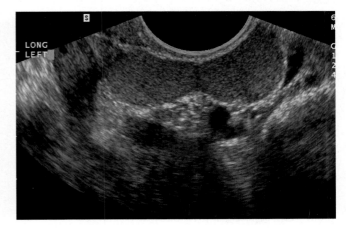

Longitudinal transvaginal views of the left adnexa. The patient has a remote history of a motor vehicle accident.

1. Describe the abnormality.

2. Can this abnormality be related to the patient's history?

3. What else should be considered in the differential diagnosis?

4. How can the diagnosis be confirmed?

Echinococcal Cyst

1. A solitary hepatic metastasis from prostate carcinoma in a patient with no evidence of metastases elsewhere is very unusual, regardless of the appearance of the lesion. In addition, the organized appearance of the lesion and the presence of calcification is very unusual for prostate cancer.

2. Given the calcification, other considerations are an old calcified hematoma or abscess, a calcified metastasis from some other primary site, a fibrolamellar hepatocellular cancer, or an echinococcal cyst.

3. Given the possibility of metastases and echinococcus, it is important to know whether the patient had a history of a primary extrahepatic malignancy other than prostate cancer or a history of travel to a part of the world where echinococcus is endemic.

4. Immunologic testing is often capable of establishing the diagnosis of echinococcal disease. Fine-needle aspiration biopsy is also acceptable. The latter was performed in this patient.

Reference

Chehida FB, Gharbi HA, Hammou A, et al: Ultrasound findings in hydatid cyst. *Ultrasound Q* 1999; 15(4):216-222.

Cross-Reference

Ultrasound: THE REQUISITES, p 15.

Comment

A tapeworm, *Echinococcus granulosus,* usually causes hydatid disease of the liver. The adult worm lives in the intestine of the definitive host, usually a dog. Eggs are excreted in the feces. The intermediate hosts, including sheep, cattle, and humans, are infected by eating contaminated plants and vegetables. Embryos travel from the intestines of the intermediate hosts into the liver and form cysts. The definitive host is infected when cyst-containing organs of the intermediate host are eaten.

In humans, the liver is the most commonly affected organ, although the lungs, spleen, bones, kidneys and central nervous system can also be affected. Cysts that form in the liver have an external membrane called the ectocyst and an internal, germinal layer called the endocyst. In addition, there is a fibrous capsule formed by the host around the cyst that is called the pericyst.

Sonographically, hydatid cysts may appear as relatively simple cysts, as cysts with multiple internal daughter cysts, as cysts with detached, floating endocystic membranes, as cysts with internal debris, and as cysts with internal or peripheral calcification.

Splenosis

1. The first image shows a homogeneous solid mass separate from a normal left ovary. The second image shows two similar-appearing solid masses.

2. With a history of significant abdominal trauma, the possibility of splenosis should be considered whenever solid peritoneal masses are seen.

3. Peritoneal carcinomatosis and mesothelioma could also have this appearance. Pedunculated fibroids are a common cause of solid extraovarian adnexal masses, but it would be very unusual for them to appear this echogenic, homogeneous, and uniform.

4. Splenosis can be confirmed with a damaged red blood cell scan or a sulfur colloid scan.

Reference

Delamarre J, Caopron JP, Drouard F, et al: Splenosis: Ultrasound and CT findings in a case complicated by an intraperitoneal implant traumatic hematoma. *Gastrointest Radiol* 1988;13:275-278.

Cross-Reference

Ultrasound: THE REQUISITES, pp 147-148.

Comment

Splenic trauma can result in dissemination of splenic tissue fragments to various parts of the body. These fragments can implant, parasitize blood flow, and enlarge. This is known as splenosis and may develop to some degree in 20% to 60% of cases of splenic trauma. The implants most often are located in the peritoneal cavity, although they can also appear in the pleura, pericardium, lung, retroperitoneum, and body wall. It is very unusual for splenosis to cause symptoms, and once the diagnosis is confirmed, treatment is rarely needed.

The diagnosis should be suspected whenever tissue similar in echogenicity to the spleen is detected outside the left upper quadrant in a patient with a history of splenic injury. The implants are frequently multiple. This patient had other implants in the pelvis and in the right upper quadrant. When the diagnosis is suspected, it can be confirmed with heat damaged Tc^{99m}-labeled red blood cell scans or sulfur colloid scans.

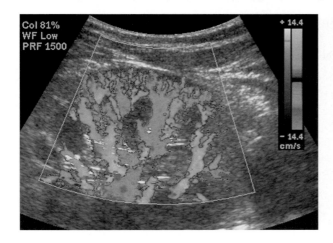
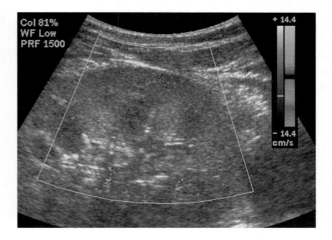

Color Doppler views of the kidney. (See color plates.)

1. Why is renal cortical flow better shown on the first image than on the second image?
2. Is the Doppler control that is responsible for the differences shown in the images a preprocessing or a postprocessing control?
3. Should this control be adjusted to a higher level for a carotid examination or a testicular examination?
4. What is the primary purpose of this Doppler control?

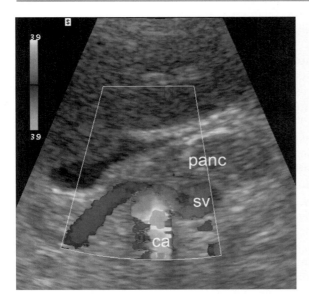
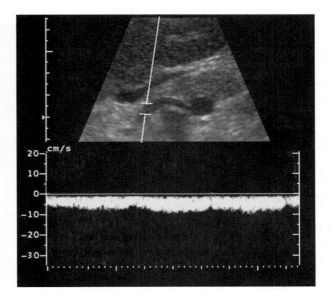

Longitudinal color Doppler view and pulsed Doppler waveform of the epigastrium at the level of the pancreas (panc), splenic vein (sv), and celiac axis (ca). (See color plates.)

1. What vessel is seen draped over the celiac axis?
2. Is diameter or flow direction more important when evaluating this vessel?
3. In this case is either the diameter or the flow direction abnormal?
4. What diagnosis can be made based on these images?

Effect of Color Priority on Color Doppler Images

1. Blood flow is poorly seen on the second image because the color priority is too low. The color priority is indicated by a horizontal green line on the grey-scale bar. Color is suppressed on any pixel in the image that has a grey-scale value above that line.

2. It is a postprocessing control, so it can be adjusted even after the image is frozen. In fact, the images shown are actually the same image with the priority set at different levels.

3. A higher setting would be more appropriate for a testicular examination.

4. The purpose of the color priority is to eliminate Doppler signals that are generated by electronic noise or moving soft tissues.

Reference

Middleton WD: Color Doppler image optimization and interpretation. *Ultrasound Q* 1998;14:194–208.

Comment

In addition to the wall filter (case 125), another control that is used to suppress color information is the color priority. This parameter establishes a grey-scale pixel value, above which color information is suppressed. It is based on the assumption that blood flow should only be demonstrated in blood vessels, and those blood vessels should appear anechoic or very hypoechoic. Therefore, any color assignment arising from a pixel that is not anechoic or very hypoechoic must be due to tissue motion or electronic noise.

When dealing with large or superficial vessels, such as the carotids, these assumptions more or less apply, and the color priority can be adjusted to mid grey-scale levels so as to prevent color assignment from overwriting the grey-scale information arising from the moderately echogenic pulsating vessel wall. However, small vessels that are not resolvable on grey-scale (such as parenchymal vessels in solid organs) have pixel echogenicity values that are similar to the values of the soft tissue around them. If the color priority is set below that tissue echogenicity, it is possible to completely suppress color from real blood flow arising from within those nonresolvable vessels. For this reason, the color priority should be raised to the higher portions of the grey-scale bar so that color suppression occurs only on the very brightest pixels. In most situations, pre-set scanning programs adjust the color priority so that it is appropriate for the vessels being scanned. Nevertheless, patient-to-patient variability sometimes makes it helpful to increase the color priority in order to increase sensitivity, or to decrease color priority in order to eliminate unwanted color signals.

Reversed Flow in the Coronary Vein

1. The vessel being imaged is the coronary vein.

2. The flow direction is more important than the diameter because Doppler can detect a change in the flow direction before there is a change in the vessel size.

3. In this case, the color assignment is blue and the venous signal is below the base line, both indicating flow away from the transducer. Given the orientation of the vessel, this also indicates flow away from the splenic vein. Normally, flow in the coronary vein is toward the splenic vein. The upper limit of normal for coronary vein diameter is 6 mm, and this vessel is approximately 3 mm in diameter.

4. Reversed flow in the coronary vein is an indication of portal hypertension.

Reference

Wachsberg RH, Simmons MZ: Coronary vein diameter and flow direction in patients with portal hypertension: Evaluation with duplex sonography and correlation with variceal bleeding. *AJR Am J Roentgenol* 1994;162:637–641.

Cross-Reference

Ultrasound: THE REQUISITES, pp 19–22.

Comment

The coronary vein (left gastric vein) normally drains venous flow from the lesser curvature of the stomach and the gastroesophageal junction into the portal system. The vein usually inserts near the confluence of the portal and splenic veins. It is easiest to identify by taking longitudinal views of the portal-splenic confluence and looking for a vessel that extends superiorly and to the left. In most patients, the coronary vein drapes over the celiac axis near the bifurcation into hepatic and splenic arteries. Occasionally, the coronary vein passes beneath the hepatic or splenic artery.

In normal patients, all veins that drain into the portal system should have flow directed toward the portal vein and the liver (hepatopetal flow). The coronary vein is no exception. Reversal of flow in any of these veins (hepatofugal flow) is a sign of portal hypertension. Because the coronary vein is one of the most common portosystemic collaterals and is relatively easy to visualize sonographically, it should be evaluated whenever there is a question of portal hypertension.

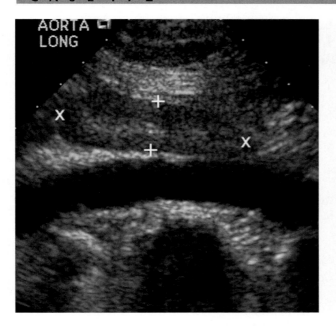
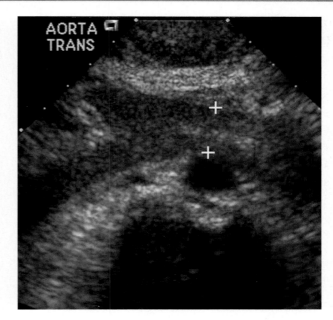

Longitudinal and transverse views of the lower abdomen.

1. What congenital anomaly is demonstrated on these two images?

2. How rare is this abnormality?

3. To what does this abnormality predispose the patient?

4. Is there a gender preference?

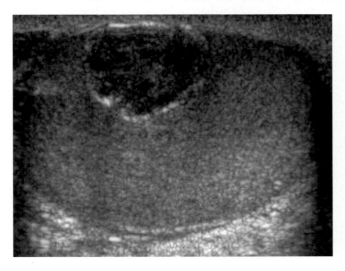
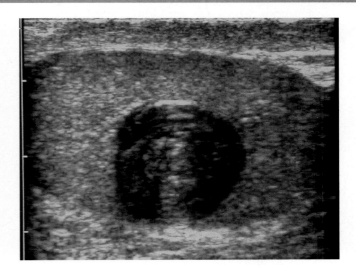

Views of the testis in two patients.

1. Describe the abnormality.

2. What is the most likely diagnosis?

3. Is this a benign or a malignant condition?

4. Is it associated with hormonal effects?

CASE 172

Horseshoe Kidney

1. Horseshoe kidney.

2. This abnormality occurs in approximately one out of every 500 births.

3. Patients are predisposed to urinary obstruction and stone formation, and are at increased risk of renal trauma. There may be an increased risk of Wilms' tumor.

4. There is a slight male predominance.

Reference

Strauss S, Duchnitsky T, Peer A, et al: Sonographic features of horseshoe kidney: Review of 34 patients. *J Ultrasound Med* 2000;19:27-31.

Cross-Reference

Ultrasound: THE REQUISITES, pp 112-115.

Comment

Horseshoe kidneys develop embryologically when there is fusion across the midline of the metanephric blastema. This almost always occurs in the lower pole region and results in a U or horseshoe-shaped kidney. The connection between the right and left lower poles is usually a band of functioning renal parenchyma, although a nonfunctioning fibrous band may be all that is present. The band of connecting tissue is located anterior to the aorta, immediately below the level of the inferior mesenteric artery. Typically there are multiple renal arteries, which may arise from the aorta, the common iliac arteries, the internal iliac arteries, or the inferior mesenteric artery.

The key to the diagnosis on sonography is detection of the bridge of connecting parenchymal tissue. This bridge appears as an oval-shaped hypoechoic structure immediately anterior to the aorta. Once this tissue is detected, it is relatively easy to document during real-time scanning that it connects to the lower pole of both kidneys. Unfortunately, the bridging parenchyma is not visualized unless a prospective search is made of the preaortic region. Since this is not a routine part of a renal sonogram, horseshoe kidneys are easy to overlook. To avoid overlooking this condition, it is important to recognize other clues to the diagnosis. The first clue that a horseshoe kidney is present is typically unusual difficulty in measuring renal lengths due to problems in profiling the lower pole. In addition, the abnormal axis of the kidneys, with the lower poles directed medial to the upper poles, is a clue.

Typically there is no differential diagnosis. On an isolated longitudinal view of the aorta, the parenchymal band may be confused with preaortic lymphadenopathy or other periaortic masses. Documentation of a connection to the lower poles of the kidneys eliminates this confusion.

CASE 173

Epidermoid Cyst

1. The first image shows a solid-appearing mass with a partially shadowing peripheral rim. The second image shows a solid-appearing mass with a lamellated appearance.

2. Both of the appearances are very characteristic of epidermoid cysts.

3. Epidermoid cysts are benign lesions.

4. Epidermoid cysts have no hormonal effects.

Reference

Moghe PK, Brady AP: Ultrasound of testicular epidermoid cysts. *Br J Radiol* 1999;72:942-945.

Cross-Reference

Ultrasound: THE REQUISITES, pp 439-440.

Comment

Epidermoid cysts of the testis are felt to be benign germ cell neoplasms that can be thought of as monodermal teratomas with only ectodermal components. They are rare, comprising less than 1% of all testicular tumors. Histologically they are composed of cystic spaces lined by squamous epithelium and filled with yellowish-white flaky-appearing desquamated keratin. They manifest in patients usually between 20 and 40 years of age as painless masses that are often chronic in nature.

On sonography, epidermoid cysts appear as well-marginated lesions that are typically hypoechoic. They may have a hyperechoic rim that completely or partially shadows, and this appearance is very typical of an epidermoid cyst. Another very typical appearance is a lamellated arrangement of concentric rings like the cut surface of an onion. In either case, the presumptive diagnosis of epidermoid cyst should be made. Since these findings are typical but not entirely diagnostic, surgical exploration is still necessary to ensure that the lesion is benign. However, in most cases a full orchiectomy can be avoided in lieu of an enucleation of the lesion.

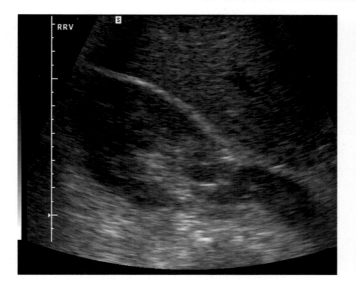
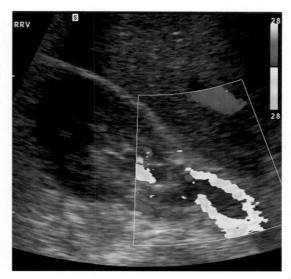

Transverse grey-scale and color Doppler view of the right upper quadrant at the level of the renal hilum. (See color plates.)

1. Describe the abnormality shown in this case.
2. Which renal vein is easiest to see in its entirety?
3. What alteration would you expect in the renal arterial flow?
4. Does detection of venous flow in the kidney exclude this diagnosis?

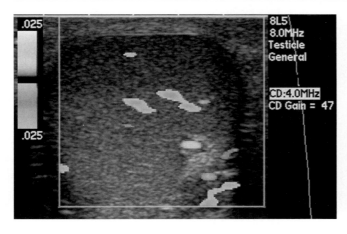
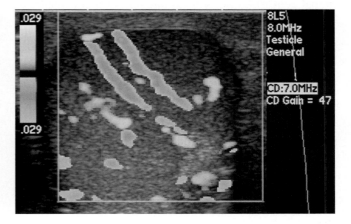

Two transverse color Doppler views of the same testis. (See color plates.)

1. Why is more blood flow shown on the second image?
2. What is the relationship between the strength of reflection from small objects such as red blood cells and the transmitted frequency?
3. What is the relationship between Doppler frequency shift and transmit frequency?
4. Under what circumstances would it be advantageous to drop the transmit frequency in order to improve Doppler sensitivity?

Renal Vein Thrombosis

1. The grey-scale image shows low-level echoes in the renal vein. These echoes could be real or artifactual. The color Doppler image shows flow around a central filling defect, confirming the presence of nonocclusive thrombosis.

2. The right renal vein is easier to see because it is shorter, and the liver can be used as a window. The left renal vein is longer and may be obscured by bowel gas from the stomach or splenic flexure.

3. Many times the arterial waveforms will be normal. If there is a change at all, the resistive index will increase.

4. Most cases of renal vein thrombosis are associated with persistent venous flow in the kidney and renal hilum, so detection of venous flow cannot be used to exclude the diagnosis.

Reference

Platt JF, Ellis JH, Rubin JM: Intrarenal arterial Doppler sonography in the detection of renal vein thrombosis of the native kidney. *AJR Am J Roentgenol* 1994; 162:1367-1370.

Cross-Reference

Ultrasound: THE REQUISITES, pp 112-115.

Comment

Renal vein thrombosis is an uncommon abnormality in adults. Although it may be idiopathic, some type of coagulopathy, such as diffuse intravascular coagulopathy or collagen vascular disease, is usually present. Renal vein thrombosis may also occur in the setting of membranoproliferative glomerulonephritis and is associated with the nephrotic syndrome. It can also be due to extension of clot from the inferior vena cava. The outcome depends on the rapidity and completeness of renal vein occlusion. Slowly progressive thrombosis allows for the development of venous collaterals, and incomplete thrombosis allows for maintained venous outflow so that effects on the kidney may be absent or minimal. On the other hand, complete and rapid thrombosis results in hemorrhagic infarction of the kidney.

Bland renal vein thrombosis appears like venous thrombosis anywhere else in the body. It produces an intraluminal defect and may enlarge the caliber of the vein. Thrombus may be hypoechoic or hyperechoic. Detection of venous outflow from the renal hilum does not exclude thrombosis because there may be persistent flow at this level in patients with partial thrombosis and collateral outflow in cases of complete thrombosis. It is also important to realize that in native kidneys, arterial inflow may be affected only minimally. This likely is related to venous collaterals that develop and provide continued venous outflow despite venous thrombosis in the main renal vein. In transplants, collateral flow is not possible, so complete renal vein thrombosis results in marked alteration in the arterial signal. This usually produces a classic to-and-fro pattern with pandiastolic flow reversal.

Effect of Transmit Frequency on Doppler Sensitivity

1. The second image was obtained with a 7 MHz transmit frequency and the first image with a 4 MHz frequency.

2. Strength of reflection is proportional to the fourth power of the transmitted frequency.

3. The Doppler frequency shift is proportional to the transmitted frequency.

4. When imaging deep vessels, it is often helpful to switch to a lower transmit frequency.

Reference

Middleton WD: Color Doppler image optimization and interpretation. *Ultrasound Q* 1998;14:194-208.

Cross-Reference

Ultrasound: THE REQUISITES, p 467.

Comment

The Doppler equation is one of the few equations in ultrasound that is worth memorizing:

$$Fd = Ft \times V \times \cos\theta \times 2 \times 1/C$$

Fd = Doppler frequency shift; Ft = Transmitted frequency; V = Velocity of blood; θ = Doppler angle; C = Speed of sound. Since the Doppler frequency shift is proportional to the transmitted frequency, higher frequency transducers cause a higher Doppler frequency shift that is easier to detect.

More importantly, the strength of the reflection from small objects such as red blood cells is proportional to the fourth power of the transmitted frequency. Therefore, higher frequency probes result in a stronger and more easily detected reflection from red blood cells. However, the improved sensitivity of higher frequency probes is counterbalanced by their poor penetration into deeper tissues. The net effect of transducer frequencies is sometimes unpredictable. In clinical practice, it is a good idea to use a variety of different probes operating at different frequencies whenever it becomes difficult to detect flow in a given vessel. For deep applications, it is often advantageous to switch to a lower frequency probe, whereas higher frequency probes are often better in superficial structures.

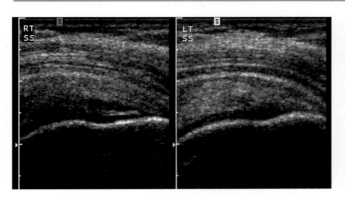
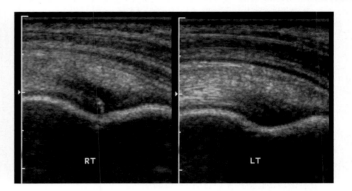

Two sets of dual longitudinal images of the rotator cuff in different patients with right shoulder pain.

1. What is the diagnosis?

2. Where does this abnormality most often occur?

3. Does this abnormality usually compress with transducer pressure?

4. Are bony changes typically associated with this abnormality?

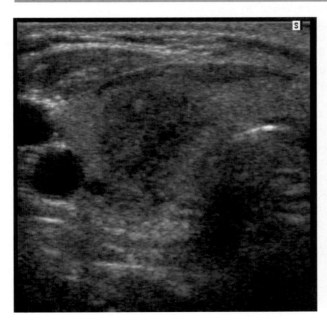
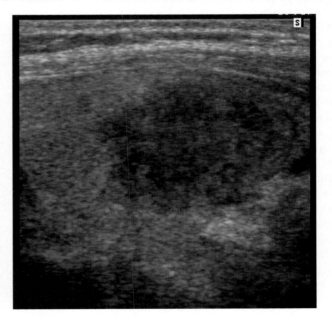

Transverse and longitudinal views of the right lobe of the thyroid in a patient with neck pain.

1. Describe the abnormality.

2. Would you expect this abnormality to resolve completely, resolve partially, or persist with medical therapy?

3. If this patient did not have neck pain, what else would you include in the differential diagnosis?

4. What is the most common type of thyroid cancer?

Partial Thickness Rotator Cuff Tear

1. Partial thickness rotator cuff tear.

2. Partial thickness tears most often occur along the deep surface of the supraspinatus insertion.

3. Partial thickness tears usually do not compress.

4. Bony pitting and irregularity is usually associated with partial thickness tears.

Reference

VanHolsbeeck MT, Kolowich PA, Eyler WR, et al: US depiction of partial thickness tear of the rotator cuff. *Radiology* 1995;197:443-446.

Cross-Reference

Ultrasound: THE REQUISITES, pp 455-457.

Comment

Tears of the rotator cuff can be divided into full thickness and partial thickness tears. Partial thickness tears are tears that do not extend all the way from the deep to the superficial surface of the cuff. They can involve either the deep surface, the superficial surface, or the internal aspect of the cuff. However, the majority arise from the deep surface and involve the supraspinatus tendon insertion.

The sonographic appearance of a partial thickness tear consists of a hypoechoic defect that remains constant despite changes in the orientation of the transducer. In most cases, there is also a bright reflector associated with the hypoechoic area. As with full thickness tears, the underlying bony cortex is usually irregular. Unlike full thickness tears, partial thickness tears are not associated with contour changes of the peribursal fat. In addition, partial thickness tears do not compress with transducer pressure.

Partial thickness tears must be distinguished from tendon anisotropy, which normally causes the deep surface of the supraspinatus insertion to appear hypoechoic. Tendon anisotropy usually becomes more echogenic when the transducer is angled upward, whereas the echogenicity of partial tears does not change. Tendon anisotropy is usually poorly marginated, while partial tears are better marginated. Finally, tendon anisotropy is usually entirely hypoechoic, whereas partial tears usually have at least a small hyperechoic component.

The reported sonographic sensitivity in detecting partial thickness tears is good, with two studies indicating a range of 93% to 96%. However, not everyone has had this degree of success, and it is clear that partial thickness tears are not as easy to identify as full thickness tears, and the criteria for partial thickness tears are less well studied. Unlike full thickness tears, partial tears are not treated with surgery unless patients fail a course of conservative management first. Therefore, the implication for missing a partial thickness tear is less than that for missing a full thickness tear.

Subacute Thyroiditis

1. The abnormality consists of a focal, poorly marginated, hypoechoic lesion in the mid right thyroid. In a patient with pain, this is highly suggestive of subacute thyroiditis.

2. With appropriate therapy, the sonographic findings should completely resolve.

3. If this patient did not have pain, thyroid cancer should be considered.

4. The most common type of thyroid cancer is papillary.

Reference

Ahuja AT, Metreweli C: Ultrasound of thyroid nodules. *Ultrasound Q* 2000;16:111-121.

Cross-Reference

Ultrasound: THE REQUISITES, pp 448-451.

Comment

The sonographic appearance in this case is nonspecific. Nevertheless, in a patient with the appropriate clinical presentation, the appearance is very typical of subacute granulomatous thyroiditis (also called de Quervain's thyroiditis). Subacute granulomatous thyroiditis is felt to be due to a viral infection. It occurs more often in women and produces an enlarged and painful thyroid and often a fever. It is often preceded by an upper respiratory infection. The entire gland may be involved, or involvement may be focal. Transient hyperthyroidism may be seen in the initial stages of the disease owing to follicular rupture. This transient hyperthyroidism may be followed by a transient phase of hypothyroidism. The process is usually diagnosed clinically and responds well to medical treatment. When sonography is performed, it typically shows a poorly marginated area of decreased echogenicity in the involved region of the thyroid. Blood flow to the area is typically normal or decreased.

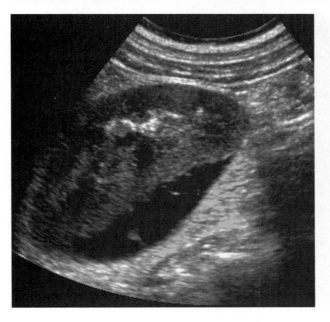
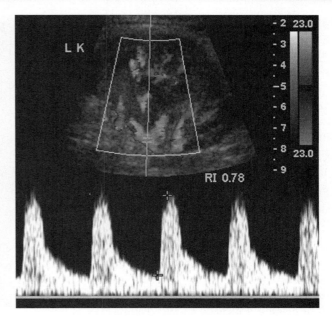

Grey-scale and Doppler views of the kidney in a patient with hypertension.

1. What is the abnormality?
2. Where is the abnormality likely to be located?
3. What is the name given to this entity?
4. What are some of the potential etiologies?

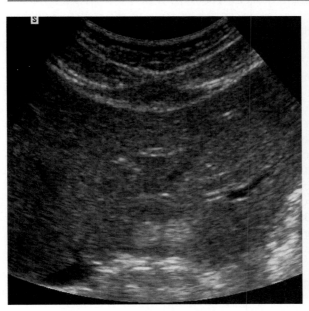
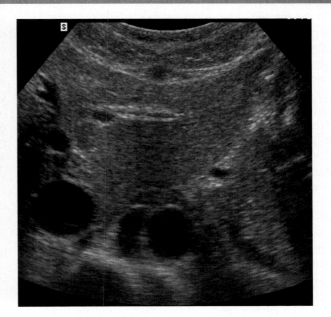

Transverse views of the left lobe of the liver and of the proximal abdominal aorta in two patients.

1. What artifact is present on both of these images?
2. What causes this artifact?
3. How can this artifact be eliminated?
4. Does sound travel faster in fat or in soft tissue?

CASE 178

Page Kidney

1. Fluid surrounding part of the kidney. The Doppler waveform shows decreased diastolic flow, with an elevated resistive index of 0.78. This suggests compression of the kidney.

2. Given the location on grey-scale scanning and the compression suggested by the increased resistive index, this lesion is almost certainly in the subcapsular space.

3. This entity is known as Page kidney.

4. Prior biopsy or other percutaneous intervention, recent lithotripsy, anticoagulation, bleeding from a tumor, and trauma are potential etiologies. This patient presented with hypertension following lithotripsy.

Reference

Chamorro HA, Forbes TW, Padowsky GO, Wholey MH: Multiimaging approach in the diagnosis of Page kidney. *AJR Am J Roentgenol* 1981;136:620–621.

Cross-Reference

Ultrasound: THE REQUISITES, pp 106–109.

Comment

In 1939, Page demonstrated that wrapping a kidney in cellophane could create hypertension. The resulting perinephritis caused compression of the kidney and altered the intrarenal hemodynamics such that ischemia developed. Activation of the renin-angiotensin-aldosterone system then resulted in hypertension. It was subsequently shown that a subcapsular hematoma could produce similar compression and could cause hypertension via the same mechanism.

Hemorrhage into the subcapsular space undergoes the same evolution that hemorrhage undergoes elsewhere in the body. In the acute period it appears echogenic. Over time, as the clot lyses and liquefies, the hematoma becomes more complex-appearing, with both cystic and solid areas. With more time, the hematoma becomes entirely liquefied and appears as a simple collection of fluid.

In the acute phase, subcapsular hematomas can be very difficult to appreciate sonographically. In most cases, the kidney looks very distorted and the normal renal architecture may be completely obliterated. This is partially due to compression of the kidney by the contained hematoma and partially due to the difficulty in determining where the hematoma stops and the kidney starts. In the latter regard, color Doppler can be helpful in distinguishing the vascular renal parenchyma from the avascular hematoma. Careful grey-scale inspection can usually find the interface between the kidney and the hematoma once the possibility of a subcapsular hematoma has been considered.

CASE 179

Midline Refraction Artifact

1. These images illustrate refraction artifact from the rectus muscles causing a duplication of a hepatic hemangioma and causing apparent widening and dissection of the aorta.

2. The rectus muscles act as an acoustic lens so that sound is bent and structures are inappropriately localized and duplicated on the image.

3. This artifact can be eliminated by scanning with the transducer to the side of the midline, away from the edge of the rectus muscle.

4. Sound travels faster in soft tissue than in fat.

Reference

Ziskin MC: Fundamental physics of ultrasound and its propagation in tissue. *Radiographics* 1993;13:105–709.

Comment

Sound waves bend when passing obliquely through an interface between two substances that transmit sound at different speeds. This is called refraction and is analogous to redirection of light by an optical lens. Since the speed of sound is least in fat (approximately 1450 m/sec) and greatest in soft tissues (approximately 1540 m/sec), refraction artifacts are most prominent at fat-soft tissue interfaces. The most widely recognized refraction artifact occurs at the junction of the rectus abdominis muscle and adjacent abdominal wall fat. Since the ultrasound computer assumes that sound travels in a straight line, structures that produce echoes after the sound pulse has been refracted will be incorrectly localized on the image. In fact, structures are typically duplicated because they reflect not only the sound pulse that has been refracted but also a sound pulse that has not been refracted. The end result is a duplication of deep abdominal and pelvic structures seen when scanning transversely through the abdominal midline.

Soft tissue and fluid interfaces can also produce refraction artifacts because the speed of sound in body fluids (1480 m/sec) is slower than in soft tissues. This can produce duplication of structures deep to the refracting interface just as with soft tissue–fat interfaces.

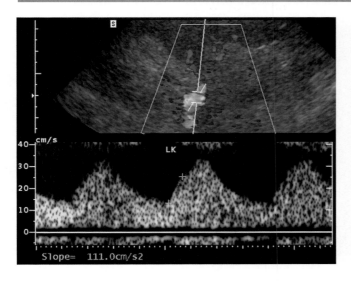

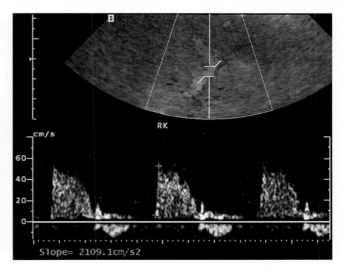

Pulsed Doppler waveforms from the left and right kidneys.

1. Which renal arterial waveform is abnormal?

2. What is a normal early systolic acceleration?

3. How severe must this condition be before acceleration values drop?

4. What term is used to describe the abnormal waveform shown in this case?

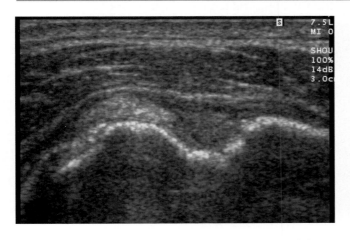

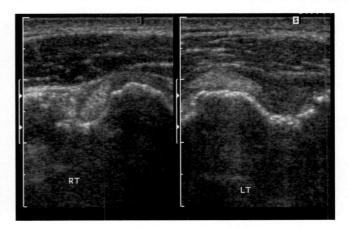

Transverse view of the anterior left shoulder and similar dual comparison views of the right and left shoulders.

1. Describe the abnormality.

2. What other abnormality would you expect in this patient?

3. Identify the greater and lesser tuberosity on the first image.

Blunted Intrarenal Artery Waveform Due to Renal Artery Stenosis

1. Neither waveform is normal. The first waveform shows a low systolic acceleration indicative of proximal arterial stenosis. The second shows diminished diastolic flow due to renal parenchymal disease.

2. A normal early systolic acceleration is greater than 3 m/sec^2.

3. Probably somewhere between 60% and 80% diameter stenosis.

4. A blunted arterial waveform is also called a parvus-tardus waveform.

Reference

Stavros T, Harshfield D: Renal Doppler, renal artery stenosis, and renovascular hypertension: Direct and indirect duplex sonographic abnormalities in patients with renal artery stenosis. *Ultrasound Q* 1994; 2(4):217–263.

Cross-Reference

Ultrasound: THE REQUISITES, pp 111–112.

Comment

A great deal of interest has been focused on the detection of renal artery stenosis in patients with hypertension. There are two basic ways to detect this abnormality using Doppler analysis. One involves evaluation of the arterial waveforms in the segmental or interlobar arteries of the kidney. The effects of a proximal stenosis have long been recognized in clinical medicine, and all medical students learn to feel the distal pulses for parvus-tardus effects in patients with aortic valve stenosis. Parvus tardus refers to decreased amplitude of the pulse and delayed time to reach the peak.

These same parvus-tardus effects can be seen in the Doppler waveform distal to a stenosis. Normally, the early systolic upstroke is extremely rapid. In patients with a proximal stenosis, the upstroke is slower. This can be quantified by determining the early systolic acceleration. Acceleration is defined as the change in velocity divided by the change in time. Both of these values can be obtained on an angle-corrected Doppler waveform by simply placing a cursor at the early and late points of the systolic upstroke.

Another effect of a proximal stenosis is a decreased systolic peak. This is harder to measure on an absolute basis but can be recognized by noting a relative change in the systolic peak compared to the diastolic flow. This change in the systolic peak compared to the diastolic flow can be quantitated with the resistive index. Since systole is reduced to a greater extent than diastole, the resistive index goes down. Therefore, asymmetry in renal resistive indexes is another way of identifying renal artery stenosis.

Biceps Tendon Dislocation

1. The biceps tendon groove is empty on the left, and the tendon is located anterior to the lesser tuberosity.

2. Patients with biceps tendon dislocation/subluxation almost always have an associated rotator cuff tear.

3. The lesser tuberosity forms the medial edge of the biceps tendon groove, and the greater tuberosity forms the lateral edge. The biceps tendon always dislocates medially. In this view, the lesser tuberosity is the tuberosity immediately posterior to the dislocated biceps tendon.

Reference

Middleton WD, Teefey SA, Yamaguchi K: Sonography of the shoulder. *Semin Musculoskeletal Radiol* 1998; 2:211–221.

Cross-Reference

Ultrasound: THE REQUISITES, pp 455–457.

Comment

The biceps tendon is normally secured in the biceps tendon groove by the transverse humeral ligament and several extensions of tissue from the supraspinatus and the subscapularis tendons. With proper transducer angulation (perpendicular to the long axis of the tendon), the biceps tendon appears as an echogenic ovoid structure in the groove. If the tendon cannot be seen in the groove, then it is either torn or dislocated, or the transducer is not angled properly. These possibilities can be distinguished by identifying the tendon inferiorly and following it superiorly. If it is intact but dislocated, the more superior tendon is seen medial to the tendon groove. It may be located anterior to the lesser tuberosity, as in this case, or medial to the lesser tuberosity.

Whenever there is a dislocated biceps tendon, it is very likely that there is an associated rotator cuff tear. When the tendon is just anterior to the lesser tuberosity, most likely there is a supraspinatus tear. When the tendon dislocates medial to the lesser tuberosity, there is usually a subscapularis tear.

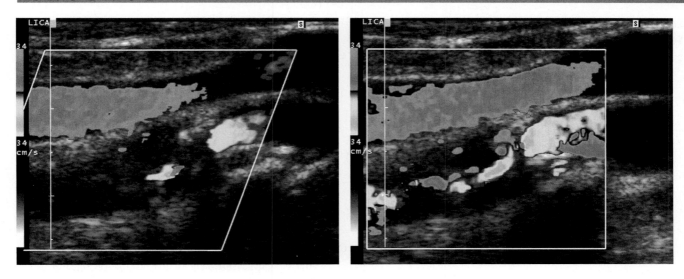

Longitudinal views of the internal carotid artery. (See color plates.)

1. Based on the different Doppler angle in the two images above, in which image would you expect the frequency shifts from the internal carotid artery to be higher?

2. Why is the internal carotid blood flow harder to detect in the first image than in the second image?

3. Is the effect responsible for the differences in these images more noticeable on linear arrays or on curved arrays?

4. When using a phased array transducer, is it better to perform Doppler analysis in the center of the sector or at the edge of the sector?

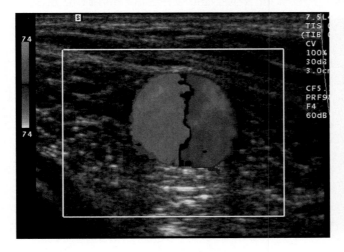 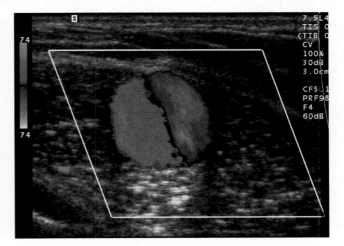

Transverse color Doppler views of the outflow vein from a dialysis fistula. (See color plates.)

1. Is aliasing present on these views?

2. Explain the color assignment on these images.

3. Why did the distribution of red and blue color assignment change when the Doppler pulse was steered to the right in the second image?

4. How accurate would you expect pulsed Doppler velocity determinations to be in this vessel?

Effect of Beam Steering on Doppler Sensitivity

1. In the first image, the beam is steered to the left so that the Doppler angle is lower. This results in a higher frequency shift from the internal carotid artery.

2. Despite the higher frequency shifts, sensitivity in the first image is reduced because of the beam steering. In the second image, the beam is directed straight down, and sensitivity improves even though there is a less favorable Doppler angle.

3. Electronic beam steering is performed on linear array transducers but not on curved array transducers, so the effect is only present on linear array images.

4. With phased array transducers, there is less beam steering in the center of the image, so it is better to perform Doppler analysis in the center, provided other angle effects are equivalent.

Reference
Middleton WD: Color Doppler image optimization and interpretation. *Ultrasound Q* 1998;14:194–208.

Comment
In the images shown in this case, the angle between the carotid artery and the transmitted Doppler pulse is greater (i.e., closer to 90 degrees) in the second image. Because of this, the blood flow in the internal carotid artery produces a smaller frequency shift in the second image and a larger shift in the first image. Consequently, it would seem to make sense that flow would be easier to detect in the first image. However, this is not the case because the transmitted Doppler pulse was steered to the left in the first image and was not steered in the second image.

Beam steering is a control that is more or less user-selectable. Whenever the Doppler pulse is directed at an angle other than perpendicular to the transducer surface, it is being electronically steered. This occurs whenever color Doppler is performed at the edge of the sector image with a phased array transducer. Beam steering is also a color and pulsed Doppler option on most linear array transducers. Whenever the Doppler beam is steered, it loses some of its focusing capabilities, and the transmitted pulse loses a greater percentage of its energy to side lobes. In addition, when the transmitted pulse is steered, the echo returns to the transducer at an angle. This produces less of an effect on the crystals and a weaker electronic impulse than when the echo returns at 90 degrees (analogous to the different force exerted on a billiard table cushion when a ball strikes the cushion at an angle compared to striking the cushion head-on). Thus, for a variety of reasons, signal strength is less when the Doppler beam is steered.

With color Doppler, the decreased signal strength may result in a loss of sensitivity sufficient enough to cause a false-positive diagnosis of vessel occlusion. Therefore, adjustment of Doppler beam steering must take into account the sometimes conflicting effects of different Doppler angles on the frequency shift as well as the signal strength.

Helical Flow

1. Aliasing is not present. The interface between red and blue in the middle of the vessel is in the dark shades, corresponding to low frequency shifts. This indicates a change in direction rather than aliasing.

2. Helical flow is present in the vessel, so that one half of the vessel has flow toward the transducer and the other half has flow away from the transducer.

3. When the Doppler pulse was steered at an angle, the division between blood flowing toward the pulse and blood flowing away from the pulse changed.

4. Pulsed Doppler velocity determinations are not accurate because flow is not parallel to the long axis of the vessel, and determination of true flow direction is impossible. Thus, determination of the true Doppler angle is not possible

Reference
Middleton WD: Color Doppler image optimization and interpretation. *Ultrasound Q* 1998;14:194–208.

Comment
We often assume that the blood flow in a vessel more or less travels in a straight line along the long axis of that vessel. In general this is true. However, there are some situations where flow is not directly straight and parallel to the axis of the vessel. In such cases, it is possible to misinterpret the direction of flow. This occurs most dramatically when there is helical flow in a vessel. With helical flow, the flow spirals in the artery in one overall axial direction. But in one half of the vessel, the flow is toward the transmitted Doppler pulse, and in the other half the flow is away from the Doppler pulse. As shown in this case, helical flow can produce the appearance of simultaneous flow in one direction in one half of the vessel and in the opposite direction in the other half of the vessel.

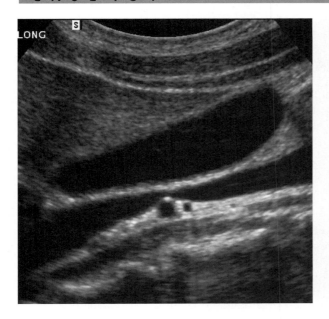
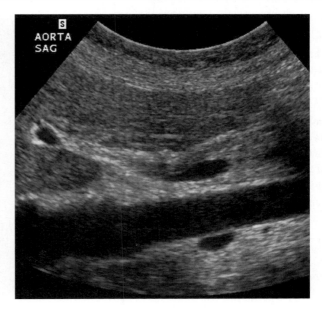

Longitudinal views of the inferior vena cava and the aorta in two patients.

1. What normal variants are shown in these views of the aorta and the inferior vena cava?

2. How common are these variants?

3. Which is seen most often on sonography?

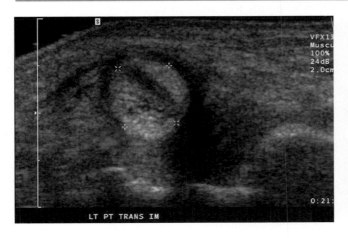
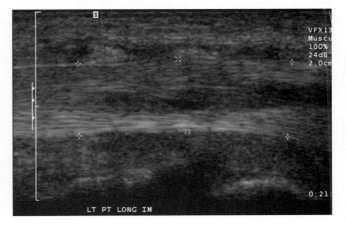

Transverse and longitudinal views of the posterior tibial tendon (cursors).

1. Describe the findings.

2. What three tendons are located posterior to the medial malleolus?

3. What two tendons are located posterior to the lateral malleolus?

4. Which of these tendons is most likely to be affected like this?

Renal Vascular Variants

1. The first image shows two right renal arteries located behind the inferior vena cava. The second image shows a retroaortic left renal vein.

2. Duplicated renal arteries occur in approximately 20% to 30% of the population. A retroaortic left renal vein occurs as an isolated finding in approximately 2% of the population and as part of a circumaortic left renal vein in approximately 10%.

3. It is much easier to see duplicated right renal arteries on sonography. Retroaortic renal veins are typically collapsed and harder to visualize with ultrasound.

Reference

Cho KJ, Thornbury JR, Prince MR: Renal arteries and veins: Normal variants. In Pollack HM, McClennan BL, Dyer RB, Kenney PJ (eds): *Clinical Urography*, 2nd ed. Philadelphia, WB Saunders, 2000, pp 2476-2489.

Cross-Reference

Genitourinary Radiology: THE REQUISITES, pp 55-59.

Comment

Multiple renal arteries are common. They usually arise from the aorta near the main renal artery. However, they occasionally arise significantly lower on the aorta and rarely from the common iliac arteries. Accessory renal arteries can enter the kidneys either through the renal hilum or directly through the renal parenchyma. Many accessory renal arteries are not detected with sonography. This is especially true of accessory left renal arteries. However, accessory right renal arteries that arise from the aorta near the main renal artery are relatively easy to see. As this case demonstrates, when accessory right renal arteries are present, longitudinal views of the inferior vena cava show two round structures behind the inferior vena cava and in front of the right diaphragmatic crus. Doppler analysis can be used to confirm the arterial nature of these structures.

Retroaortic left renal veins are another common renal vascular variant. Like accessory renal arteries, they are easily overlooked on sonography. Normally there are no vascular structures located between the abdominal aorta and the spine. When present, a retroaortic left renal vein appears as a vascular structure communicating with the inferior vena cava and passing posterior to the aorta. On longitudinal scans it appears as an anechoic or hypoechoic oval-shaped structure behind the aorta, as shown in this case. It is usually associated with a normally located left renal vein (i.e., a vein that passes between the superior mesenteric vein and the aorta) and in such a case is termed a circumaortic left renal vein.

Partial Longitudinal Tendon Tear

1. An elongated, hypoechoic defect along the long axis of the tendon is seen on the longitudinal view, and a central defect is seen on the transverse view.

2. The three tendons are the Posterior Tibial, the flexor Digitorum longus, and the flexor Hallucis longus. Mnemonic—Tom, Dick, and Harry.

3. The peroneus longus and brevis tendons are located posterior to the lateral malleolus.

4. The posterior tibial tendon is the most likely to develop partial tears such as this one.

References

Fessell DP, Vanderschueren GM, Jacobson JA, et al: US of the ankle: Technique, anatomy, and diagnosis of pathologic conditions. *Radiographics* 1998;18:325-340.

Waitches GM, Rockett M, Brage M, Sudakoff G: Ultrasonographic-surgical correlation of ankle tendon tears. *J Ultrasound Med* 1998;17:249-256.

Cross-Reference

Ultrasound: THE REQUISITES, pp 455-456.

Comment

The normal posterior tibial tendon runs immediately posterior and then inferior to the medial malleolus. It passes into the foot and fans out to insert on the navicular as well as on the cuneiforms and the proximal metatarsals of the second, third, and fourth toes. Immediately posterior to the posterior tibial tendon is the flexor digitorum longus tendon. Further posterior and medial is the flexor hallucis longus. Like other tendons, these three tendons have a fibrillar echo pattern that varies in echogenicity depending on the angle between them and the sound pulse.

The scans that are shown in this case demonstrate a focal, elongated hypoechoic area within an enlarged posterior tibial tendon. This is the typical appearance of a partial tear. Sonography is an excellent means of diagnosing tears of the ankle tendons. In one study, sonography predicted the condition of the tendon (intact, partially torn, or completely torn) with 90% accuracy when compared to surgery.

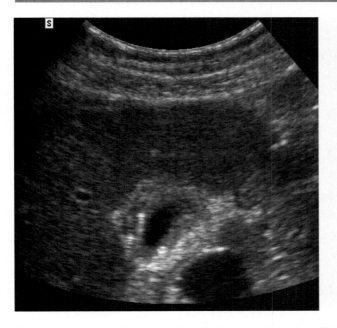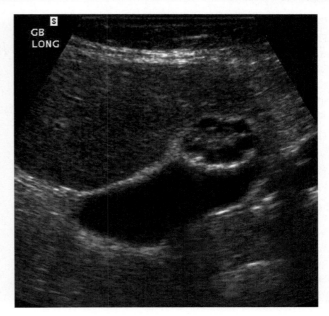

Transverse and longitudinal views of the gallbladder in two patients.

1. Describe the abnormal findings in these images.
2. Do gallstones cause this condition?
3. What is the treatment of choice?
4. What is the characteristic pathologic finding in this condition?

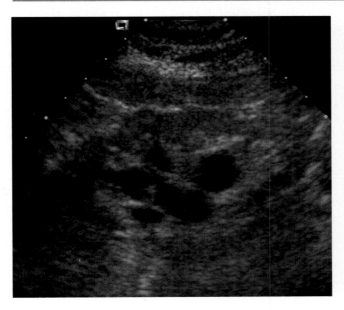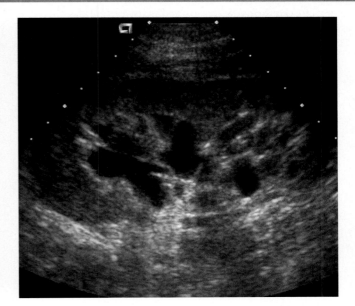

Longitudinal views of the kidney in two patients.

1. Describe the abnormality in these kidneys.
2. What are the two major conditions that should be considered in the differential diagnosis?
3. How is it possible to distinguish these conditions?
4. What is the origin of the abnormality shown in this case?

Adenomyomatosis of the Gallbladder

1. The first image shows gallbladder wall thickening and several short, bright comet-tail artifacts arising from the gallbladder wall. The second image shows a fundal mass that contains multiple internal cystic spaces. All of these findings are seen in adenomyomatosis.

2. This condition is not caused by gallstones.

3. No treatment is required. This is generally an asymptomatic condition.

4. The characteristic finding on pathology is Rokitansky-Aschoff sinuses.

Reference

Raghavendra BN, Subramanyam BR, Balthazar EJ, et al: Sonography of adenomyomatosis of the gallbladder: Radiologic-pathologic correlation. *Radiology* 1983; 146:747–752.

Cross-Reference

Ultrasound: THE REQUISITES, pp 48–49.

Comment

Adenomyomatosis is a hyperplastic condition of the gallbladder wall. It is characterized by small mucosal diverticula that protrude into a thickened layer of muscle. The mucosal diverticula are called Rokitansky-Aschoff sinuses. Adenomyomatosis is not related to gallstones and occurs equally in men and women. It is a benign condition with no malignant potential.

Adenomyomatosis occurs in three forms. It can involve the gallbladder diffusely, segmentally, or focally. The diffuse form may or may not cause enough wall thickening to be detected on sonography. The segmental form of adenomyomatosis causes an annular region of wall thickening that may separate the lumen into two different compartments. In such cases, bile stasis in the fundal compartment predisposes to gallstone formation. The focal form most often appears as a mass in the gallbladder fundus. Although the Rokitansky-Aschoff sinuses are well visualized as cystic spaces in the second image, they are usually too small to be resolved. However, it is not uncommon for cholesterol crystals to accumulate in the Rokitansky-Aschoff sinuses, and these crystals are frequently associated with comet-tail artifacts that can be seen sonographically.

In most cases, the diagnosis of adenomyomatosis can be made with confidence based on the sonographic findings. When there is extensive wall thickening and the characteristic comet-tail artifacts or Rokitansky-Aschoff sinuses are not seen, the possibility of gallbladder cancer should also be considered. In such cases, an oral cholecystogram may be helpful to better visualize the Rokitansky-Aschoff sinuses and thus confirm the diagnosis of adenomyomatosis.

Peripelvic Cysts Simulating Hydronephrosis

1. Both images show fluid-filled structures separating the renal sinuses.

2. The differential diagnosis is hydronephrosis and peripelvic cysts.

3. Look for communication between the fluid-filled structures and each other and with the renal pelvis.

4. Peripelvic cysts are believed to be lymphatic in origin.

Reference

Koelliker SL, Cronan JJ: Acute urinary tract obstruction: Imaging update. *Urol Clin North Am* 1997;24:571–582.

Cross-Reference

Ultrasound: THE REQUISITES, pp 85–86.

Comment

A number of abnormalities can simulate hydronephrosis. Perhaps the most common is peripelvic cysts. These cysts are believed to be congenital and arise from lymphatics in the renal sinus. Although they are filled with simple fluid, it is generally more difficult to clear them out of all internal echoes than it is to clear simple cortical cysts. They may be single, but they are often multiple. Single cysts are usually easy to diagnose with sonography. When multiple peripelvic cysts are present, they may become elongated and ovoid and herniate out into the renal hilum. Under these conditions, they are often mistaken for hydronephrosis.

The best way to distinguish multiple peripelvic cysts from hydronephrosis is to obtain a coronal view. In such a view, true hydronephrosis usually appears very typical, with a dilated renal pelvis that extends into dilated infundibulae that extend into the upper, mid, and lower zones of the kidney. With peripelvic cysts, this typical appearance is lacking. Whenever there is doubt, intravenous urography is a good method to distinguish between the two possibilities. If the patient has renal dysfunction, gadolinium-enhanced MRI or nuclear scintigraphy can be used.

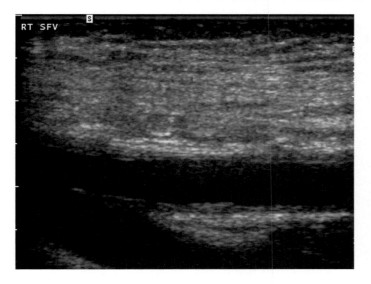
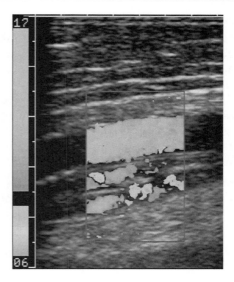

Longitudinal grey-scale view of the superficial femoral vein in one patient and longitudinal color Doppler view of the superficial femoral artery and vein in another patient. (See color plates.)

1. What is the abnormality in these two different patients with the same condition?
2. What is the significance of these findings?
3. Is clot echogenicity a reliable way of distinguishing acute from chronic deep vein thrombosis (DVT)?
4. Is vein diameter a reliable way to distinguish acute from chronic DVT?

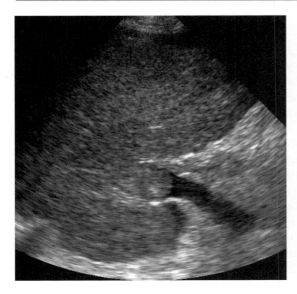
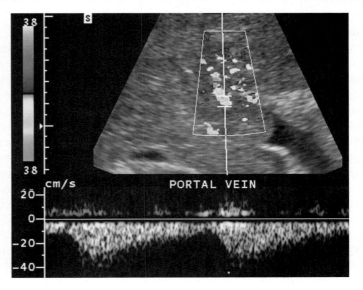

Longitudinal grey-scale view of and color Doppler view and pulsed Doppler waveform from the portal vein. (See color plates.)

1. What is the significance of an expanded portal vein lumen filled with echogenic material?
2. What is the significance of the vascularity shown on the color Doppler image?
3. What is the most likely etiology of this abnormality?
4. Is it safe to biopsy an abnormality such as this?

Chronic Deep Vein Thrombosis

1. On grey-scale imaging, normal vein walls are so thin that they are visualized as an echogenic interface with no measurable thickness. In this case, the grey-scale image shows a wall that is easily resolvable. On color Doppler, normal venous blood flow is seen as a single channel of color extending from one wall to the other wall. In this case, multiple irregular channels are present in the lumen of the vein.

2. Both of these findings represent chronic changes from prior episodes of acute deep vein thrombosis (DVT).

3. Acute thrombus tends to be hypoechoic, and chronic thrombus tends to be more echogenic. However, there is a moderate amount of overlap, so that echogenicity is not a useful way to determine the age of the clot.

4. Acute DVT often expands the lumen of the vein. The lumen is usually contracted or normal with chronic DVT. As with echogenicity, there is enough overlap between acute and chronic DVT that vein diameter is not a reliable distinguishing characteristic.

Reference
Cronan JJ, Leen V: Recurrent deep venous thrombosis: Limitations of US. *Radiology* 1989;170:739–742.

Cross-Reference
Ultrasound: THE REQUISITES, pp 483–485.

Comment
Following an episode of acute DVT, clot may resolve in several ways. In the fortunate patient, it will completely resolve, and the vein will return to a normal appearance and normal function. This occurs in approximately 60% of patients, most often when the thrombosis is relatively limited to begin with. In less fortunate patients, clot resorption leaves various sequelae that may compromise valvular function and lead to the postphlebitic syndrome. One sequela is a focal eccentric thickening of the vein wall. Another is diffuse thickening of the vein wall, occasionally with associated wall calcification. A third change is development of irregular channels within the partially recanalized vein lumen. These changes usually occur and stabilize within 6 months of the initial thrombosis. Since these chronic changes can be difficult to distinguish from acute changes, some experts advocate a repeat ultrasound after 6 months in order to establish a new base line. This type of comparison scan can be extremely valuable when the patient returns with recurrent symptoms and the question of acute versus chronic DVT is raised.

Tumor Thrombus in the Portal Vein

1. Echogenic material within the portal vein indicates venous thrombosis. When the lumen is expanded by the thrombus, it is much more likely to be tumor thrombus than bland thrombus.

2. Detection of internal vascularity within a portal vein thrombus indicates that the thrombus is vascularized tissue and is not bland thrombus. This represents a sign of tumor invasion of the portal vein.

3. The most common cause of tumor thrombus in the portal vein is hepatocellular cancer. Other possibilities include metastatic disease of the liver, cholangiocarcinoma, and islet cell tumors of the pancreas.

4. Biopsy of portal vein thrombus is safe and can simultaneously establish the diagnosis as well as the stage of the tumor.

Reference
Dodd GD III, Memel DS, Baron RL, et al: Portal vein thrombosis in patients with cirrhosis: Does sonographic detection of intrathrombus flow allow differentiation of benign and malignant thrombus? *AJR Am J Roentgenol* 1995;165:573.

Cross-Reference
Ultrasound: THE REQUISITES, p 24.

Comment
Up to 30% of hepatocellular carcinomas invade the portal veins. The thrombus starts in the peripheral veins and then grows into the more central portal veins. As the thrombus grows toward the central portal veins, it drags its arterial supply with it. For this reason, the arterial flow in tumor thrombus is usually in the opposite direction as the portal venous flow. In some patients, it is relatively easy to see the internal blood vessels in tumor thrombus on color Doppler and to obtain an arterial signal on pulsed Doppler. However, in other patients this may not be possible. Therefore, inability to detect internal Doppler signals does not necessarily mean that the thrombus is bland. Certain grey-scale findings can also be helpful. Tumor thrombus often expands the lumen of the portal vein, while bland thrombus rarely does. In addition, tumor thrombus may contain small cystic spaces, and this is uncommon in bland thrombus.

When it is necessary to obtain a tissue diagnosis in a patient with suspected hepatocellular carcinoma and tumor thrombus, it is safe to biopsy the thrombus in the portal vein. At our institution, this is done as a fine-needle aspiration with a 22- to 25-gauge needle.

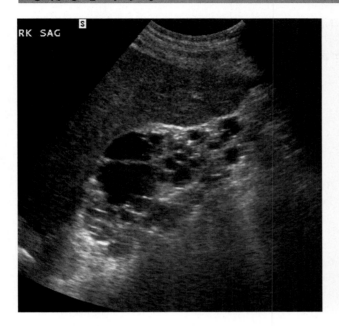
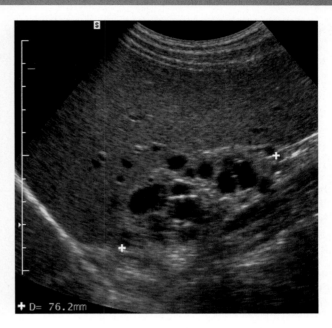

Longitudinal views of the right kidney in two patients.

1. What is the likely etiology of the cysts in these patients' kidneys?

2. Are these patients at increased risk for renal tumors?

3. Will renal transplantation alter the natural history of this condition?

4. Are cysts more likely in other organs?

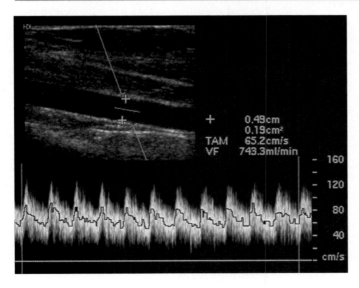

Measurement of flow volume in a patient following placement of an arteriovenous fistula for hemodialysis.

1. What is the standard method of measuring blood flow volume using pulsed Doppler?

2. What does the line in the center of the waveform indicate?

3. What does TAM stand for?

4. Does this method work best in large vessels with high flow or in small vessels with low flow?

Acquired Cystic Disease

1. Multiple cysts are seen in atrophic, echogenic kidneys. This is typical of acquired cystic disease (ACD).

2. ACD predisposes patients to renal tumors.

3. Transplantation improves the natural history of ACD.

4. Cysts are isolated in the kidneys. Other organs are not involved.

Reference

Levine E, Slusher SL, Grantham JJ, Wetzel LH: Natural history of acquired renal cystic disease in dialysis patients: A prospective longitudinal CT study. *AJR Am J Roentgenol* 1991;156:501–506.

Cross-Reference

Ultrasound: THE REQUISITES, pp 87–88.

Comment

Acquired cystic disease (ACD) is a condition that is commonly seen in patients with chronic renal failure. It is especially prevalent in patients on dialysis and increases with the duration of dialysis. After 3 years of dialysis, the incidence is approximately 80%. The genesis of the cysts is believed to be hyperplasia of the tubular epithelium with resulting nephron dilatation. The cause of the epithelial hyperplasia has not been discovered. Successful treatment of the renal failure with transplantation has been shown to reverse the development of these cysts.

One of the complications of ACD is hemorrhage into the cysts, the perinephric space, or the subcapsular space. This hemorrhaging can cause significant morbidity and even mortality. The other potential complication is the development of renal cell carcinoma. The incidence of renal cancer is estimated at approximately 10% in patients with ACD.

On sonography, the typical appearance is that of small echogenic kidneys with multiple cortical-based cysts. Early in the process, the cysts are small, and, therefore, it may be difficult to demonstrate all of the classic characteristics of simple cysts. With time, the cysts become more numerous and larger. In fact, ACD may result in overall enlargement of the kidneys to the point where they can be confused with kidneys with polycystic kidney disease.

Renal cell cancer can be recognized as a solid mass contrasted to all of the adjacent cysts. Because the differential diagnosis includes a hemorrhagic cyst, use of color Doppler can be helpful if internal vascularity is detected in a mass. Although contrast enhanced CT and MRI are superior to sonography in detecting renal cancers in patients with ACD, sonography remains a valuable problem solving tool when CT or MRI is inconclusive.

Measurement of Flow Volume

1. Multiply the cross-sectional area of the vessel by the average flow velocity.

2. The line in the center of the waveform is the mean flow velocity.

3. TAM stands for Time Averaged Mean velocity.

4. This method works best in large vessels with high flow volumes.

Reference

Taylor KJW, Holland S: Doppler US: Part I. Basic principles, instrumentation, and pitfalls. *Radiology* 1990;174:297–307.

Comment

Flow volume measurements are possible with Doppler techniques. They are calculated by multiplying the velocity by the cross-sectional area of the vessel. In most cases, the area of the vessel is obtained by measuring a diameter and using the equation for area, assuming that the vessel is circular in cross section. The velocity is obtained from a standard angle-corrected pulsed Doppler waveform. At any point in time, the waveform displays a range of velocities from a maximum to a minimum. In order to avoid overestimation of flow (by using the maximum velocity) or underestimation of flow (by using the minimum velocity), one must multiply the area of the vessel by the mean velocity. Internal software is provided so that the mean velocity can be determined at each point in time. It is also important to realize that the flow velocity in a vessel varies in different parts of the lumen. Therefore, one must open up the Doppler sample volume so that it includes the entire diameter of the lumen.

If the flow is constant and nonpulsatile, then a single mean velocity obtained at any point in time is adequate to measure flow volume. If the flow is pulsatile, such as the arterial flow in this case, then the mean velocity has to be averaged over time to obtain a time averaged mean velocity (TAM). It is the TAM that is multiplied by the cross-sectional area to calculate flow volume.

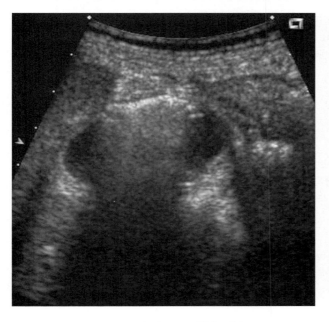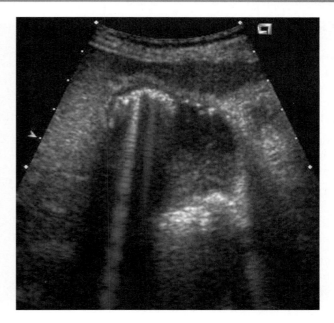

Transverse views of the gallbladder.

1. Describe the abnormal findings.
2. Is this abnormality more common in men or in women?
3. Is this a medical or a surgical condition?
4. What other gallbladder abnormalities can simulate this condition?

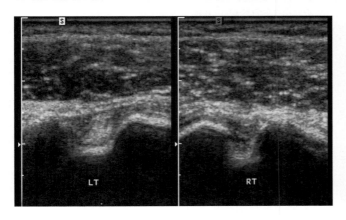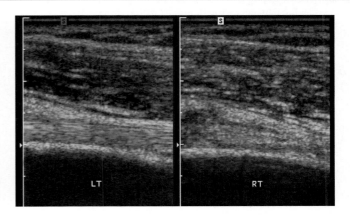

Dual transverse and longitudinal views of the left and right biceps tendon groove.

1. Describe the abnormality.
2. Is this diagnosis difficult to make clinically?
3. Which head of the biceps muscle is involved?
4. Are there other conditions that should be considered?

Emphysematous Cholecystitis

1. The first image shows an echogenic reflection along the nondependent wall of the gallbladder that casts a dirty shadow. The second image shows ring-down artifact arising from the same area. These findings indicate air and are consistent with emphysematous cholecystitis.

2. Emphysematous cholecystitis is more common in men, presumably because they have a higher incidence of vascular disease than women.

3. This condition represents a severe form of cholecystitis and should be treated surgically, or, if the patient is not an operative candidate, with percutaneous cholecystostomy.

4. Other causes of increased echogenicity in the nondependent wall include porcelain gallbladder and a gallbladder full of stones

Reference

Middleton WD: The gallbladder. In Goldberg BB (ed): *Diagnostic Ultrasound.* Baltimore, Williams & Wilkins, 1993, pp 116–142.

Cross-Reference

Ultrasound: THE REQUISITES, pp 44–45.

Comment

Emphysematous cholecystitis represents a rare and advanced form of complicated cholecystitis. It occurs in elderly patients with underlying vascular disease. It is believed that infection with gas-forming organisms results from gallbladder ischemia. Therefore, many of these patients have diabetes and many do not have gallstones. The risk of perforation is significantly increased in patients with emphysematous cholecystitis. Therefore, surgery should be performed unless there are contraindications to surgery. Percutaneous catheter drainage is an alternative if the patient cannot tolerate surgery.

The sonographic appearance of emphysematous cholecystitis can overlap that of porcelain gallbladder and a gallbladder completely filled with stones. All appear as an echogenic curvilinear reflector with posterior shadowing. In most cases, the shadow is dirty with emphysematous cholecystitis and clean with the other two conditions. In addition, gas generally produces a brighter reflection than calcification or stones. Finally, gas often produces a ring-down artifact, and stones and calcification do not. In this case, a ring-down artifact is seen on the second image; thus, the diagnosis of emphysematous cholecystitis can be made with confidence.

Biceps Tendon Rupture

1. The transverse views show an empty biceps tendon groove on the right. The longitudinal views show lack of the normal fibrillar pattern in the tendon groove.

2. In most patients, the tendon and muscle belly retract and produce a bulge in the anterior arm that is easy to see and feel on physical examination.

3. The long head is involved.

4. In addition to tendon rupture, the differential diagnosis for an empty biceps tendon groove includes tendon dislocation and anisotropic effects due to improper transducer angulation.

Reference

Middleton WD: Shoulder pain. In Bluth EI, Benson C, Arger P, et al (eds): *The Practice of Ultrasonography.* New York, Thieme, 1999.

Cross-Reference

Ultrasound: THE REQUISITES, p 455.

Comment

Patients with impingement syndrome of the shoulder may have symptoms related to the rotator cuff, the biceps tendon, or both. The origin of these symptoms can be difficult to sort out clinically. For this reason, it is important to scan the biceps in patients suspected of having a rotator cuff tear.

Rupture of the biceps tendon is usually readily detected on physical examination because the retracted muscle belly forms a lump in the upper arm that becomes more prominent when the biceps is flexed. On sonography, biceps tendon rupture is one of the causes of an empty-appearing groove. Biceps tendon dislocation is the other cause. One must also be aware that if the transducer is not oriented perpendicular to the tendon, the anisotropic properties of the tendon cause it to appear hypoechoic, and the result is an empty-appearing groove.

In some cases, a ruptured biceps tendon becomes scarred to the tendon groove or just below the tendon groove. This is referred to as autotenodesis, and in such cases there is minimal or no retraction of the muscle belly, and the diagnosis is less apparent on physical examination. Sonographically, the tendon appears attenuated at the level of the groove, but there are usually some detectable fibers, especially on longitudinal views. In most cases, the diagnosis is still possible because the intra-articular portion of the biceps is absent.

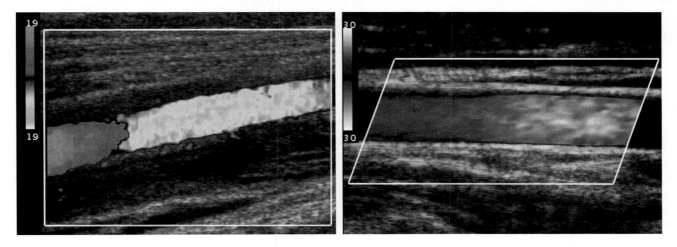

Longitudinal view of the superficial femoral artery and the common carotid artery. (See color plates.)

1. Assuming that at any point in time, there is a similar blood flow velocity and direction along the length of these vessels, why is the color assignment different in the proximal and distal segments?

2. Can the peak systolic flow velocity be determined from these images?

3. Other than blood flow velocity, what determines the color shading?

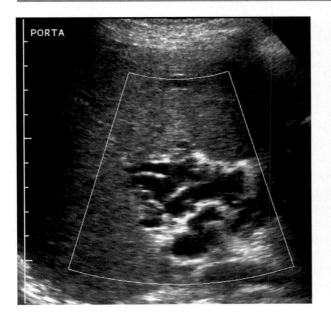 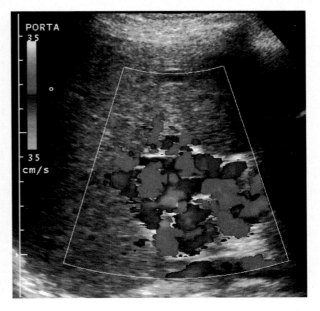

Grey-scale and color Doppler views of the porta hepatis. (See color plates.)

1. What is the cause of the multiple channels seen in the porta hepatis?

2. Is the blood flow in these vessels toward the liver or away from the liver?

3. Are these vessels arterial or venous?

4. Do they form anterior or posterior to the portal vein and hepatic artery?

Effect of Frame Rate on Color Doppler Images

1. Each image takes a certain amount of time to create. If the frame rate is 10 frames/sec, each image takes one tenth of a second to make. The first image, of the superficial femoral artery, was created between the time of antegrade systolic flow, producing the red segment, and retrograde early diastolic flow, producing the blue segment. The second image, of the common carotid artery, was created between end-diastole and early systole, so that the darker red segment of the vessel reflects slower diastolic flow, and the lighter red segment reflects faster systolic flow.

2. Color Doppler images are encoded based on mean velocity. A pulsed Doppler waveform is required to measure peak velocity.

3. Color shading is determined by the mean frequency shift. In addition to velocity, mean frequency shift is dependent on the Doppler angle, the transmitted frequency, and the amount of filtering of low-frequency shifts.

Reference

Middleton WD: Color Doppler image optimization and interpretation. *Ultrasound Q* 1998;14:194–208.

Comment

In analyzing color assignments, it is important to remember that it takes a finite amount of time to generate each frame of a real-time scan. If the flow velocity or the flow direction in a vessel varies with time, different segments of the vessel may have different color assignments because they were generated at a different point in time. This is seen frequently in arteries where there is a rapid change in flow velocities between diastole and peak systole.

Another important point to recognize is that at any point in time, there is a range of frequency shifts within any pixel in the image. This occurs because red blood cells are moving at different velocities and in slightly different directions. If one looks at a Doppler waveform, at any point in time it is possible to determine a maximum, a minimum, and a mean frequency shift. The color that is assigned to a pixel during color Doppler scanning depends on the *mean* frequency shift. In many clinical applications (such as estimating carotid stenoses), it is important to measure the *maximum* frequency shift. This is not possible using conventional color Doppler and can only be done with pulsed Doppler waveform analysis.

Cavernous Transformation of the Portal Vein

1. The channels seen in the porta hepatis represent collateral vessels that have developed because of portal vein thrombosis.

2. Overall flow in these collaterals is toward the liver (hepatopetal).

3. These vessels represent venous collaterals.

4. Portal collaterals typically form anterior to the portal vein and hepatic artery.

Reference

Weltin G, Taylor KJW, Carter AR, Taylor CR: Duplex Doppler: Identification of cavernous transformation of the portal vein. *AJR Am J Roentgenol* 1985; 144:999–1001.

Cross-Reference

Ultrasound: THE REQUISITES, pp 26–27.

Comment

In the setting of portal vein thrombosis, periportal collaterals often form and supply venous flow to the liver. If these collaterals are large enough, they can be seen on grey-scale and on color or power Doppler images of the porta hepatis. They appear as multiple tortuous vessels. Although it is unusual, it is possible to see periportal collaterals when the portal vein is compromised but not completely thrombosed.

In most cases, the thrombosed portal vein is also seen in the setting of cavernous transformation. However, if the thrombosed portal vein is thin and fibrosed, or if it is filled with thrombus that is isoechoic to the adjacent liver, it may be hard to identify and/or recognize. If the portal vein thrombus is not appreciated, and there is a single periportal collateral, this collateral may be mistaken for a patent main portal vein. One way to avoid this mistake is to look at the relationship of the vessel to the hepatic artery. The normal portal vein travels deep to the hepatic artery. Periportal collaterals travel anterior to the hepatic artery. Another potential pitfall in the proper interpretation of cavernous transformation is an enlarged, tortuous hepatic artery. Arterial enlargement usually occurs in the setting of cirrhosis and portal hypertension and can be distinguished from venous collaterals by Doppler waveform analysis. In the majority of cases, the collaterals form in the hepatoduodenal ligament. Recently, cases have been observed where the collaterals form in the wall of the common bile duct, producing marked duct wall thickening.

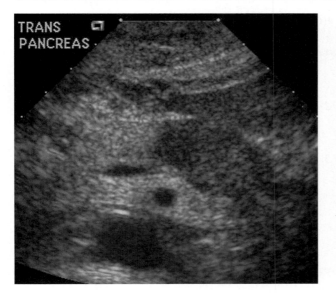

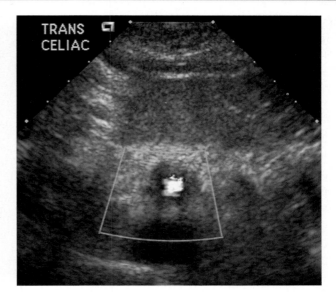

Transverse views of the pancreas and of the celiac axis. (See color plates.)

1. Describe the abnormalities.
2. Should this patient see a surgeon?
3. What other sites should be evaluated sonographically while the patient is being scanned?
4. What is the best way to establish the diagnosis?

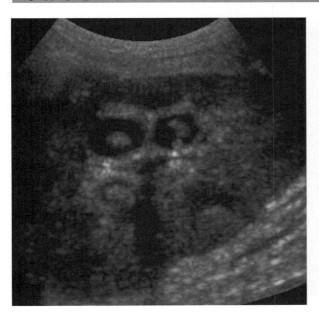

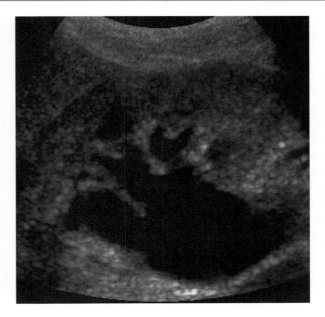

Longitudinal views of the kidney in slightly different obliquities.

1. What is the differential diagnosis of nonshadowing soft tissue masses in the renal calyces?
2. What is the most likely diagnosis in this case?
3. Does this finding require further evaluation?
4. How often is this finding seen in the absence of hydronephrosis?

Vascular Invasion from Pancreatic Cancer

1. The first image shows a hypoechoic mass at the junction of the pancreatic body and tail. The second image shows a concentric soft tissue mass surrounding the celiac axis. These findings are consistent with pancreatic cancer that has encased the celiac axis.

2. Because of the vascular involvement, this patient is not a surgical candidate.

3. Other sites of metastases that would make the patient unresectable include the liver and the peritoneum.

4. Biopsy can be performed with endoscopic ultrasound guidance, percutaneous ultrasound guidance, or CT guidance.

Reference

E Angeli, M Venturini, A Vanzulli: Color Doppler imaging in the assessment of vascular involvement by pancreatic carcinoma. *AJR Am J Roentgenol* 1997;168:193–197

Cross-Reference

Ultrasound: THE REQUISITES, pp 135–136.

Comment

Patients with ductal adenocarcinoma of the pancreas frequently present with jaundice or with nonspecific abdominal pain. Because of their presentation, many of these patients are first imaged with ultrasound. Once the tumor is detected, the next aspect of the patient's evaluation is to determine the resectability of the tumor. Common factors that render a tumor nonresectable include liver metastases, invasion of the peripancreatic vessels, and spread to the peritoneum. Sonography is capable of detecting all of these modes of metastases.

The vessels that are most frequently invaded include the superior mesenteric artery, the celiac axis and its branches, and the portal, splenic, and superior mesenteric veins. Normally the peripancreatic arteries are surrounded circumferentially by dense, echogenic, fibrofatty tissue. Invasion of the arteries is indicated when this echogenic tissue is interrupted by hypoechoic soft tissue. Complete encasement of the artery by soft tissue is essentially diagnostic of invasion and makes the patient nonresectable. Encasement of less than 360 degrees is less reliable but nevertheless significantly reduces the chance of resection with clear surgical margins. Venous invasion is more difficult to detect because the veins are normally in direct contact with the pancreas without intervening fat. Thrombosis and narrowing of the peripancreatic veins are signs of venous invasion. Development of peripancreatic venous collaterals is a secondary sign of venous obstruction.

Prominent Papillary Tips

1. Blood clots, sloughed papillae, fungus balls, transitional cell cancer, malakoplakia, leukoplakia, cholesteatoma, and prominent papillary tips can potentially cause nonshadowing calyceal defects.

2. The fact that the lesions are seen in multiple calyces and appear similar in all is very typical of prominent papillary tips.

3. This appearance is so characteristic of prominent papillary tips that no further evaluation is needed.

4. The papillary tips appear prominent because the calyx is slightly distended by the hydronephrosis. This finding is almost never seen in the absence of hydronephrosis.

Reference

Dillard JP, Talner LB, Pinckney L: Normal renal papillae simulating calyceal filling defects on sonography. *AJR Am J Roentgenol* 1987;148:895–896.

Cross-Reference

Ultrasound: THE REQUISITES, pp 94–96.

Comment

The normal renal pyramids are cone-shaped, with the apex of the cone directed toward the calyx. The rounded apex, or papillary tip, protrudes into the calyx, producing the typical cuplike appearance seen on intravenous urograms. In the normal situation, the angles of the calyceal fornices are acute, and there is not enough urine in the calyces to make the outline of the papillary tip visible. However, in the setting of hydronephrosis, the calyx may distend with urine, and the papillary tip can become surrounded by the urine in the calyceal fornices. When viewed in long axis, the morphology of the papillary tip is usually easily visible, and its origin is recognizable. When viewed in short axis, the papillary tip can simulate a pathologic filling defect in the collecting system. This pitfall is very unusual in native kidneys and slightly more common in renal transplants.

Characteristic features include the similar appearance seen in several calyces and the presence of mild to moderate hydronephrosis. Obtaining views in various obliquities can help in distinguishing this pitfall from true filling defects, but simple awareness of this pitfall is usually enough to avoid misinterpretation.

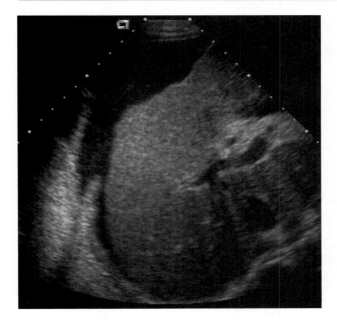

Transverse view of the liver.

1. What artifact is demonstrated on this image?

2. What causes this appearance?

3. Is this finding seen in the absence of ascites?

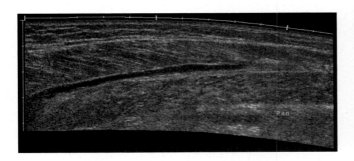

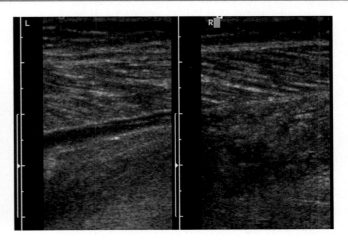

Longitudinal extended field of view of the left calf and dual longitudinal images of the left and right gastrocnemius and soleus muscles.

1. Which leg is abnormal?

2. What is the most likely diagnosis?

3. Which muscle is usually affected?

4. What conditions is this abnormality frequently confused with clinically?

Diaphragmatic Duplication Artifact

1. Both images show artifactual duplication of the diaphragm.

2. This artifact is caused by refraction of sound between the edge of the liver and the ascites.

3. In the absence of ascites there would be soft tissue around the liver, and refraction would not occur, so this artifact would not be seen.

Reference

Middleton WD, Melson GL: Diaphragmatic discontinuity associated with perihepatic ascites: A sonographic refractive artifact. *AJR Am J Roentgenol* 1988; 151:709-711.

Cross-Reference

Ultrasound: THE REQUISITES, pp 112-115.

Comment

The subject of sound refraction in the abdominal midline has been covered in a previous case (case 179). This case is an example where sound is refracted at the oblique interface between a solid structure (the liver), in which sound travels more rapidly, and a liquid (ascites), in which sound travels more slowly. Interfaces such as this act as an acoustic lens and cause sound waves to bend. According to Snell's law, the angle of incidence in the first tissue divided by the speed of sound in the first tissue equals the angle of transmission in the second tissue divided by the speed of sound in the second tissue.

When an ultrasound pulse is transmitted, the computer assumes that it travels in a straight line and that all reflections arise from that line. When the sound wave is bent, the reflections no longer arise from the original line of transmission, so the computer misplaces all of those echoes along the line that it assumes the sound is traveling. Therefore, the net result of refraction is mislocalization of structures. In fact, structures become duplicated because they are insonated once by a sound wave that is not bent and a second time by a sound wave that has been bent. Therefore the computer thinks the echoes are arising from two different locations.

Refraction causes duplication artifacts where the duplicated structures are located side by side at the same depth in the image. The other common duplication artifact is caused by mirror images, and in that case, the duplication artifact is always deeper in the image than the original structure.

Muscle Tear and Hematoma

1. Abnormal separation of the gastrocnemius and soleus muscles is observed on the left side. The right side is normal.

2. The findings are typical of a tear of the gastrocnemius muscle at its attachment to the aponeurosis with the soleus.

3. This finding is sometimes referred to as tennis leg and occurs at the distal aspect of the medial head of the gastrocnemius.

4. Patients with this condition frequently are referred for imaging to rule out deep vein thrombosis or ruptured Baker's cyst.

Reference

Bianchi S, Martinoli C, Abdelwahab IF, et al: Sonographic evaluation of tears of the gastrocnemius medial head ("tennis leg"). *J Ultrasound Med* 1998;17:157-162.

Cross-Reference

Ultrasound: THE REQUISITES, pp 112-115.

Comment

Tears of the medial head of the gastrocnemius muscle are a common problem in middle-aged amateur athletes who are physically active. This tear is sometimes referred to as tennis leg. It occurs when the knee is extended (producing stretching of the gastrocnemius) and the calf muscles are forcefully contracted. This injury generally results in acute pain and swelling of the calf. Tenderness is usually localized to the medial aspect of the mid calf. Although the history and clinical findings are usually characteristic, other abnormalities are often considered. Imaging is therefore used to establish a definitive diagnosis and to determine the extent of the injury.

The normal gastrocnemius muscle inserts into an aponeurosis located between the gastrocnemius and the soleus. Normally, the fibers of the gastrocnemius can be visualized extending directly to this aponeurosis. A tear is diagnosed by identifying a hematoma between the muscle fibers and the aponeurosis. If this injury is imaged acutely, the hematoma may appear hyperechoic. However, with time, the clotted blood starts to lyse, and the hematoma develops areas of liquefaction. Ultimately, the hematoma converts into a simple-appearing fluid collection. This evolution takes several days to weeks to occur.

Once the correct diagnosis is established, these patients are usually managed conservatively with various degrees and durations of rest and immobilization.

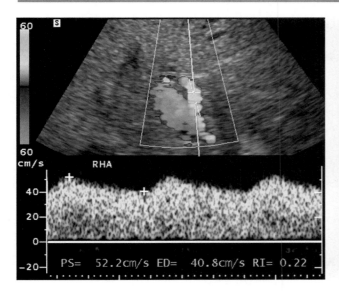 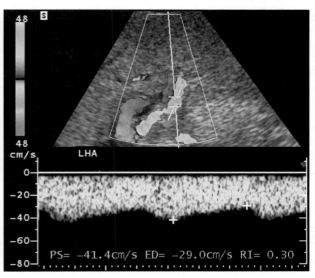

Pulsed Doppler waveform from the intrahepatic portion of the right hepatic artery and the left hepatic artery in a liver transplant patient. (See color plates.)

1. What do both of these waveforms have in common?
2. What else is abnormal about the left hepatic artery?
3. What test would you recommend next?
4. What would you expect to see on a cholangiogram?

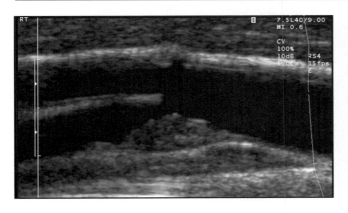 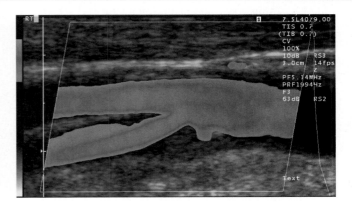

Longitudinal grey-scale view and power Doppler scan of the carotid bifurcation. (See color plates.)

1. Describe the abnormalities.
2. How good is ultrasound at making this diagnosis?
3. What is the significance of this finding?
4. How does intraplaque hemorrhage appear?

Hepatic Artery Thrombosis Status Post Liver Transplant

1. Both arteries demonstrate a blunted (parvus-tardus) pattern with decreased resistive indices.

2. Flow in the left hepatic artery is reversed, indicating that it is serving as a collateral.

3. The next test should be an arteriogram. This test was performed and confirmed complete hepatic artery thrombosis with reconstitution of the left hepatic artery via the left gastric artery.

4. Since the bile ducts in a liver transplant are dependent on hepatic arterial supply, arterial thrombosis causes biliary ischemia and can produce strictures or complete necrosis of the ducts.

Reference
Wachsberg RH: Sonography of liver transplants. *Ultrasound Q* 1998;14(2):76-94.

Cross-Reference
Ultrasound: THE REQUISITES, pp 30-31.

Comment
Hepatic artery stenosis or thrombosis is the most common vascular complication following liver transplantation. It occurs in approximately 10% of cases. Significant hepatic artery stenosis and hepatic artery thrombosis with collateral flow can be detected with Doppler scanning by noting a blunted arterial waveform distal to the stenosis. Blunting can be quantitated in several ways. The easiest is by measuring the resistive index. If the resistive index is less than 0.4, the waveform should be considered severely blunted, and a diagnosis of hepatic artery stenosis or thrombosis should be made. If the resistive index is between 0.4 and 0.5, then hepatic artery stenosis/thrombosis should be considered. If the resistive index is above 0.5, hepatic artery stenosis/thrombosis is very unlikely. Stenosis, thrombosis, or severely diminished flow may also cause an inability to detect flow. Realize, however, that lack of detectable flow may also be due to technical factors. Therefore, if the scan is difficult or limited in some way, inability to confirm arterial flow should be correlated carefully with clinical parameters. If the examination is not limited and no flow is detectable, then arterial compromise should be suggested.

Ulcerated Carotid Plaque

1. The grey-scale view shows a hypoechoic plaque at the origin of the internal carotid artery. The power Doppler scan shows an area of blood flow extending into the mid aspect of the plaque. These findings are typical of plaque ulceration.

2. Ultrasound is not very sensitive at detecting plaque ulceration.

3. Ulceration indicates a higher risk of emboli regardless of the degree of stenosis.

4. Intraplaque hemorrhage appears as a focal hypoechoic area in the plaque or as areas of heterogeneity.

Reference
Bluth EI: Evaluation and characterization of carotid plaque. *Semin US CT MRI* 1997;18:57-65.

Cross-Reference
Ultrasound: THE REQUISITES, pp 476-477.

Comment
Some plaques that produce minimal stenosis can still produce clinical symptoms by serving as a source of emboli. This occurs when the intimal surface of the plaque breaks down and exposes the plaque to intraluminal blood. One of the first stages in this process is the development of intraplaque hemorrhage. Detection of intraplaque hemorrhage on sonography is controversial. Some believe that sonographic resolution is generally not sufficient to identify intraplaque hemorrhage. Others believe that intraplaque hemorrhage is reliably seen as focal areas of decreased echogenicity, while stable plaques (i.e., plaques that do not break down and produce emboli) appear homogeneous.

Plaque ulceration also appears as a focal area of decreased echogenicity. On color or power Doppler, ulceration appears as a defect in the plaque that communicates with the lumen and has detectable internal flow. With large ulcers, a swirling pattern of flow is seen. Although some ulcers are certainly detectable with color Doppler, many ulcers are not. In fact, many ulcers that are found pathologically are not even detectable with arteriography. Partially because of the limitations in detecting ulceration and in characterizing plaque, the major focus of carotid Doppler scanning is to identify and estimate the severity of stenoses.

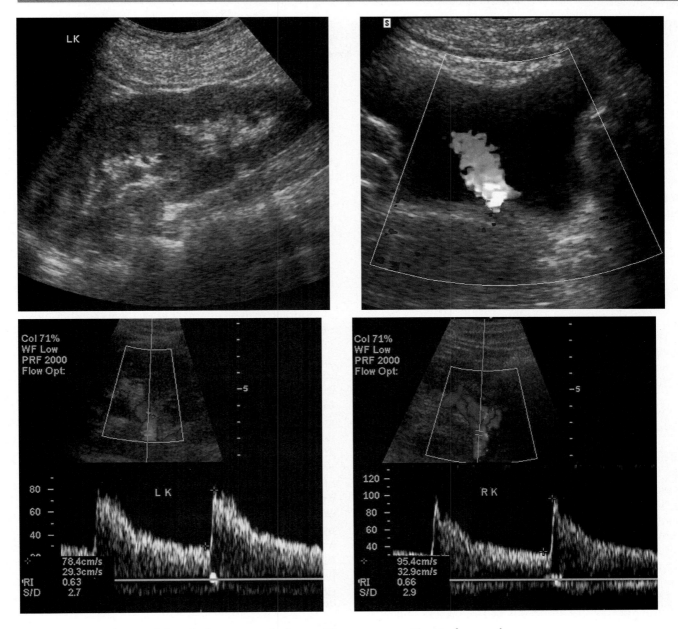

Pregnant patient with a left ureteral stone (the same patient shown in case 27). The figures include a longitudinal view of the left kidney, transverse color Doppler view of the bladder, and pulsed Doppler waveforms from the left and right kidney.

1. What is a normal resistive index (RI) for an intrarenal artery?

2. Are RI measurements a reliable means of determining the presence or absence of urinary obstruction?

3. What is being shown on the color Doppler view of the bladder?

4. In the setting of acute high-grade urinary obstruction, which becomes abnormal first, RI measurements or ureteral jets?

Urinary Obstruction

1. A normal resistive index (RI) ranges from 0.5 to 0.7.

2. This is a controversial topic, but RI measurements seem to have significant limitations in the evaluation of urinary obstruction.

3. The color Doppler view shows a ureteral jet arising from the left ureteral orifice.

4. Ureteral jets become abnormal before the RI becomes abnormal.

References

Baker S, Middleton WD: In vivo color Doppler sonographic analysis of ureteral jets in normal volunteers: Importance of the relative specific gravity of urine in the ureter and bladder. *AJR Am J Roentgenol* 1992;159:773-775.

Burge JH, Middleton WD, McClennan BL, Hildeboldt CF: Ureteral jets in healthy subjects and in patients with unilateral ureteral calculi: Comparison with color Doppler ultrasound. *Radiology* 1991;180:437-442.

Koelliker SL, Cronan JJ: Acute urinary tract obstruction: imaging update. *Urol Clin North Am* 1997;24:571-582.

Cross-Reference

Ultrasound: THE REQUISITES, pp 77-81.

Comment

On sonography, the detection of urinary obstruction depends primarily on the identification of hydronephrosis. Unfortunately, urinary tract obstruction is not synonymous with hydronephrosis. For this reason, a fair amount of effort has been directed toward developing ways that can help sort out kidneys that are obstructed but not hydronephrotic and kidneys that are hydronephrotic but not obstructed.

One relatively direct way of looking at this is to monitor the flow of urine out of the ureters and into the bladder. This can be done in a qualitative manner by watching for ureteral jets. For many years, it was known that grey-scale ultrasound was capable of identifying echogenic jets of urine periodically entering the bladder from the ureteral orifices. However, detection of ureteral jets on grey-scale imaging is intermittent and often subtle, and ureteral jets were never used to analyze urinary obstruction. When color Doppler became available, ureteral jets became much easier to recognize, and it became possible to obtain useful information from the analysis of ureteral jets. In particular, studies showed that ureteral jets were eliminated by moderate and high-grade obstruction, and a useful characteristic of ureteral jets is that they disappear immediately in the setting of obstruction and reappear immediately when

the obstruction is relieved. One limitation is that low-grade, partial obstructions may not cause a detectable change in ureteral jets.

In order for ureteral jets to be analyzed, they must be detectable. For this reason, it is important to realize that ureteral jets are detected only when there is a difference in the density between the urine in the bladder and the urine in the ureters. This is usually the case because density of urine in the bladder is an average of the density of urine that has accumulated over time and thus is slightly different from the density of urine exiting the ureter at any particular point in time. However, when someone is well hydrated and empties his or her bladder immediately prior to the examination, there will be dilute urine in both the bladder and the ureters, and jets may not be seen even when there is very active diuresis. Therefore, patients should be instructed to avoid completely emptying the bladder prior to the analysis of ureteral jets.

Doppler analysis of renal blood flow is another means of studying renal dysfunction. This is generally done by measuring the RI of intrarenal arterial waveforms. Many different underlying renal diseases will affect the RI value. Urinary obstruction is no exception. This is likely due to the release of vasoactive substances that cause vasoconstriction. Since diastolic flow is affected to a greater extent than systolic flow, the effect can be identified by noting an increase in the RI measurement. Studies have shown that the best value to use as the upper limit of normal for the RI is 0.70. In the clinical setting of suspected unilateral obstruction, an RI value greater than 0.70 on the affected side should raise the suspicion of obstruction even if there is no grey-scale evidence of hydronephrosis. If there is underlying renal parenchymal disease that causes bilateral elevation of the RI, then RI asymmetry of greater than 0.08 to 0.10 should prompt increased consideration of unilateral obstruction.

While a unilateral elevation in the RI can be helpful, it is important to realize that the RI may remain elevated for a variable length of time after obstruction has been relieved. A normal RI is not very useful and should not be used as a way of excluding obstruction. Part of the problem is that in the setting of acute obstruction, it takes time for the RI to become abnormal. In addition, partial obstruction may not cause an abnormality in the RI value.

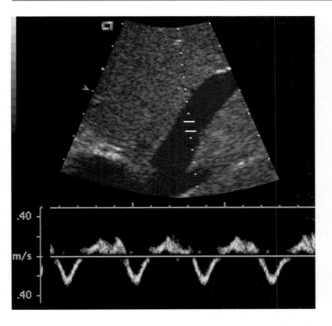
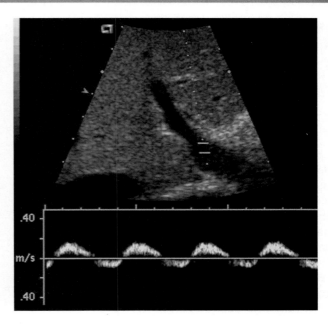

Grey-scale views and accompanying pulsed Doppler waveforms from the hepatic vein and the portal vein.

1. What is wrong with the hepatic venous waveform?
2. What does this indicate?
3. What is wrong with the portal venous waveform?
4. What does this indicate?

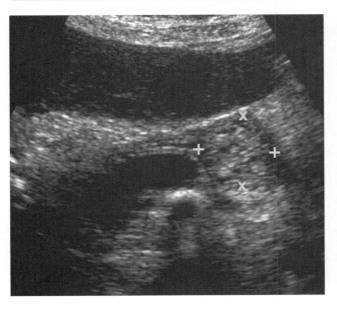
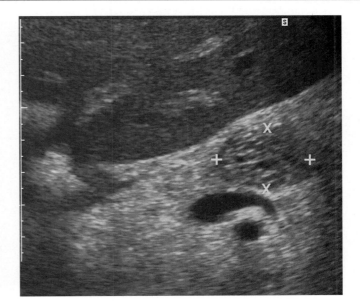

Views of the pancreas in two patients.

1. Describe the abnormality seen in these patients.
2. Is this lesion most likely benign or malignant?
3. What type of fluid would you expect to aspirate?
4. Is this patient more likely to be 20 or 60 years old?

Passive Hepatic Congestion

1. The hepatic vein waveform shows inversion of the normally antegrade systolic pulse so that there is only one antegrade pulse, which occurs during diastole.

2. Inversion of the systolic peak indicates the presence of tricuspid regurgitation.

3. The portal vein waveform is abnormally pulsatile.

4. Portal vein pulsatility to this degree indicates passive congestion.

References

Abu-Yousef MM: Duplex Doppler sonography of the hepatic vein in tricuspid regurgitation. *AJR Am J Roentgenol* 1991;156:79-83.

Duerinckx A, Grant E, Perrella R, et al: The pulsatile portal vein: Correlation of duplex Doppler with right atrial pressures. *Radiology* 1990;176:655-658.

Gallix BP, Taourel P, Dauzat M, et al: Flow pulsatility in the portal venous system: A study of Doppler sonography in healthy adults. *AJR Am J Roentgenol* 1997;169:141-144.

Cross-Reference

Ultrasound: THE REQUISITES, pp 29-30.

Comment

The appearance of the normal hepatic vein waveform has been described in a previous case (case 112). Recall that there should be antegrade flow out of the liver at all times except for during right atrial contraction. In fact, the antegrade flow is divided into a systolic component, which is usually larger, and a diastolic component, which is usually smaller. In this case, there is only one antegrade component. During most of the cardiac cycle there is retrograde flow in the hepatic veins. This means the effective venous outflow from the liver is reduced. Consequently, the hepatic sinusoids become congested.

In the normal liver, the portal venous system is isolated from the right atrial pulsations by the hepatic parenchyma. Therefore, the portal venous waveform is normally flat with minimal pulsatility. However, when the sinusoids become congested, the right atrial pulsations can be transmitted to the portal vein, and the portal vein waveform becomes pulsatile. It is important to realize that some degree of portal vein pulsatility can be normal. This is especially true in otherwise healthy thin patients. The point at which a pulsatile portal vein should be called abnormal is not precisely defined. However, if the maximum velocity drops below zero, then the possibility of right-side heart dysfunction should be considered.

Microcystic Serous Cystadenoma of the Pancreas

1. Both images show a mass that is predominantly solid-appearing but that contains multiple tiny cystic spaces. This is a typical appearance of microcystic (serous) cystadenomas.

2. These are benign lesions with no malignant potential.

3. The cyst fluid is glycogen-rich serous fluid.

4. This lesion is typically seen in elderly women.

Reference

Buck JL, Hayes WS: Microcystic adenoma of the pancreas. *Radiographics* 1990;10:313-322.

Cross-Reference

Ultrasound: THE REQUISITES, pp 137-139.

Comment

Microcystic serous neoplasms of the pancreas are benign lesions that consist of multiple small cystic spaces. The individual cysts typically range from less than 1 mm to 20 mm in diameter. On cut section, they have a honeycomb or spongy appearance. The cyst fluid, and particularly the cellular cytoplasm, is rich in glycogen. These cysts may contain a central stellate scar, and central calcification occurs in up to 40% of lesions. There is no significant predilection to any part of the pancreas. It is uncommon for these tumors to produce symptoms or to cause obstruction of the bile duct or pancreatic duct unless they are very large. Together with mucinous cystic neoplasms, they account for approximately 10% of pancreatic cysts.

On sonography, the lesion usually appears solid with some small cystic areas. Depending on the size of the internal cystic spaces and the number of reflecting interfaces between the cysts, the lesion may range in echogenicity from hyperechoic to hypoechoic. In some cases, the appearance is of a cystic mass composed of multiple small cysts. The central scar is rarely seen on sonography. It is not uncommon for the lesion to appear very cystic on CT and very solid on ultrasound. This combination should suggest the diagnosis of microcystic serous cystadenoma. These tumors are typically very vascular, and this is occasionally reflected on color Doppler scans.

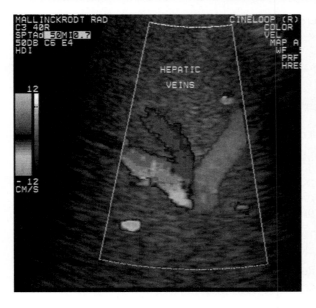
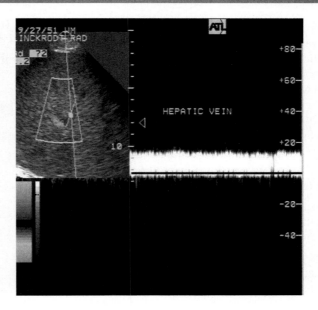

Color Doppler view of hepatic vein branches and pulsed Doppler waveform from one of these veins. (See color plates.)

1. How sensitive is sonography in establishing the diagnosis of the condition shown in this case?

2. What happens to portal venous flow in the condition shown here?

3. Is normal hepatic venous flow hepatofugal or hepatopetal?

4. What causes flattening of the hepatic venous waveform?

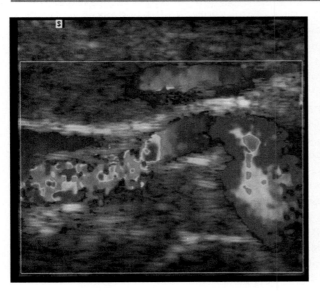
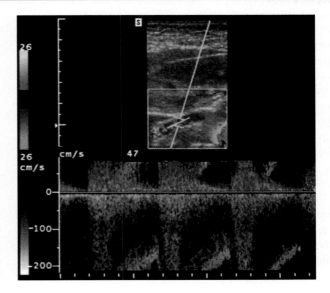

Magnified transverse color Doppler view and pulsed Doppler waveform of the right renal artery. (See color plates.)

1. What is the abnormality?

2. Is this the most common site for renal artery stenosis?

3. Is this patient most likely male or female?

4. What is the treatment of choice for this condition?

Hepatic Vein Thrombosis

1. Sonography is a relatively sensitive way to diagnose hepatic vein thrombosis, and it is a reasonable way to start the imaging evaluation. However, there are cases where the hepatic veins cannot be seen well on ultrasound (e.g., end stage cirrhotic livers and extremely enlarged livers), and alternative modalities such as MRI may be required.

2. Hepatic vein thrombosis is one of the posthepatic causes of portal hypertension. Therefore, all of the signs of portal hypertension can occur.

3. Normal hepatic venous flow is hepatofugal (away from the liver). In this case, the flow in one of the branches is hepatopetal (toward the liver).

4. Anything that isolates the hepatic vein from the right atrium can cause flattening of the normal venous pulsatility. Possibilities include hepatic vein thrombosis, inferior vena cava or hepatic vein webs, extrinsic compression, and tumor invasion. Cirrhosis can also cause flattening of the normal venous pulsatility because regenerating nodules compress the hepatic veins and cause strictures.

Reference

Kane R, Eustace S: Diagnosis of Budd-Chiari syndrome: Comparison between sonography and MR angiography. *Radiology* 1995;195:117–121.

Cross-Reference

Ultrasound: THE REQUISITES, pp 27–29.

Comment

Hepatic vein thrombosis (HVT) can be either bland or due to tumor thrombus. Bland thrombus appears like thrombus elsewhere in the body. It can range from hyperechoic to anechoic. In the acute setting, extensive hepatic vein thrombosis can manifest as a Budd-Chiari syndrome with hepatic failure, liver enlargement, and massive ascites. In such cases, visualization of the hepatic veins may be very difficult. In chronic cases, the hepatic veins may be small and fibrotic and difficult to see. Therefore, it is important to look for the hemodynamic consequences of HVT in addition to looking for the thrombosis itself.

Because HVT isolates the hepatic vein from the right atrium, the pressure fluctuations in the right atrium do not get transferred to the patent portions of the hepatic vein. Therefore, the hepatic vein waveform loses its pulsatility and becomes monophasic. Since hepatic venous flow from obstructed segments cannot flow to the inferior vena cava in the normal way, it seeks collateral pathways, usually via unobstructed hepatic veins (such as accessory hepatic veins) or via subcapsular veins. In both cases, there are segments of hepatic veins where the flow is reversed as it travels toward the collateral.

This produces the typical appearance shown in this case where one hepatic vein branch is flowing in a hepatofugal direction and a communicating vein is flowing in a hepatopetal direction.

Fibromuscular Dysplasia

1. The color Doppler image shows very disordered flow localized to the mid right renal artery. The Doppler waveform shows increased velocity, with the arterial signal aliased from the negative side of the base line to the positive side of the base line.

2. This is not a common site for stenosis. Usually the narrowing is closer to the origin of the renal artery.

3. Renal artery fibromuscular dysplasia is more common in women.

4. Angioplasty is the treatment of choice.

Reference

Luscher TF, Lie JT, Stanson AW, et al: Arterial fibromuscular dysplasia. *Mayo Clin Proc* 1987;62:931–952.

Cross-Reference

Genitourinary Radiology: THE REQUISITES, p 395.

Comment

Fibromuscular dysplasia can affect the intima, media, or adventitia of the artery. Medial fibroplasia is the most common type in adults. After atherosclerosis, fibromuscular dysplasia is the most common cause of renovascular hypertension. It occurs most often in middle-aged women. Unlike atherosclerosis, fibromuscular dysplasia affects the mid and distal renal artery and spares the proximal segment. It may extend into the branch vessels.

The classic "string of beads" appearance seen angiographically is produced by fibromuscular ridges alternating with areas of arterial wall thinning and aneurysm formation. Percutaneous angioplasty is very effective in restoring the patient's normal blood pressure.

The morphologic changes in the artery are almost never visible sonographically. However, as in this case, the disturbed flow can be detected as marked heterogeneity in color assignment on color Doppler scanning. This case is unusual because the patient was quite thin and could be scanned with a linear array transducer, allowing for resolution not typically seen. Because of the location of the lesion, renal artery fibromuscular dysplasia is more difficult to detect with Doppler scanning than is atherosclerosis. When dealing with hypertensive middle-aged or young adult women without a history of vascular disease, it is very important to visualize the mid renal artery.

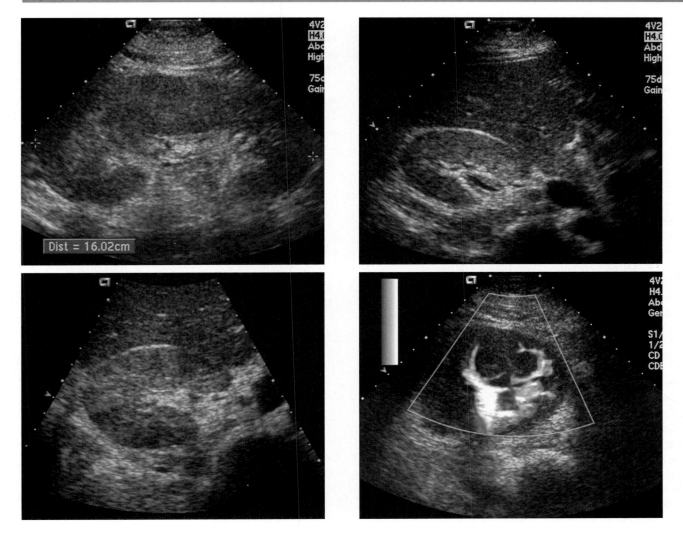

Longitudinal and two transverse grey-scale views and transverse power Doppler view of the kidney in a patient with flank pain.

1. Describe the abnormalities.

2. How good is ultrasound at making this diagnosis?

3. What is the role of ultrasound in managing these patients?

Pyelonephritis

1. The kidney is enlarged (16 cm), there is thickening of the renal pelvis, there is a patchy area of increased cortical echogenicity, and there is a focal area of decreased vascularity seen on power Doppler. These findings are typical of pyelonephritis.

2. Many patients with pyelonephritis have sonographically normal kidneys. Ultrasound is not a good way of making the diagnosis.

3. Since ultrasound is not sensitive at diagnosing pyelonephritis, its role is more to look for complications in patients who are not responding to treatment.

Reference

Baumgarten DA, Baumgartner BR: Imaging and radiologic management of upper urinary tract infections. *Urol Clin North Am* 1997;24:545–569.

Cross-Reference

Ultrasound: THE REQUISITES, pp 99–100.

Comment

Pyelonephritis usually arises as a result of the ascent of infection from the bladder, or less commonly from a hematogenous route. In adults, pyelonephritis is usually diagnosed clinically, patients are treated with antibiotics, and symptoms improve within 48 to 72 hours. In this group of patients, radiologic imaging is not necessary. However, patients with pyelonephritis may be imaged for other reasons, or may be imaged prior to the proper clinical diagnosis. Therefore, the appearance of pyelonephritis should be recognized when it is encountered.

On sonography, the most common finding is usually mild urothelial thickening of the renal pelvis, the ureter, or the intrarenal collecting system. This is usually a subtle finding and typically is not seen unless a directed search is made. Normally the wall of the collecting system is visualized as a single bright line that represents the reflection between the surface of the wall and the adjacent urine in the lumen. When the wall becomes thick, the substance of the wall can be seen as a hypoechoic layer adjacent to the normal surface reflection. This produces a layered appearance with a bright central layer and a hypoechoic peripheral layer. In this respect, thickened urothelium appears similar to thickened bile duct walls (case 156). In addition to infection, stones in the ureter or renal pelvis can cause wall thickening, as can indwelling stents. Urothelial thickening may also appear after bouts of obstruction due to redundancy of the wall. In kidney transplants, rejection and ischemia are additional causes.

Other findings seen with pyelonephritis include renal enlargement, patchy areas of either increased or decreased echogenicity (often in a somewhat wedge shape), loss of central sinus echogenicity, loss of corticomedullary distinction, and tiny amounts of perinephric fluid usually seen best around the poles of the kidney. Color Doppler may show areas of decreased perfusion that correspond to areas of decreased enhancement on CT scans. All of these findings are more difficult to see in adults than in children.

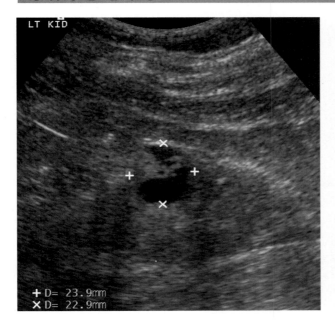
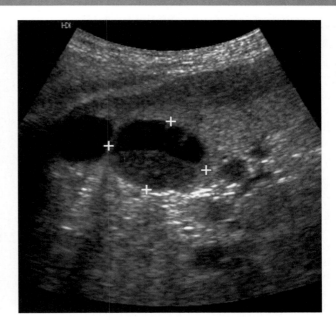

Views of the kidney in two patients.

1. Describe the renal masses shown on these images.
2. What is the differential diagnosis?
3. What would the most likely diagnosis be if these patients also had pheochromocytomas?
4. What else can be done sonographically to assist in this differential diagnosis?

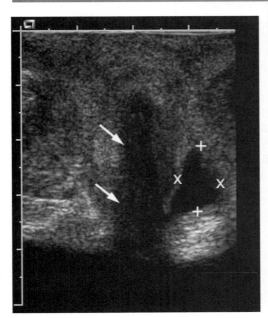
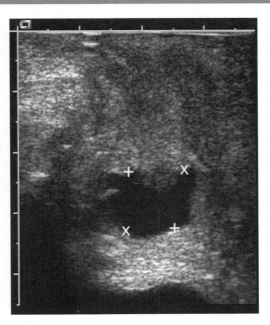

Transperineal views of the urethra. The first image is in a coronal plane and the second image is in a sagittal plane just to the left of the midline.

1. What is the differential diagnosis?
2. To what are the arrows pointing?
3. The wall of this lesion is lined with what?
4. Are these abnormalities more commonly seen in men or in women?

C A S E 2 0 8

Complex Renal Cysts

1. Both masses are predominantly cystic but contain significant solid-appearing internal components.

2. The primary possibilities include hemorrhagic cysts and cystic renal cell cancer. Complex cystic masses can also be due to infected cysts or abscesses, multilocular cystic nephroma, partially thrombosed aneurysms, echinococcal cysts, or urinomas.

3. The presence of complex renal masses and pheochromocytomas suggests von Hippel-Lindau disease and renal cell cancer.

4. Color Doppler scanning would indicate a cystic renal cell cancer if vascularity were seen in the solid components. This was the case in the first image. If the solid component were mobile when the patient changed position, then the diagnosis would be a hemorrhagic cyst with mobile clot. This was the case with the second image.

Reference

Kawashima A, Goldman SM, Sandler CM: The indeterminate renal mass. *Radiol Clin North Am* 1996;34:997–1015.

Cross-Reference

Ultrasound: THE REQUISITES, pp 81–84.

Comment

Benign renal cysts are the most common incidental lesion detected during abdominal sonography. When cysts have an anechoic lumen, a well-defined back wall, and produce posterior acoustic enhancement, they require no further evaluation. A limited number of thin septations also require no further evaluation. However, when they have a thick or irregular wall, thick septations, or obvious solid elements similar to those seen in these images, cysts should not be considered simple, and further evaluation is necessary. As mentioned in the answer to question 4, looking for motion or vascularity may help in further characterization. Intravenous ultrasound contrast agents will almost certainly help to sort out many of these lesions by detecting the presence or absence of enhancing components similar to the principles used with CT or MRI.

In this case, the first image was of a cystic renal cell cancer. Approximately 15% of renal cell cancers have significant cystic components or are predominantly cystic. Cystic changes may be due to hemorrhage or necrosis (often seen in larger lesions), or to true cystic elements.

C A S E 2 0 9

Urethral Diverticulum

1. The differential diagnosis is urethral diverticulum or periurethral abscess.

2. The arrows are pointing to the urethra.

3. The wall is lined with fibrous tissue, not urothelium.

4. Urethral diverticulae are much more common in women.

Reference

Siegel C, Middleton WD, Teefey SA, et al: Sonography of the female urethra. *AJR Am J Roentgenol* 1998;170:1269–1272.

Cross-Reference

Genitourinary Radiology: THE REQUISITES, pp 244–245.

Comment

These images are obtained from a transperineal approach. They show a fluid collection posterior to the urethra. This is the most common location for a urethral diverticulum. These diverticulae frequently dissect around the left and right lateral aspects of the urethra.

It is believed that most female urethral diverticulae develop from an infected paraurethral gland that erodes into the urethra and maintains a persistent patent neck between the urethra and the cavity. Because these lesions do not contain elements of the urethral wall, they are really pseudodiverticulae.

Sonography is an excellent way to evaluate women with suspected urethral diverticulae. Sonography is better tolerated than urethrography, and it is just as accurate. In fact, ultrasound also visualizes periurethral lesions that do not communicate with the urethra, and in that respect it is superior to urethrography. MRI with a transvaginal or transrectal probe is also an excellent way of evaluating patients with suspected urethral diverticulae.

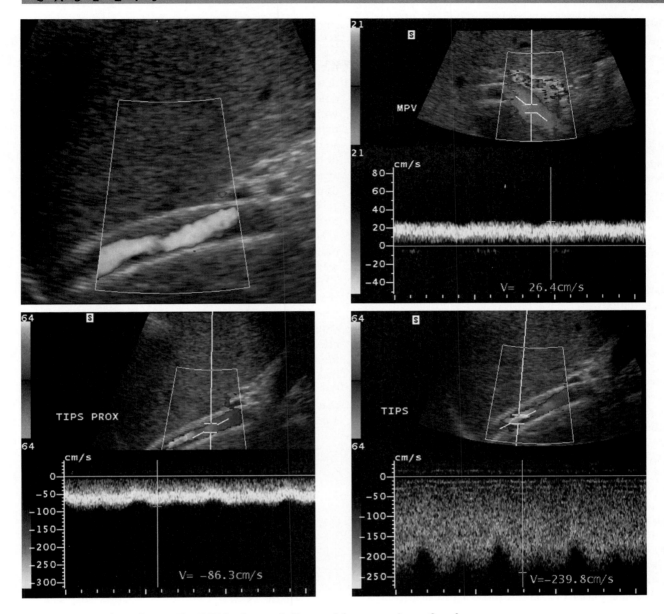

Power Doppler view of a TIPS shunt followed by a series of color Doppler views and pulsed Doppler waveforms from the main portal vein, proximal stent, and mid stent. (See color plates.)

1. What are the important findings on these scans?

2. What happens to the portal vein velocity after a successful TIPS shunt?

3. What happens to the flow in the right and left portal vein after a successful TIPS shunt?

4. What is the significance of focal color Doppler aliasing in a TIPS stent?

Stenosis of a TIPS Stent

1. The power Doppler view shows incomplete color fill-in of the stent due to hypoechoic tissue along the wall of the stent. The portal vein waveform shows an abnormally low velocity in the main portal vein (less than 30 cm/sec). The stent waveforms show an elevated velocity in the mid stent (greater than 190 cm/sec) and a discrepancy of velocities in the proximal and in the mid stent (velocity difference of greater than 100 cm/sec is abnormal).

2. Normally, the portal vein velocity increases following placement of a TIPS stent.

3. Usually, flow in the right and left portal veins reverses after TIPS so that blood flow is directed toward the stent.

4. Focal aliasing in a TIPS often identifies the site of peak velocity.

References

Feldstein VA, Patel MD, LaBerge JM: TIPS shunts: Accuracy of Doppler US in determination of patency and detection of stenoses. *Radiology* 1996;201:141–147.

Kanterman RY, Darcy MD, Middleton WD, et al: Doppler sonographic findings associated with transjugular intrahepatic portosystemic shunt (TIPS) malfunction. *AJR Am J Roentgenol* 1997;168:467–472.

Cross-Reference

Ultrasound: THE REQUISITES, pp 31–32.

Comment

The transjugular intrahepatic portosystemic shunt (TIPS) has become a well-accepted treatment of portal hypertension and its complications. Although the technical success rate for placement of TIPS shunts is greater than 90%, a number of complications can cause shunt malfunction. These include stenosis of the stent or hepatic vein and shunt thrombosis. The 1-year primary patency rate is 25% to 60%. However, with radiologic intervention, the 1-year patency rate increases to approximately 85%. Because of this, there is much incentive to monitor these stents so that stenosis can be detected and treated early, prior to development of clinical symptoms. Although the use of ultrasound as a screening test in this patient population is controversial, multiple centers have shown that Doppler scanning can be an effective means of following patients after TIPS.

Normally, the portal vein velocity increases after a TIPS has been placed. We expect the post-TIPS portal vein velocity to be greater than 30 cm/sec. Lower velocities should raise the suspicion of a stenosis. Flow velocity in the TIPS itself should be rapid. In our experience, the normal range for stent velocity is 90 to 190 cm/sec. Higher and lower velocities should both raise the suspicion of a stenosis. In the area of the stenosis, the velocities increase. This increase can sometimes be detected as a focal area of color aliasing in the stent on color Doppler scanning. Such areas should be sampled with pulsed Doppler scanning so that velocities can be measured from the waveform. Another sign of TIPS stenosis is a change in direction of flow in the right and/or left portal vein from toward the stent (hepatofugal) to away from the stent (hepatopetal). This change in flow direction tends to be a late finding.

We have found it difficult to rely on a single parameter to make the diagnosis of TIPS stenosis. For instance, a portal vein velocity of 28 cm/sec would not be an indication for venography unless other abnormalities were present. Likewise, a slightly elevated maximum stent velocity or a slightly depressed minimum stent velocity would not be indications for venography if they were isolated abnormalities. However, we have found that combining the results of multiple parameters is effective in predicting the need for venography and intervention. It is worth noting that some centers have had success in predicting stenosis by measuring only the minimum stent velocity. These groups have found that a stent velocity below 50 to 60 cm/sec is a sign of a failing stent.

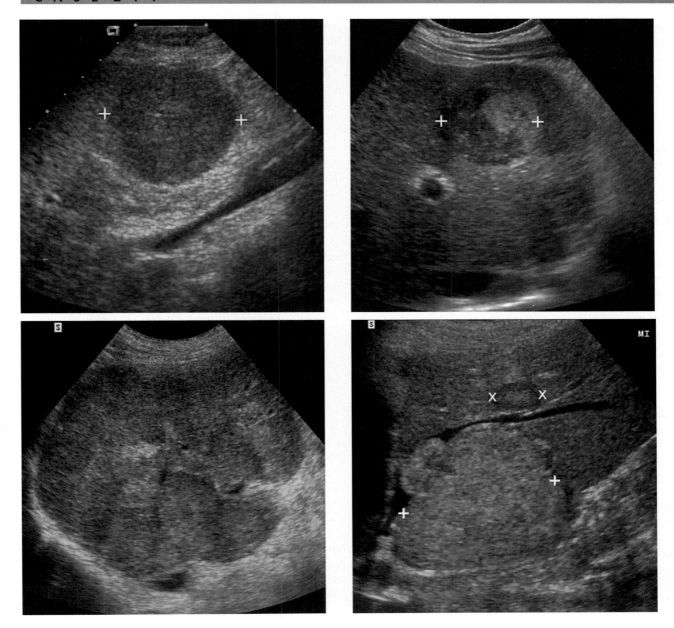

Views of the liver in four patients with the same condition.

1. What are the two most likely diagnoses in these patients?

2. Which image allows you to strongly suggest one diagnosis over the other?

3. What history are these patients likely to have?

4. What would you expect these lesions to look like on color Doppler?

Hepatocellular Carcinoma

1. The most likely possibilities are metastatic disease and hepatocellular carcinoma.

2. The last image shows tumor invading the adjacent hepatic vein. This behavior is much more consistent with hepatocellular carcinoma than with metastatic disease.

3. All of these patients had a history of cirrhosis or hepatitis.

4. Hepatocellular carcinoma is usually a hypervascular lesion with disorganized, chaotic vascular pattern. The ability to detect and visualize this vascularity on color Doppler depends on the location of the lesion. Superficial lesions are more successfully interrogated with color Doppler than deep lesions. Intravenous contrast agents improve the sonographic analysis of vascularity in hepatocellular cancer.

Reference

El-Serag HB, Mason AC: Rising incidence of hepatocellular carcinoma in the United States. *N Engl J Med* 1999:340:745–750.

Cross-Reference

Ultrasound: THE REQUISITIES, pp 12–14.

Comment

Hepatocellular carcinoma (HCC) is the fourth most common cancer in the world, and its incidence is increasing in the United States. It affects patients with underlying chronic liver disease. The most common causes are alcoholic cirrhosis and chronic hepatitis B and C. Cirrhosis develops during the first 10 years after transmission in 20% of patients with chronic hepatitis C. Once cirrhosis has occurred, HCC develops at a rate of 1% to 4% per year in patients with chronic hepatitis C infection. In cirrhosis, it is believed that regenerating nodules undergo dysplastic changes and that dysplastic nodules progress to HCC. In patients with end-stage liver disease undergoing liver transplantation, this progressive dysplastic process results in HCC in approximately 25% of patients with hepatitis B and C and in 10% of patients with alcoholic cirrhosis. HCC is especially common in Asia and sub-Saharan Africa because of the high incidence of hepatitis B and C. Other predisposing causes are hemochromatosis, liver flukes, exposure to aflatoxins, Wilson's disease, and use of anabolic steroids.

As the images in this case show, the sonographic appearance of HCC is quite variable. Lesions can be hypoechoic (first image) or hyperechoic (large lesion on last image). Some will have a target appearance (small lesion on last image). Large lesions are more frequently heterogeneous. Occasionally, lesions will be mixed with organized nodular areas of increased echogenicity in a background of decreased echogenicity (second image), or vice versa. Calcification and cystic changes occur but are distinctly unusual. Because cirrhotic liver parenchyma may attenuate the ultrasound beam more than the tumor, increased through transmission is occasionally seen posterior to HCC.

The pattern of HCC also varies and is dependent on the population of patients being scanned. In groups of patients who are being screened, tumors are detected when they are relatively small and solitary. In unscreened populations, tumors tend to be larger and are often mutifocal. One pattern seen often in unscreened patients is a large, dominant mass with multiple smaller satellite lesions (last image). A final pattern is a diffuse infiltrative appearance that can affect entire segments and lobes of the liver (third image). In many cases, the lesions that infiltrate large portions of the liver are more difficult to detect sonographically than the smaller lesions.

Sonographically visible portal vein invasion is also common with the larger masses (see case 189). It is believed that many of the satellite lesions are metastases that arise from the tendency of HCC to invade the portal veins. Hepatic vein invasion also occurs (last image) but is less common than portal vein invasion.

In most patients, the key to the diagnosis of HCC is the clinical history of chronic liver disease. Elevated alpha-fetoprotein levels may suggest the diagnosis, but false negative results are common, particularly with small tumors. False positive results are also seen in otherwise uncomplicated cirrhosis and during flares of hepatitis. In a cirrhotic patient, HCC should be the primary consideration whenever a solid liver mass is detected on sonography. In my institution, such patients undergo CT and in most cases subsequently have an ultrasound guided percutaneous liver biopsy. My approach is to start with fine needle aspiration (FNA) using a 25-gauge needle. With experienced cytopathologists, this can provide a diagnosis in approximately 50% of cases. If the FNA is nondiagnostic, I proceed immediately to a core biopsy using 18- to 20-gauge needles. Many radiologists do not do FNA for HCC but rather start initially with core biopsies.

Note: Page numbers followed by the letter f refer to figures.